# Sperm Chromatin for the Clinician

Armand Zini • Ashok Agarwal
Editors

# Sperm Chromatin for the Clinician

## A Practical Guide

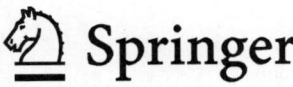 Springer

*Editors*
Armand Zini, MD
Department of Surgery
Division of Urology
McGill University
St. Mary's Hospital Center
Montreal, QC, Canada

Ashok Agarwal, PhD, HCLD (ABB)
Director, Center for Reproductive Medicine
Glickman Urological and Kidney Institute
Cleveland Clinic
Cleveland, OH, USA

ISBN 978-1-4614-7842-3
Springer New York Heidelberg Dordrecht London

Library of Congress Control Number: 2013944560

Printed on acid-free paper

Springer is part of Springer Science+Business Media (www.springer.com)

# Preface

The evaluation of sperm DNA and chromatin abnormalities has gained significant importance in the past several years, mainly as a result of the recent advances in assisted reproductive technologies (ARTs). *In vitro* fertilization (IVF) and, intra-cytoplasmic sperm injection (ICSI) have revolutionized the treatment of male-factor infertility. However, we have come to realize that the genetic integrity of the sperm is a key aspect of the paternal contribution to the offspring, particularly, in the context of ARTs. With the growing concerns about the long-term safety of ARTs (especially ICSI) we have seen an increasing number of studies on the male genome's influence on reproductive outcomes. These studies now shed some light on the influence of sperm chromatin and DNA abnormalities on reproductive outcomes. Along with these clinical studies, we also have made real advances in our understanding of the basic aspects of sperm chromatin and DNA integrity. We are now starting to better understand the unique organization of the sperm chromatin, as well as, the nature and etiology of sperm DNA damage.

We have assembled this textbook with the idea of bringing together the key practical elements of this rapidly evolving field. The authors were carefully selected based on their expertise and proven track record of high quality research in the field. Our book is primarily intended for clinicians and laboratory andrologists as it mainly focuses on the etiology of sperm chromatin and DNA damage and the effect of this damage on male reproductive potential. For clinicians and laboratory andrologists, this book will help guide clinical practice in this area.

We would like to thank Richard Lansing, executive editor, for his support and advice and Margaret Burns, publishing manager, for her tireless efforts in reviewing and editing each of the manuscripts. Furthermore, we would like to thank all of the outstanding contributors for sharing their knowledge and for submitting their manuscripts on time. Finally, we are indebted to our families who have endured many long nights when we were working late on this book.

Montreal, QC, Canada                                            Armand Zini
Cleveland, OH, USA                                         Ashok Agarwal

# Editor Biographies

**Dr**. **Armand Zini** is Associate Professor of Surgery and Director of the Andrology Fellowship program at McGill University. Dr. Zini received his Medical degree and completed his urologic training at McGill University in Montreal. He then completed a fellowship in Male Infertility at the New York Hospital-Cornell Medical Centre and The Population Council in New York, working with Drs. Marc Goldstein and Peter Schlegel. Dr. Zini's main expertise is in clinical male infertility. Over the past 10 years, he has focused his research activity on the study of human sperm chromatin and DNA integrity, and, he has published numerous important papers on the influence of sperm DNA damage on reproductive outcomes. In 2005, he gave the John Collins lecture entitled "Sperm DNA damage and Male Infertility" at the annual meeting of the American Society for Reproductive Medicine. In 2006, he was invited to present on the "Tests of sperm DNA damage" at the Canadian Fertility and Andrology Society (CFAS) annual meeting and in 2008 was invited to present on the "Clinical importance of sperm DNA damage" at both the Canadian Fertility and Andrology Society (CFAS) and the American Society of Andrology (ASA) annual meetings. Dr. Zini has recently presented on the "Role of antioxidants and sperm DNA damage" (Sperm DNA Symposium in Rome, Italy, March 2009) and at the 2009 European Society for Human Reproduction and Embryology (ESHRE) consensus workshop on sperm DNA testing in Sweden. Dr. Zini is currently funded for studies on sperm physiology and the epigenetic effects of vitamin supplements.

**Dr**. **Ashok Agarwal** is the Director of Research at the Center for Reproductive Medicine at Cleveland Clinic Foundation and a Professor at the Lerner College of Medicine of Case Western Reserve University. His current research interests include studies on molecular markers of oxidative stress, DNA integrity, apoptosis in the pathophysiology of male and female reproduction, and effect of radio frequency radiation on fertility and fertility preservation in patients with cancer. Dr. Agarwal has published over 500 scientific articles and reviews in peer reviewed scientific journals, authored over 50 book chapters, and presented over 700 papers at scientific meetings. He is on the editorial board of over a dozen scientific journals. His laboratory has trained more than 100 basic scientists and clinical researchers from the United States and abroad. He is the Program Director of the highly successful Summer Internship Course in Reproductive Medicine. In the last 4 years, over 100 premed and medical students from across the United States and overseas have graduated from this highly competitive program. Dr. Agarwal has been invited as a guest speaker to over 20 countries for important international meetings. He has directed more than a dozen Andrology Laboratory and ART Workshops in recent years.

# Contents

# Contributors

**Ashok Agarwal** Director, Center for Reproductive Medicine, Glickman Urological and Kidney Institute, Cleveland Clinic, Cleveland, OH, USA

**R. John Aitken** Discipline of Biological Sciences, School of Environmental and Life Sciences, University of Newcastle, Callaghan, NSW, Australia

ARC Centre of Excellence in Biotechnology and Development, Priority Research Centre in Reproductive Science, University of Newcastle, Callaghan, NSW, Australia

**Naif Al-Hathal** Division of Urology, Department of Surgery, Royal Victoria Hospital, McGill University, Montreal, QC, Canada

**Rod Balhorn** Department of Applied Science, University of California, Davis, CA, USA

**Guylain Boissonneault** Department of Biochemistry, Université de Sherbrooke, Sherbrooke, QC, Canada

**Jason Matthew Boman** Division of Urology, Department of Surgery, Centre Hospitalier Régional du Suroît, Montreal, QC, Canada

**Mona Bungum** Reproductive Medicine Centre, Skåne University Hospital Malmö, Lund University, Sodra Forstadsgatan, Malmö, Sweden

**Alexandra Calle** Department of Animal Reproduction and Animal Genetic Resources Conservation, National Research Institute for Agriculture and Food Technology (INIA), Madrid, Spain

**Aldo E. Calogero** Section of Endocrinology, Andrology and Internal Medicine, and Master in Andrological, Human Reproduction and Biotechnology Sciences, Department of Internal Medicine and Systemic Diseases, University of Catania, Policlinico "G. Rodolico", Catania, Italy

**Peter Chan** Department of Surgery, McGill University and
the Research Institute of the MUHC, Montréal, QC, Canada

**Rosita A. Condorelli** Section of Endocrinology, Andrology
and Internal Medicine, Human Reproduction and Biotechnology Sciences,
Department of Biomedical Sciences, University of Catania, Catania, Italy

**Rosario D'Agata** Section of Endocrinology, Andrology and Internal Medicine,
Human Reproduction and Biotechnology Sciences, Department of Biomedical
Sciences, University of Catania, Catania, Italy

**Geoffry N. De Iuliis** Department of Biological Sciences,
ARC Centre of Excellence in Biotechnology and Development,
Priority Research Centre in Reproductive Science,
University of Newcastle, Newcastle, NSW, Australia

**Hasan M. El-Fakahany** Department of Dermatology,
STD's and Andrology, Al-Minya University, Al-Minya, Egypt

**Raúl Fernández-González** Department of Animal Reproduction and
Animal Genetic Resources Conservation, National Research Institute
for Agriculture and Food Technology (INIA), Madrid, Spain

**Maria San Gabriel** Division of Urology, Department of Surgery,
McGill University, St. Mary's Hospital Center, Montreal, QC, Canada

**Aleksander Giwercman** Reproductive Medicine Centre,
Skåne University Hospital Malmö, Lund University, Malmö, Sweden

**Marie-Chantal Grégoire** Department of Biochemistry,
University of Sherbrooke, Sherbrooke, QC, Canada

**Alfonso Gutiérrez-Adán** Department of Animal Reproduction
and Animal Genetic Resources Conservation, National Research
Institute for Agriculture and Food Technology (INIA), Madrid, Spain

**Sandro La Vignera** Section of Endocrinology, Andrology and Internal Medicine,
Human Reproduction and Biotechnology Sciences, Department of Biomedical
Sciences, University of Catania, Catania, Italy

**Frédéric Leduc** Department of Biochemistry,
Université de Sherbrooke, Sherbrooke, QC, Canada

**Sheena E.M. Lewis** Centre for Public Health, Institute of Clinical Science,
Queen's University of Belfast, Belfast, Northern Ireland, UK

**Eleonora B. Pasqualotto** Department of Gynecology,
University of Caxias do Sul, Caxias do Sul, RS, Brazil

**Fábio F. Pasqualotto** Department of Urology, University of Caxias do Sul,
Bairro São Pelegrino, Caxias do Sul, RS, Brazil

**Miriam Pérez-Crespo** Department of Animal Reproduction
and Animal Genetic Resources Conservation, National Research
Institute for Agriculture and Food Technology (INIA), Madrid, Spain

**Eva Pericuesta** Department of Animal Reproduction and Animal Genetic
Resources Conservation, National Research Institute for Agriculture
and Food Technology (INIA), Madrid, Spain

**Miguel Ángel Ramírez** Department of Animal Reproduction and Animal
Genetic Resources Conservation, National Research Institute
for Agriculture and Food Technology (INIA), Madrid, Spain

**Bernard Robaire** Department Pharmacology and Therapeutics,
Department of Obstetrics and Gynecology, McGill University,
Montréal, QC, Canada

**Denny Sakkas** Department of Obstetrics, Gynecology and Reproductive
Sciences, Yale University School of Medicine, New Haven, CT, USA

**Rakesh Sharma** Andrology Laboratory and Center for Reproductive Medicine,
Glickman Urological and Kidney Institute, OB-GYN and Women's Health
Institute, Cleveland Clinic, Cleveland, OH, USA

**Luke Simon** Centre for Public Health, Queens University Belfast,
Institute of Clinical Sciences, Belfast, Northern Ireland, UK

**Marcello Spanò** Laboratory of Toxicology, Unit of Radiation Biology
and Human Health, Italian National Agency for New Technologies,
Engery, and Sustainable Economic Development,
Casaccia Research Centre, Casaccia, Rome, Italy

**Enzo Vicari** Department of Internal Medicine and Systemic Diseases,
University of Catania, Catania, Italy

**Dan Yu** Centre for Public Health, Institute of Clinical Science, Queens University
Belfast, Belfast, Northern Ireland, UK

**Armand Zini** Department of Surgery, Division of Urology, McGill University,
St. Mary's Hospital Center, Montreal, QC, Canada

# Part I
# Biological Determinants of Sperm Chromatin Damage

# Chapter 1
# Sperm Chromatin: An Overview

**Rod Balhorn**

## Origins of Sperm Chromatin Research

The first research conducted on sperm chromatin, which dates back almost 150 years, began with the discovery of its two primary molecular components – DNA and protamine. Only a year after Gregor Mendel reported his work on the laws of heredity in 1865 [1], Ernst Haeckel suggested that the nuclei of cells must contain the material responsible for the transmission of genetic traits [2]. Friedrich Miescher, working in Felix Hoppe Seyler's laboratory in Germany, had become intrigued by cells and began conducting experiments to determine their chemical composition. Working initially with lymphocytes obtained from blood and later enriched populations of leukocytes he obtained from hospital bandages, Miescher noticed a precipitate that formed when he added acid to extracts of cells he was using to isolate proteins [3]. While he and the rest of the scientific community were unaware that this material, which he called nuclein, was the genetic material Mendel and Haeckel had referred to, he became fascinated by and continued to study its properties [4]. Walther Flemming's work over the next decade introduced the scientific community to the cellular substructures called chromosomes and the concept of mitosis, and Flemming was the first to introduce the term *chromatin* [5]. It took the next 30 years, however, before cellular biologists began to realize the importance of individual chromosomes as the carriers of genetic information.

Miescher, who began his research career isolating and characterizing proteins, spent the majority of his time investigating nuclein (DNA). When he discovered he could not obtain enough of the nuclein from human cells to properly examine its properties, he turned to working with fish sperm. Salmon provided an abundance of sperm, and the sperm cells were considered ideal because they had almost no

R. Balhorn, PhD
Department of Applied Science,
University of California, Davis, CA, USA
e-mail: rodbalhorn@hughes.net

A. Zini, A. Agarwal (eds.), *Sperm Chromatin for the Clinician*,
© Springer Science+Business Media New York 2013

cytoplasm to contaminate his nuclear preparations with protein. In addition to being the first to isolate DNA, Miescher was also the first to isolate protamine, which he called protamin, and to discover its highly basic nature [6]. He discovered that nuclein and protamin made up the majority of the mass of the sperm head, and he also provided the first insight into the fundamental interaction that bound these two components together inside the sperm nucleus – that nuclein was bound in a salt-like state to protamin. As the interest in DNA and protamine grew, other researchers began to examine the molecules present in sperm. The majority of the initial work characterizing the composition of protamine molecules was carried out by Kossel and his group, not Miescher, over several decades spanning from about 1890–1920 [7–10]. The proteins bound to DNA in sperm were distinguished from those found in other cells very early on, but the real significance of this difference was not appreciated until almost half a century later when more detailed studies of spermatogenesis and spermiogenesis revealed significant differences in DNA packaging and sperm chromatin compaction. Up until this time, sperm chromatin was considered by many to be similar to the chromatin found in somatic cells.

## Spermatogenesis: A Special Form of Terminal Differentiation

In species that reproduce sexually, testicular cells undergo a radical transformation as they progress through a process of differentiation called spermatogenesis. Diploid somatic cells that contain two complements of the genome divide in meiosis to produce haploid cells containing only a single copy of each chromosome. The nuclei and chromatin inside these haploid cells also undergo a series of structural and functional changes. In mammals, specific genes within the male genome are imprinted to identify their "parent of origin" [11, 12], and the chromatin is transformed from a highly functional, genetically active state characteristic of the somatic testis cell it was derived from to a quiescent or completely inactive state found in the fully mature sperm cell.

One might think of this transformation as the testicular cell embarking on a path of terminal differentiation similar to the differentiation of a stem cell into a liver, kidney or brain cell. The final cell not only differs structurally from the stem cell but also performs very different functions. Unlike the genome in most stem cells, however, the genome of most maturing vertebrate spermatids undergo an additional step in the process, a transient stage in which the entire genome is deprogrammed and shut down. This genome-wide inactivation bears some similarity to processes of heterochromatinization that have been observed to occur with one X-chromosome in vertebrates [13, 14], the entire genome in avian erythrocytes [15], and one set of chromosomes in mealy bugs [16]. These changes, which are induced by modifying or replacing the proteins that bind to and package DNA, enable the male genome of the sperm to be deprogrammed and maintained in a quiescent state until it enters the oocyte and is ready to be combined with the genome of the female to create a diploid embryonic cell. The process provides a mechanism by which the genes contributed by the male can be reactivated in the proper combinations to ensure the first cells function as embryonic stem cells, subpopulations of which later redifferentiate into the other types of cells that are required for the development of a fully functional organism.


## Variability in the Composition of Sperm Chromatin

Both Miescher's and Kossel's studies of sperm focused on the morphological and compositional differences they observed between sperm and other cells. Kossel examined the proteins found in the sperm head, using the properties and composition of the proteins as indicators of the differences or similarities that might distinguish these cells in different species. The majority of the fish protamines analyzed by Kossel and others were found to be small proteins with unusually high contents of the two amino acids arginine and lysine. While these two amino acids were known to be present in all proteins at a low level (typically ~5%), the arginine-rich fish protamines were found to contain 50–90% arginine and the lysine-rich fish protamines contained as much as 28% lysine. Because the fish protamines appeared to be comprised mostly of arginine and lysine, Kossel proposed that the protamines might be one of the simplest proteins.

As researchers began examining the sperm chromatin proteins of other species, it became clear that there was a great deal of variability in the types of proteins used to package DNA in sperm. Sea urchins also proved to be an easy source from which sperm could be obtained in large numbers, and analyses of sea urchin sperm revealed that protamines were not present in the sperm chromatin of this organism. Instead, the DNA was found to be packaged by histones [17, 18]. Each of the five histones is larger (by a factor of two) than protamines and significantly less basic. In contrast to the protamines, the histones contain a great deal less arginine (2–10% of the total amino acids) and more lysine (13–28%). Subsequent analyses of sperm chromatin proteins isolated from the sperm of other invertebrates and vertebrates have shown that the size and amino acid sequences of the proteins used to package sperm DNA vary considerably [19]. Many of these proteins are smaller and substantially more basic than the histones and larger and less basic than protamines.

Amphibian and fish sperm provide one of the best examples of this variability. Sperm produced by frogs in the genus *Rana*, for example, have their DNA packaged entirely by histones [20]. Both histones and protamine-like intermediate proteins are found in the sperm chromatin of the clawed African frog (*Xenopus*) [21], while histones and protamines package the DNA in toad (*Bufo*) sperm [22]. Similar observations have been made in studies of fish sperm. Different species of fish, even within the same order, have been shown to use histones, protamine-like proteins, or protamines to condense their sperm chromatin, demonstrating that these differences do not correspond strictly with phylogeny. In addition, the particular type of protein used to package sperm DNA does not appear to be linked to mode of fertilization, as had been suggested based on the studies conducted with amphibian sperm. While several internally fertilizing fish such as *Xiphophorus helleri guentheri* (swordtail), *Xiphophorus maculatus* (platyfish), *Poecilia reticulata* (guppy), *Poecilia picta* (guppy), and *Cymatogaster aggregata* (shiner perch) all produce sperm containing protamines [23], several externally fertilizing species such as the grass carp (*Ctenopharyngodon idella*) [24], tub gurnard (*Trigla lucerna*) [25], and sea bream (*Sparus aurata*) [26] produce sperm containing DNA packaged by histones. However, this relationship between the mode of fertilization and type of protein used to package DNA in sperm does not extend to all species of fish. The sperm produced by salmon, herring, and many other species of fish that spawn and fertilize externally contain DNA that is packaged by protamines.

What these studies and those of chromatin in the sperm of other vertebrates and invertebrates have demonstrated is an evolutionary pattern in which the sperm chromatin proteins transition from histones to protamine-like proteins to protamines [27]. The variation observed in amphibians show that sporadic reversions are possible [28], and the fish studies [29] are consistent with this idea and provide additional examples that show the change from protamine to histone (or alternatively histone to protamine) has occurred independently several times during evolution.

## Spermatid Differentiation and Chromatin Remodeling

Prior to meiosis, the chromatin in the spermatocyte nucleus is diffusely organized and appears structurally similar to that found in the nuclei of all other somatic cells. The predominant chromatin proteins are the somatic histones and a wide variety of other proteins that interact with DNA to regulate gene activity, anchor the genome to the nuclear matrix, and contribute to chromatin function. As the cell proceeds through meiosis and enters the early stages of spermiogenesis, several new DNA-binding proteins are synthesized that bind to DNA and initiate a series of subtle transformations in the organization and activity of the spermatid's chromatin. The nature of these proteins and their impact on chromatin organization and function differ widely among species.

The changes that have been characterized in the greatest detail are those that occur in placental mammals. The first new proteins to appear are four histone variants that replace some or the majority of their somatic H2B, H3, H2A, and H1 histone counterparts [30]. These proteins were originally referred to as testis specific histones with a "T" designation being added to the histone's name. More recently, the same histone variants have been referred to as sperm-specific histones because they are frequently retained at some level in mature sperm. TH3 histone appears very early in spermatogenesis in spermatogonia. TH2B and TH2A histone variants are synthesized and integrated into the chromatin of pachytene spermatocytes just prior to meiosis, and a new H1 histone variant, H1t or TH1, appears near the end of meiotic prophase. Up to 90% of H2B is replaced by TH2B. The proportion of replacement for H3 and H2A is unknown. Seven H1 variants or subtypes have been identified in mice and men. In the case of the spermatid H1 variant, H1t, it replaces approximately half of the other H1 subtypes. However, some of these subtypes, such as H1a, actually increase in abundance and are not replaced. While these sperm histone variants are thought to play some role in altering the functionality of the chromatin, the basic structural subunit of chromatin organization, the nucleosome, is retained.

Electron microscopy studies have shown that the first noticeable change in chromatin structure occurs when the sperm specific histone H1t variant is deposited in spermatid chromatin. Prior to H1t deposition, the chromatin appears more diffuse and contains regions that are more clumped than others. When H1t appears, the chromatin is transformed into a more uniform and granular state. H1t remains bound to DNA for a relatively short period of time and then begins to disappear in elongating spermatids. Following its loss, the chromatin takes on a more filamentous organization [31].

In mammals, the majority of the histones are replaced after meiosis by three smaller, more basic proteins that have been designated "transition proteins" because they only remain associated with DNA for a relatively short period of time. The mammalian transition proteins TP1, TP2, and TP4 appear in the chromatin of mid-stage spermatids at the same time the majority of the histones are removed from the chromatin. Studies in human and rat spermatids have shown that TP2 synthesis and deposition in spermatid chromatin precedes that of TP1 [32, 33]. With the appearance of TP1 and TP2, the chromatin begins to condense somewhat with condensation progressing in the nucleus from an apical to caudal direction [31, 34]. Very little is currently known about TP4. While a great deal remains to be learned about the function of these proteins, it is clear that they play important roles in replacing histones (TP1 has been reported to destabilize nucleosomes by preventing DNA bending [35]), initiating the termination of gene transcription by TP2 binding to CpG sites [35], enabling or facilitating the repair of DNA strand breaks [36], and contributing to chromatin condensation. By the time TP1, TP2, and TP4 deposition are completed, the chromatin becomes uniformly condensed and no longer appears to retain the subunit structure characteristic of nucleosomes. A fourth protein, TP3, was also considered to be a member of this group when it was first observed in spermatid chromatin. Once the protein was sequenced, however, TP3 was identified to be the precursor form of protamine 2 [37]. Instead of being displaced from late-spermatid DNA, the protein is simply processed to a smaller form (protamine 2) that remains bound to DNA throughout the remainder of spermiogenesis.

These transition proteins are replaced by a set of positively charged proteins called protamine in late-step spermatids as the chromatin is reorganized one final time before the sperm becomes fully mature. The mammalian protamines are small proteins rich in cysteine and the basic amino acids arginine, lysine, and histidine. Considerable variation in amino acid sequence has been observed within the protamines of mammals [38–41], but all the proteins examined fall into one of two protamine families, protamine P1 or protamine P2. The nature of protamine binding to DNA and the consequences of the synthesis and incorporation of the protamines into spermatid chromatin suggest that these proteins may perform a number of functions. These include protecting the DNA from physical and chemical damage while the chromatin is in a state in which it cannot repair DNA damage and compacting the genomic material to produce a smaller, more hydrodynamically shaped cell. The compaction of the genome that occurs when protamine binds to DNA also ensures the entire genome is retained in a genetically inactive state until fertilization, and it may even aid in the shaping of the sperm head by generating the forces needed to shape the nucleus from within [42].

## Higher Ordered Organization of Chromatin in Mature Sperm

In contrast to the variability that has been observed in the composition of sperm chromatin in many vertebrates and invertebrates, there appears to be remarkably little variation in the final modes of DNA packaging that have been observed in sperm produced by different species of mammals. The sperm of all mammals examined to date, including monotremes, marsupials, and placental mammals, use protamines to package the majority of their DNA into the sperm head. In several mammalian species, a small fraction of the sperm genome has been observed to retain its histone packaging. This histone-containing fraction, which is currently thought to be present in all mammalian sperm, is small, comprising not more than a fraction to 1% of the genome. In human sperm, however, the fraction of DNA bound by histones is significantly larger, possibly as high as 10–15% [43–47].

Recent studies have identified a number of DNA sequences or genes that remain associated with histones in mammalian sperm. These include telomeric DNA [48], genes for epsilon and gamma globin [49], a paternally imprinted IGF-2 gene [50], microRNA clusters, the promoters of a number of genes expressing signaling proteins important for early embryonic development, and genes that produce transcription factors such as those in the Hox family [51]. Based on the types of genes that have been identified in histone associated sperm chromatin, it has been suggested that one function for the retention of these histones may be to maintain a subset of genes contributed by the male in a quiescent but accessible state so they can be activated immediately after fertilization and prior to the removal of the protamines. The histone-associated genes were also found to be highly enriched in a variety of imprinted genes, indicating another function of these histones may also be to play a role in epigenetic programming.

The chromatin in monotreme and marsupial spermatids is condensed during spermiogenesis in a fashion similar to that observed in other species that use only protamines to package their DNA, but the nature of the nuclear protein–DNA interactions that lead to this condensation in monotreme sperm have not yet been characterized. Chromatin condensation in platypus sperm is initiated by the formation of a layer of electron dense chromatin granules under the nucleolemma [52]. As the spermatids continue to mature, foci of condensing chromatin are observed throughout the nucleus. These studies have not, however, provided much information about either the organization or subunit structure of mature sperm chromatin in monotremes. A combination of EM and AFM studies of sperm chromatin in two marsupials, the fat tailed dunnart (*Sminthopsis crassicaudata*) and brush-tailed possum (*Trichosurus vulpecula*), has indicated the DNA is organized in nodular subunits [53]. Those regions of the chromatin that appear to be packaged by protamines have nodules with diameters of 50–80 nm, while other regions believed to contain histones bound to DNA contained much larger clusters (120–160 nm) of smaller nodules.

Chromatin reorganization and compaction occurs in a similar manner in placental mammals. The chromatin is transformed from the diffuse, genetically active state to a highly electron dense, compact form of chromatin that is completely inactive. Both electron and atomic force microscopy studies of spermatid chromatin and partially decondensed sperm chromatin have provided insight into the higher ordered structure of sperm chromatin in placental mammals. EM images of the chromatin in differentiating late-step spermatids have shown that the DNA starts off organized with features characteristic of somatic chromatin (~11 nm nodules and 30 nm fibers [54]), which are subsequently transformed into nodular structures or fibers with diameters (50–100 nm) much larger than individual nucleosomes. As chromatin condensation progresses, these nodules coalesce into increasingly larger masses or fibers that eventually become so electron dense and tightly packed that they can no longer be distinguished.

Similar structural information has been derived from high resolution microscopy studies of sperm chromatin that has been partially decondensed by treatment with polyanions, reducing agents, or high ionic strength or by partial digestion by nucleases [55–62]. Analyses of partially decondensed sperm chromatin by electron microscopy have shown that at least two different sized structural units are present, small nodules similar in size to nucleosomes and much larger globular structures. Atomic force microscopy images of decondensed human sperm also revealed the presence of two types of structures: small subunits similar in diameter (~10 nm) and thickness (~5 nm) to somatic nucleosomes and lifesaver shaped larger structures approximately 60–100 nm in diameter and 20 nm thick with a hole or depression in the center [56]. Toroids with lifesaver-like features and similar dimensions have also been generated in vitro when protamine or other polycations were added to dilute solutions of DNA or to individual DNA molecules [63–65]. These toroids, which contain approximately 50,000 bp of DNA complexed with protamine, are spontaneously generated when protamine binds to and neutralize the phosphodiester backbone of double-stranded DNA [56, 66]. Closely packed beads with diameters similar to these toroids were found by Koehler to comprise the lamellar sheets of chromatin packed inside rat, rabbit, bull, and human sperm [59, 60, 67].

## Mammalian Protamines

While the unusually high arginine content of protamine was recognized by both Miescher and Kossel to be a unique feature of fish sperm nuclear proteins more than 100 years ago, it took more than 50 years for researchers to begin to understand and appreciate the structural and functional differences between the protamines and histones. Structurally, the two families of DNA-binding proteins are very different. The four core histones interact with each other to form a well-defined octamer core of protein around which almost two turns of DNA are wrapped [68]. The DNA bound to the histones remains accessible to polymerases and other proteins and the genes packaged by histone remain active or can be readily activated. By marked contrast, the protamines contain so many positively charged amino-acid side chains that when protamine binds to DNA, it wraps around the DNA helix, neutralizing the negatively charged phosphodiester backbone of DNA and creating a maximally compact form of chromatin [56]. This prevents the genes packaged by protamines from being accessed by other proteins and modified, transcribed or repaired.

Two different types of protamines package DNA in mammalian sperm, P1 and P2. The smaller protein, protamine P1, is found in the sperm of all mammals [69]. The P1 protamine of placental mammals is a single peptide chain containing only 50 amino acids [70]. The one known exception is stallion P1, which contains 51 amino acids. The P1 protamines in marsupials and monotremes are larger (57–70 residues). The platypus and echidna protamines also differ from the P1 protamines of placental mammals in that they do not contain any cysteine residues [71]. This is also the case for most marsupial protamines [41]. One exception has been reported, however, in the family of Dasyuridae. Shrew-like marsupials in the genus *Planigales* produce protamines that containing 5–6 cysteines [72], a number similar to the number of cysteines that are typically found in the P1 protamines of placental mammals.

The P1 protamine of placental mammals is unstructured in solution and only adopts a specific conformation when bound to DNA [73]. Protamine P1 sequences are typically divided into three small domains, a central DNA-binding domain comprised of a series of $(Arg)_n$ DNA-binding domains interspersed with one or two uncharged amino acids and two short N- and C-terminal peptide domains that do not bind to DNA [70, 74]. Only the DNA-binding domain appears to be present in monotreme and marsupial P1 molecules [41, 71]. The two short terminal peptide domains in placental mammal P1 molecules contain serine and threonine residues that are phosphorylated shortly after the protein is synthesized, and this modification is thought to facilitate the protein's binding correctly to DNA. Similar phosphorylatable residues appear to be distributed throughout the monotreme and marsupial P1 sequences. These domains in placental mammal P1 molecules also contain multiple cysteine residues that form inter- and intraprotamine disulfide bonds and link each protamine molecule to its neighbor when the maturing spermatid passes through the epididymis [74].

Protamine P2, which is slightly larger than P1 (63 amino acids in mouse) is only expressed in the differentiating spermatids of a subset of placental mammals. These include primates, most rodents, lagomorphs, and perissodactyls [69]. Unlike protamine P1, P2 is synthesized as a larger precursor protein (106 residues in mouse) that is deposited onto DNA and subsequently shortened over a period of several days [75]. This processing of the precursor protein occurs by progressive and sequential cleavage of short peptide fragments from the amino terminus of the precursor

[76–78]. The function of this processing remains unknown. P2 also appears to be phosphorylated transiently. How the final processed form of P2 interacts with DNA has not yet been determined, but studies of P1 and P2 in several species suggest the majority of the length of the P2 molecule binds to DNA. The "footprint" of P1 when bound to DNA is 10–11 base pairs, or one full turn of DNA, while the "footprint" of P2 appears to be larger (15 bp) [43]. The final processed form of P2 also appears to use a series of $(Arg)_n$ anchoring peptide segments to bind to DNA. These segments are shorter and less well defined than those found in the DNA-binding domain of P1, and they are distributed throughout the entire length of the P2 sequence. P2 also contains multiple cysteine residues that participate in the formation of the disulfide bonds that interconnect all the protamines late in spermiogenesis.

## Structure of the DNA–Protamine Complex

While the relative proportion of the two protamines in sperm chromatin varies widely between mammalian genera, the proportion appears to be conserved among the species within a genus [69]. P2 is believed to bind to DNA in a manner similar to P1, but the evidence for this is limited and primarily circumstantial. Beyond the knowledge that both protamines P1 and P2 bind along the DNA in some manner that allows the two proteins to be cross-linked together by disulfide bridges during the final stage of sperm maturation, very little is known about the details of P2 binding to DNA or the distribution of the two protamines along a segment of DNA.

Because it has not been possible to determine the structure of a native or artificial protamine–DNA complex by X-ray crystallography or NMR spectroscopy, most of the information that has been learned about how the protamines interact with DNA has been determined using lower resolution techniques. Low-angle X-ray scattering experiments performed on intact sperm heads confirmed the close packing of the DNA within sperm chromatin, showing the center to center distance between adjacent DNA molecules is approximately 2.7 nm [79]. To achieve this tight packing, the molecules must be organized in a hexagonal arrangement with only 7 Å distance of separation between the surfaces of adjacent molecules. High-resolution EM studies of individual toroidal subunits [80] have shown that the individual DNA molecules coiled into the toroid are tightly packed in a hexagonal arrangement, consistent with what has been observed by low-angle X-ray scattering. Such a packing arrangement for DNA is also consistent with the microscopy data obtained from stallion sperm heads [81], particularly if the toroidal structures are stacked tightly together as lifesavers and organized in layers similar to the lamellae reported by Koehler [59, 60, 67].

At the molecular level, the protamines bind to duplex DNA in a manner that is independent of base sequence [66, 82]. The primary interactions are electrostatic and involve the binding of the positively charged guanidinium groups in the arginine residues present in the DNA anchoring domains of protamine to the negatively charged phosphates that comprise the DNA phosphodiester backbone. The high affinity of binding is derived from two aspects of these interactions, the formation of a salt bridge and hydrogen bond between the guanidinium group and the phosphate and the binding of every arginine residue in the DNA-binding domain of protamine to every phosphate group in one turn of DNA. Both computer modeling and X-ray scattering and other experimental studies [73, 83–85] have shown that the DNA-binding domain of protamine P1 wraps in an extended conformation around the DNA helix, partially filling the major groove. By interacting in this way, adjacent arginine residues in the $(Arg)_n$ anchoring domains would be expected to bind to phosphates on opposite strands of the duplex DNA molecule, interlocking the relative positions of the bases together and preventing strand separation or changes in DNA conformation throughout the period that the protamines remain bound to DNA. This would result in the production of a neutral, highly insoluble complex that allows the DNA strands to be packed tightly together without charge repulsion.

## Chromosome Territories, Loop Domains, and Matrix Attachment Regions

Three important structural features of somatic chromatin organization appear to be retained by mammalian sperm chromatin even after all the nuclear protein transitions and condensation have been completed. Confocal microscopy of somatic cells hybridized to fluorochrome-tagged DNA probes have shown that the DNA of individual chromosomes are not randomly distributed throughout the nucleus, but each is confined to a specific domain or territory inside the interphase nucleus [86–90]. Not only is there evidence that the chromosomal DNA molecules occupy a reproducible position, but there is also evidence that the domains are folded into shapes characteristic of a particular chromosome [91]. Similar observations have been made regarding the distribution of chromosomal DNA in mammalian sperm nuclei. Fluorescence in situ hybridization has been used to demonstrate that the DNA of individual chromosomes are also localized to specific domains inside the heads of human, bull, mouse, echidna, and platypus sperm [48, 91–94]. While these studies have not provided strong evidence that the chromosomes are arranged in any particular order relative to each other in the sperm heads of placental mammals, there is some evidence for a particular arrangement in echidna and platypus sperm.

Two other organizational features that are retained in sperm cell nuclei are the chromatin loop domains and the attachment of the chromatin to a nuclear protein scaffold or nuclear matrix [95–98]. The protein content of the nuclear matrix changes as the spermatid differentiates [95], but the DNA remains bound to the matrix at a very large number of sites (~50,000). This matrix appears by EM to be a network of dense protein filaments filling the interior of the head of the spermatid and sperm bounded by a peripheral structure, the lamina. The DNA in between the sites of attachment to the matrix appears to retain the loop organization present in somatic cells [99, 100]. These loops, which contain 40,000–50,000 bp of DNA in both the somatic and sperm nucleus, are anchored to a matrix through specific chromatin domains, called nuclear scaffold/matrix attachment regions (SARs/MARs). The retention of the matrix and its associations with DNA in sperm are important to maintain because their presence would facilitate and speed up the process of genome reactivation following fertilization and the initiation of the first cycle of DNA replication in the male pronucleus [101, 102]. The loop domains are believed to play an essential role in transcriptional regulation, DNA replication, and chromosome organization both prior to spermiogenesis and after fertilization. In sperm, these loops may also aid in the packing of the DNA by protamines into toroids, which also contain ~50,000 bp of DNA.

The retention of these particular features of chromosome and chromatin organization appears to preserve important genome organizational information critical to both germinal and somatic cell function. Clearly, the primary function of spermiogenesis is to produce a package of genomic information, the sperm cell, that will facilitate the transport of one complement of the male's chromosomes to and into the oocyte for the purpose of generating an embryo containing genomic contributions from both the male and female of the species. Once this is accomplished, the genome must be quickly reactivated so that it can begin functioning as a somatic cell, with subsets of genes being turned on and off as the cells are transformed from embryonic stem cells into the cells of the various tissues and organs.

## Reorganization of Sperm Chromatin Following Fertilization

The formation of the male pronucleus and other processes associated with early embryonic development that occur immediately after fertilization have been well characterized by light microscopy. However, remarkably little is known at the molecular level about the early events that contribute to the unpackaging of sperm chromatin following fertilization. The current hypothesis is that the protamines are actively removed from the DNA by a histone chaperone similar to the nucleoplasmin first identified in frogs [103–105]. This protein chaperone has been shown to bind and carry core histones and, in the presence of DNA, is able to load the histones onto the DNA and generate nucleosomes. Sequence analyses of the frog and related mammalian proteins have shown that these proteins contain a series of polyglutamic acid sequences. Experiments conducted with sperm chromatin have also shown that the protein is able to remove protamine from the DNA prior to loading it with histones [106]. One possible mechanism of protamine removal may involve these segments of polyglutamic acid. The polyglutamic acid regions in nucleoplasmin-like proteins could form a series of salt bridges with the $(Arg)_n$ DNA-binding domains of the protamines and remove the protamines from DNA intact prior to depositing the histones and reestablishing the nucleosomal organization required to reactivate the new embryo's genome.

Another early event associated with the unpacking of the sperm chromatin that occurs almost immediately after removing the protamines is the initiation of a period of DNA synthesis associated with DNA damage repair [107–110]. This repair synthesis is required to repair DNA strand breaks and remove DNA adducts or other damage that is acquired during spermiogenesis and epididymal transit and storage when repair activities could not be performed due to the packaging of the genome by protamines. Studies have shown that the majority of the damage brought into the oocyte by the sperm is repaired during this period of DNA synthesis, and this process is considered to be critical for maintaining the integrity of the male genome and for ensuring normal embryonic development.

## Consequences of Disrupting Sperm Chromatin Remodeling

Several changes associated with the reorganization of spermatid chromatin have been shown to be important for male fertility. One involves the removal of the majority of the histones and their replacement by protamines. Numerous studies have suggested that there is a positive correlation between male subfertility or infertility and elevated levels of histone in mature human sperm [77, 111–117]. It is not known, however, whether the problems encountered relate to the lack of removal of somatic histones from genes that need to be packaged by protamines, deficiencies in expression and incorporation of the sperm specific histone variants into subsets of nucleosomes, or errors in imprinting that may involve histone packaging.

Alterations in the expression and/or translation of the protamine genes have also been linked to infertility. Changes in the proportion of the P1 or P2 proteins present in sperm chromatin have been shown to not only be linked to infertility [118–124] but also adversely impact in vitro fertilization outcome and early embryonic development [125–129]. The observed differences in protamine content ranged from having very little protamine, to having too little protamine P1 or too little protamine P2. By contrast, analyses of sperm obtained from fertile human males have shown repeatedly that the sperm contain a specific proportion (1:1) of P1 and P2 [118–120, 130]. The primary cause for the observed changes in sperm protamine content appears to involve errors in gene expression, although incomplete processing of the P2 precursor may also contribute to decreased levels of the mature P2 protein.

Other studies have shown that the timely formation of the protamine disulfide cross-links that occur during the final stages of sperm maturation are important. In mammals, both protamines P1 and P2 contain multiple cysteine residues. The thiol groups of these cysteines are in the reduced form (free thiols) when the protamines are synthesized and deposited onto DNA, and they remain reduced until the final stage of spermiogenesis when they participate in the formation of both inter-and intramolecular protamine disulfides as the sperm pass through the epididymis [74, 131–134]. Cases of human, stallion, and bull infertility have been correlated with what appear to be errors in disulfide cross-linking among the protamines. What role these disulfide bonds play is still not known, but one theory is that the formation of interprotamine disulfide bonding stabilizes the chromatin and protects it from physical damage. An equally feasible possibility is that these disulfide bonds not only stabilize the chromatin but also prevent the thiol groups from being oxidized or alkylated during the long period of time required for spermatid maturation and sperm storage prior to fertilization. This might be important if the cysteine residues in mammalian protamine also play some other role in sperm chromatin, such as participating in protamine removal from DNA after fertilization. If the thiols were required for efficient protamine removal, the oxidation or alkylation of even a few cysteines could potentially complicate or prevent the efficient removal of the modified protamine from the male genome, and its retention would block the gene it was bound to from being transcribed or replicated later in development. Mice exposed to alkylating agents such as methyl methanesulfonate and ethylene oxide at a time prior to protamine disulfide bond formation have been shown to produce sperm with alkylated protamine thiols [135–137]. Matings conducted with the treated males resulted in the production of embryos that died early in development from dominant lethal mutations [136]. The sperm containing the protamines with alkylated cysteines succeeded in fertilizing oocytes and inducing embryonic development, but at some point after fertilization the embryo died when a key gene could not be turned on.

Male infertility has also been linked to deficiencies in sperm chromatin-associated zinc. Zinc is known to be essential for several aspects of sperm development, ranging from contributions to structural elements in the tail to roles in chromatin organization and protamine structure and function [138]. A deficiency in zinc can affect the developing sperm directly, or it can impact the function of other testicular cells that contribute to or play a role in spermatid maturation, such as sertoli cells. Because zinc plays multiple roles in spermatogenesis and testicular function, it has been difficult to decipher how sperm chromatin bound zinc impacts the functionality of the sperm cell. Chromatin associated zinc is almost exclusively bound to protamine P2 in mammals [139]. In human, bull, mouse, and hamster sperm, a single zinc atom is bound to each P2 molecule. Zinc does not appear to bind to protamine P1. Zinc ion coordination by P2 occurs sometime after the synthesis of P2 and its deposition onto DNA, long before the sperm cell enters the seminal fluid and the sperm chromatin can be impacted by seminal fluid zinc. Where the zinc binds in P2 has not been determined, but the amino acids in protamine P2 that coordinate the zinc appear to change during sperm maturation. In sonication resistant spermatids, the zinc is coordinated only by cysteines, while in mature sperm, both histidine and cysteine residues participate in the coordination (unpublished results). The function of this P2 bound zinc is not known, but it has been suggested that the coordination of the zinc by protamine may influence the binding of the protamine to DNA [140, 141] or to other protamines [138]. An alternative possibility is that zinc coordination by cysteine residues in protamine might also protect the thiol groups and prevent their oxidation until it is time for the cysteines to form inter- and intramolecular disulfide bonds. Several studies have also suggested that exposures to other metals, such as copper and lead, may result in these metals binding to the cysteines in protamine in place of zinc (or prior to disulfide bond formation) and their being transported into the oocyte upon fertilization [133, 142, 143]. In addition to potentially disrupting the function of sperm by altering chromatin decondensation or protamine P2 function, the delivery of these and other toxic metals into the oocyte would also be expected to have an adverse impact on early embryonic development.

# Future Research and Practical Applications

The dramatic changes in the structure and function of sperm chromatin that occur during spermatogenesis have continued to intrigue researchers for more than a century. In addition to wanting to understand how these changes in chromatin organization affect genome function, many of the studies conducted in placental mammals have been driven by a desire to understand the relationship between sperm chromatin organization and sperm function (fertility) or dysfunction (subfertility or infertility). While we have learned a great deal, many important questions still remain unanswered. Major technological advances in imaging techniques, transgenic animal production, gene function disruption, molecular and compositional analysis at the single cell and sub-cellular level as well as the development of many new molecular probes now make it possible to design and carry out studies that examine structure and function at the level of the individual cell in ways that have not been previously possible. Studies to be conducted in the next decade using these tools should advance our understanding of sperm chromatin structure and function quickly while providing new information that can be used to diagnose and treat male infertility, develop new male contraceptives, and contribute to other unrelated areas of research such as improving the efficiency of creating transgenic animals or targeted genome silencing for cancer therapy.

# References

1. Mendel G. Experiment in plant hybribization. Paper presented at: Brunn Natural History Society; March, 1865, 1865; Brunn, Czechoslovakia.
2. Haeckel E. Generelle Morphologie der Organismen. Berlin: Reimer; 1866.
3. Miescher F. Letter I to Wilhelm His; Tubingen, February 26th, 1869. In: His W, ed. Die Histochemischen und Physiologischen Arbeiten von Friedrich Miescher – Aus dem sissenschaft – lichen Briefwechsel von F. Miescher. Vol 1. Liepzig: F. C. W. Vogel; 1869:pp. 33–8.
4. Miescher F. Uber die chemische Zusammensetzung der Eiter – zellen. Med Chem Unters. 1871;4:441–60.
5. Flemming W. Uber das Verhalten des Kern bei der Zellltheilung und uber dei Bedeutung mekrkerniger Zellen. Arch Pathol Anat Physiol. 1879;77:1–29.
6. Miescher F. Das Protamin – Eine neue organishe Basis aus den Samenssden des Rheinlachses. Ber Dtesch Chem Ges. 1874;7:376.
7. Kossel A. Ueber die Constitution der einfachsten Eiweissstoffe. Z Pysiologische Chemie. 1898;25:165–89.
8. Kossel A, Dakin HD. Uber Salmin und Clupein. Z Pysiologische Chemie. 1904;41:407–15.
9. Kossel A, Dakin HD. Weitere Beitrage zum System der einfachsten Eiweisskorper. Z Pysiologische Chemie. 1905;44:342–6.
10. Kossel A, Edlbacher F. Uber einige Spaltungsprodukte des Thynnins und Pereins. Z Pysiologische Chemie. 1913;88:186–9.
11. Reik W, Walter J. Genomic imprinting: parental influence on the genome. Nat Rev Genet. 2001;2(1):21–32.
12. Solter D. Differential imprinting and expression of maternal and paternal genomes. Annu Rev Genet. 1988;22:127–46.

13. Gartler SM, Goldman MA. X-chromosome inactivation, Encyclopedia of life. New York: Wiley Interscience; 2005. p. 1–6.
14. Heard E, Clerc P, Avner P. X-chromosome inactivation in mammals. Annu Rev Genet. 1997; 31:571–610.
15. Ney PA. Gene expression during terminal erythroid differentiation. Curr Opin Hematol. 2006; 13(4):203–8.
16. Berlowitz L. Chromosomal inactivation and reactivation in mealy bugs. Genetics. 1974;78(1): 311–22.
17. Bloch D. Handbook of Genetics, vol. 5. New York: Plenum Press; 1976.
18. Palau J, Ruiz-Carrillo A, Subirana JA. Histones from sperm of the sea urchin *Arbacia lixula*. Eur J Biochem. 1969;7(2):209–13.
19. Eirin-Lopez JM, Ausio J. Origin and evolution of chromosomal sperm proteins. Bioessays. 2009;31(10):1062–70.
20. Kasinsky HE, Huang SY, Mann M, Roca J, Subirana JA. On the diversity of sperm histones in the vertebrates: IV. Cytochemical and amino acid analysis in Anura. J Exp Zool. 1985;234(1):33–46.
21. Mann M, Risley MS, Eckhardt RA, Kasinsky HE. Characterization of spermatid/sperm basic chromosomal proteins in the genus Xenopus (Anura, Pipidae). J Exp Zool. 1982;222(2):173–86.
22. Takamune K, Nishida H, Takai M, Katagiri C. Primary structure of toad sperm protamines and nucleotide sequence of their cDNAs. Eur J Biochem. 1991;196(2):401–6.
23. Su H. Characterization of nuclear basic proteins in sperm and erythrocytes of vertebrates. Vancouver: Department of Zoology, University of British Columbia; 2004.
24. Kadura SN, Khrapunov SN, Chabanny VN, Berdyshev GD. Changes in chromatin basic proteins during male gametogenesis of grass carp. Comp Biochem Physiol B. 1983;74(2):343–50.
25. Saperas N, Lloris D, Chiva M. Sporadic appearance of histones, histone-like proteins, and protamines in sperm chromatin of bony fish. J Exp Zool. 2005;265(5):575–86.
26. Kurtz K, Saperas N, Ausio J, Chiva M. Spermiogenic nuclear protein transitions and chromatin condensation. Proposal for an ancestral model of nuclear spermiogenesis. J Exp Zool B Mol Dev Evol. 2009;312B(3):149–63.
27. Ausio J. Histone H1 and evolution of sperm nuclear basic proteins. J Biol Chem. 1999;274(44): 31115–8.
28. Kasinsky HE, Gutovich L, Kulak D, et al. Protamine-like sperm nuclear basic proteins in the primitive frog *Ascaphus truei* and histone reversions among more advanced frogs. J Exp Zool. 1999;284(7):717–28.
29. Saperas N, Chiva M, Pfeiffer DC, Kasinsky HE, Ausio J. Sperm nuclear basic proteins (SNBPs) of agnathans and chondrichthyans: variability and evolution of sperm proteins in fish. J Mol Evol. 1997;44(4):422–31.
30. Churikov D, Zalenskaya IA, Zalensky AO. Male germline-specific histones in mouse and man. Cytogenet Genome Res. 2004;105(2–4):203–14.
31. Oko RJ, Jando V, Wagner CL, Kistler WS, Hermo LS. Chromatin reorganization in rat spermatids during the disappearance of testis-specific histone, H1t, and the appearance of transition proteins TP1 and TP2. Biol Reprod. 1996;54(5):1141–57.
32. Kistler WS, Henriksen K, Mali P, Parvinen M. Sequential expression of nucleoproteins during rat spermiogenesis. Exp Cell Res. 1996;225(2):374–81.
33. Steger K, Klonisch T, Gavenis K, Drabent B, Doenecke D, Bergmann M. Expression of mRNA and protein of nucleoproteins during human spermiogenesis. Mol Hum Reprod. 1998;4(10): 939–45.
34. Alfonso P, Kistler WS. Immunohistochemical localization of spermatid nuclear transition protein 2 in the testes of rats and mice. Biol Reprod. 1993;48(3):522–9.
35. Pradeepa MM, Rao MR. Chromatin remodeling during mammalian spermatogenesis: role of testis specific histone variants and transition proteins. Soc Reprod Fertil Suppl. 2007;63:1–10.
36. Caron N, Veilleux S, Boissonneault G. Stimulation of DNA repair by the spermatidal TP1 protein. Mol Reprod Dev. 2001;58(4):437–43.

37. Unni E, Zhang Y, Meistrich ML, Balhorn R. Rat spermatid basic nuclear protein Tp3 is the precursor of protamine 2. Exp Cell Res. 1994;210(1):39–45.

38. Queralt R, Adroer R, Oliva R, Winkfein RJ, Retief JD, Dixon GH. Evolution of protamine P1 genes in mammals. J Mol Evol. 1995;40(6):601–7.

39. Retief JD, Dixon GH. Evolution of pro-protamine P2 genes in primates. Eur J Biochem. 1993;214(2):609–15.

40. Retief JD, Krajewski C, Westerman M, Dixon GH. The evolution of protamine P1 genes in dasyurid marsupials. J Mol Evol. 1995;41(5):549–55.

41. Retief JD, Krajewski C, Westerman M, Winkfein RJ, Dixon GH. Molecular phylogeny and evolution of marsupial protamine P1 genes. Proc Biol Sci. 1995;259(1354):7–14.

42. Cree LH, Balhorn R, Brewer LR. Single molecule studies of DNA-protamine interactions. Protein Pept Lett. 2011;18(8):802–10.

43 Bench GS, Friz AM, Corzett MH, Morse DH, Balhorn R. DNA and total protamine masses in individual sperm from fertile mammalian subjects. Cytometry. 1996;23(4):263–71.

44. Gatewood JM, Cook GR, Balhorn R, Schmid CW, Bradbury EM. Isolation of four core histones from human sperm chromatin representing a minor subset of somatic histones. J Biol Chem. 1990;265(33):20662–6.

45. Gusse M, Sautière P, Bélaiche D, et al. Purification and characterization of nuclear basic proteins of human sperm. Biochim Biophys Acta. 1986;884(1):124–34.

46. Tanphaichitr N, Sobhon P, Taluppeth N, Chalermisarachai P. Basic nuclear proteins in testicular cells and ejaculated spermatozoa in man. Exp Cell Res. 1978;117(2):347–56.

47. Wykes SM, Krawetz SA. The structural organization of sperm chromatin. J Biol Chem. 2003;278(32):29471–7.

48. Zalenskaya IA, Zalensky AO. Non-random positioning of chromosomes in human sperm nuclei. Chromosome Res. 2004;12(2):163–73.

49. Gardiner-Garden M, Ballesteros M, Gordon M, Tam PP. Histone- and protamine-DNA association: conservation of different patterns within the beta-globin domain in human sperm. Mol Cell Biol. 1998;18(6):3350–6.

50. Banerjee S, Smallwood A. Chromatin modification of imprinted H19 gene in mammalian spermatozoa. Mol Reprod Dev. 1998;50(4):474–84.

51. Hammoud SS, Nix DA, Zhang H, Purwar J, Carrell DT, Cairns BR. Distinctive chromatin in human sperm packages genes for embryo development. Nature. 2009;460(7254):473–8.

52. Lin M, Jones RC. Spermiogenesis and spermiation in a monotreme mammal, the platypus, Ornithorhynchus anatinus. J Anat. 2000;196(Pt 2):217–32.

53. Soon LL, Bottema C, Breed WG. Atomic force microscopy and cytochemistry of chromatin from marsupial spermatozoa with special reference to Sminthopsis crassicaudata. Mol Reprod Dev. 1997;48(3):367–74.

54. Horowitz RA, Agard DA, Sedat JW, Woodcock CL. The three-dimensional architecture of chromatin in situ: electron tomography reveals fibers composed of a continuously variable zig-zag nucleosomal ribbon. J Cell Biol. 1994;125(1):1–10.

55. Allen MJ, Lee C, Lee JDt, et al. Atomic force microscopy of mammalian sperm chromatin. Chromosoma. 1993;102(9):623–30.

56. Balhorn R, Cosman M, Thornton K, et al. Protamine mediated condensation of DNA in mammalian sperm. In: Gagnon C, editor. The male gamete: from basic knowledge to clinical applications: Proceedings of the 8th International Symposium of Spermatology. Vienna, IL: Cache River; 1999.

57. Evenson DP, Witkin SS, de Harven E, Bendich A. Ultrastructure of partially decondensed human spermatozoal chromatin. J Ultrastruct Res. 1978;63(2):178–87.

58. Koehler JK. Fine structure observations in frozen-etched bovine spermatozoa. J Ultrastruct Res. 1966;16(3):359–75.

59. Koehler JK. A freeze-etching study of rabbit spermatozoa with particular reference to head structures. J Ultrastruct Res. 1970;33(5):598–614.

60. Koehler JK, Wurschmidt U, Larsen MP. Nuclear and chromatin structure in rat spermatozoa. Gamate Res. 1983;8:357–77.

61. Sobhon P, Chutatape C, Chalermisarachai P, Vongpayabal P, Tanphaichitr N. Transmission and scanning electron microscopic studies of the human sperm chromatin decondensed by micrococcal nuclease and salt. J Exp Zool. 1982;221(1):61–79.
62. Wagner TE, Yun JS. Fine structure of human sperm chromatin. Arch Androl. 1979;2(4): 291–4.
63. Allen MJ, Bradbury EM, Balhorn R. AFM analysis of DNA-protamine complexes bound to mica. Nucleic Acids Res. 1997;25(11):2221–6.
64. Bloomfield VA. Condensation of DNA by multivalent cations: considerations on mechanism. Biopolymers. 1991;31(13):1471–81.
65. Marquet R, Wyart A, Houssier C. Influence of DNA length on spermine-induced condensation. Importance of the bending and stiffening of DNA. Biochim Biophys Acta. 1987;909(3): 165–72.
66. Brewer LR, Corzett M, Balhorn R. Protamine-induced condensation and decondensation of the same DNA molecule. Science. 1999;286(5437):120–3.
67. Koehler JK. Human sperm head ultrastructure: a freeze-etching study. J Ultrastruct Res. 1972; 39(5):520–39.
68. Finch JT, Lutter LC, Rhodes D, et al. Structure of nucleosome core particles of chromatin. Nature. 1977;269(5623):29–36.
69. Corzett M, Mazrimas J, Balhorn R. Protamine 1: protamine 2 stoichiometry in the sperm of eutherian mammals. Mol Reprod Dev. 2002;61(4):519–27.
70. Balhorn R. The protamine family of sperm nuclear proteins. Genome Biol. 2007;8(9):227.
71. Retief JD, Winkfein RJ, Dixon GH. Evolution of the monotremes. The sequences of the protamine P1 genes of platypus and echidna. Eur J Biochem. 1993;218(2):457–61.
72. Retief JD, Rees JS, Westerman M, Dixon GH. Convergent evolution of cysteine residues in sperm protamines of one genus of marsupials, the Planigales. Mol Biol Evol. 1995;12(4):708–12.
73. Hud NV, Milanovich FP, Balhorn R. Evidence of novel secondary structure in DNA-bound protamine is revealed by raman spectroscopy. Biochemistry. 1994;33(24):7528–35.
74. Balhorn R. Mammalian protamines: structure and molecular interactions. In: Adolph KW, editor. Molecular biology of chromosome function. New York: Springer; 1989. p. 366–95.
75. Yelick PC, Balhorn R, Johnson PA, et al. Mouse protamine 2 is synthesized as a precursor whereas mouse protamine 1 is not. Mol Cell Biol. 1987;7(6):2173–9.
76. Carré-Eusèbe D, Lederer F, Lê KH, Elsevier SM. Processing of the precursor of protamine P2 in mouse. Peptide mapping and N-terminal sequence analysis of intermediates. Biochem J. 1991;277(Pt 1):39–45.
77. Chauviere M, Martinage A, Debarle M, Sautiere P, Chevaillier P. Molecular characterization of six intermediate proteins in the processing of mouse protamine P2 precursor. Eur J Biochem. 1992;204(2):759–65.
78. Elsevier SM, Noiran J, Carre-Eusebe D. Processing of the precursor of protamine P2 in mouse. Identification of intermediates by their insolubility in the presence of sodium dodecyl sulfate. Eur J Biochem. 1991;196(1):167–75.
79. Schellman JA, Parthasarathy N. X-ray diffraction studies on cation-collapsed DNA. J Mol Biol. 1984;175(3):313–29.
80. Hud NV, Vilfan ID. Toroidal DNA condensates: unraveling the fine structure and the role of nucleation in determining size. Annu Rev Biophys Biomol Struct. 2005;34:295–318.
81. Livolant F. Cholesteric organization of DNA in the stallion sperm head. Tissue Cell. 1984;16(4):535–55.
82. Bianchi F, Rousseaux-Prevost R, Bailly C, Rousseaux J. Interaction of human P1 and P2 protamines with DNA. Biochem Biophys Res Commun. 1994;201(3):1197–204.
83. Feughelman M, Langridge R, Seeds WE, et al. Molecular structure of deoxyriboncleic acid and nucleoprotein. Nature. 1955;175:834–8.
84. Prieto MC, Maki AH, Balhorn R. Analysis of DNA-protamine interactions by optical detection of magnetic resonance. Biochemistry. 1997;36(39):11944–51.
85. Wilkins MFH. Physical studies of the molecular structure of deoxyribonucleic acid and nucleoprotein. Cold Spring Harb Symp Quant Biol. 1956;21:75–90.

86. Cremer T, Cremer C. Chromosome territories, nuclear architecture and gene regulation in mammalian cells. Nat Rev Genet. 2001;2(4):292–301.
87. Lichter P, Cremer T, Borden J, Manuelidis L, Ward DC. Delineation of individual human chromosomes in metaphase and interphase cells by in situ suppression hybridization using recombinant DNA libraries. Hum Genet. 1988;80(3):224–34.
88. Savage JR. Interchange and intra-nuclear architecture. Environ Mol Mutagen. 1993;22(4): 234–44.
89. Schardin M, Cremer T, Hager HD, Lang M. Specific staining of human chromosomes in Chinese hamster × man hybrid cell lines demonstrates interphase chromosome territories. Hum Genet. 1985;71(4):281–7.
90. Weierich C, Brero A, Stein S, et al. Three-dimensional arrangements of centromeres and telomeres in nuclei of human and murine lymphocytes. Chromosome Res. 2003;11(5):485–502.
91. Manuelidis L. Individual interphase chromosome domains revealed by in situ hybridization. Hum Genet. 1985;71(4):288–93.
92. Manvelyan M, Hunstig F, Bhatt S, et al. Chromosome distribution in human sperm – a 3D multicolor banding-study. Mol Cytogenet. 2008;1:25.
93. Mudrak O, Tomilin N, Zalensky A. Chromosome architecture in the decondensing human sperm nucleus. J Cell Sci. 2005;118(Pt 19):4541–50.
94. Zalensky A, Zalenskaya I. Organization of chromosomes in spermatozoa: an additional layer of epigenetic information? Biochem Soc Trans. 2007;35(Pt 3):609–11.
95. Chen JL, Guo SH, Gao FH. Nuclear matrix in developing rat spermatogenic cells. Mol Reprod Dev. 2001;59(3):314–21.
96. Santi S, Rubbini S, Cinti C, et al. Ultrastructural organization of the sperm nuclear matrix. Ital J Anat Embryol. 1995;100 Suppl 1:39–46.
97. Ward WS, Coffey DS. DNA packaging and organization in mammalian spermatozoa: comparison with somatic cells. Biol Reprod. 1991;44(4):569–74.
98. Yaron Y, Kramer JA, Gyi K, et al. Centromere sequences localize to the nuclear halo of human spermatozoa. Int J Androl. 1998;21(1):13–8.
99. Heng HH, Goetze S, Ye CJ, et al. Chromatin loops are selectively anchored using scaffold/ matrix-attachment regions. J Cell Sci. 2004;117(Pt 7):999–1008.
100. Heng HH, Krawetz SA, Lu W, Bremer S, Liu G, Ye CJ. Re-defining the chromatin loop domain. Cytogenet Cell Genet. 2001;93(3–4):155–61.
101. Shaman JA, Yamauchi Y, Ward WS. Function of the sperm nuclear matrix. Arch Androl. 2007;53(3):135–40.
102. Shaman JA, Yamauchi Y, Ward WS. The sperm nuclear matrix is required for paternal DNA replication. J Cell Biochem. 2007;102(3):680–8.
103. Frehlick LJ, Eirin-Lopez JM, Jeffery ED, Hunt DF, Ausio J. The characterization of amphibian nucleoplasmins yields new insight into their role in sperm chromatin remodeling. BMC Genomics. 2006;7:99.
104. McLay DW, Clarke HJ. Remodelling the paternal chromatin at fertilization in mammals. Reproduction. 2003;125(5):625–33.
105. Philpott A, Leno GH. Nucleoplasmin remodels sperm chromatin in Xenopus egg extracts. Cell. 1992;69(5):759–67.
106. Katagiri C, Ohsumi K. Remodeling of sperm chromatin induced in egg extracts of amphibians. Int J Dev Biol. 1994;38(2):209–16.
107. Derijck A, van der Heijden G, Giele M, Philippens M, de Boer P. DNA double-strand break repair in parental chromatin of mouse zygotes, the first cell cycle as an origin of de novo mutation. Hum Mol Genet. 2008;17(13):1922–37.
108. Generoso WM, Cain KT, Krishna M, Huff SW. Genetic lesions induced by chemicals in spermatozoa and spermatids of mice are repaired in the egg. Proc Natl Acad Sci USA. 1979;76(1):435–7.
109. Matsuda Y, Seki N, Utsugi-Takeuchi T, Tobari I. Changes in X-ray sensitivity of mouse eggs from fertilization to the early pronuclear stage, and their repair capacity. Int J Radiat Biol. 1989;55(2):233–56.

110. Matsuda Y, Yamada T, Tobari I. Studies on chromosome aberrations in the eggs of mice fertilized in vitro after irradiation. I. Chromosome aberrations induced in sperm after X-irradiation. Mutat Res. 1985;148(1–2):113–7.
111. Blanchard Y, Lescoat D, Le Lannou D. Anomalous distribution of nuclear basic proteins in round-headed human spermatozoa. Andrologia. 1990;22(6):549–55.
112. de Yebra L, Ballesca JL, Vanrell JA, Bassas L, Oliva R. Complete selective absence of protamine-P2 in humans. J Biol Chem. 1993;268(14):10553–7.
113. Foresta C, Zorzi M, Rossato M, Varotto A. Sperm nuclear instability and staining with aniline blue: abnormal persistence of histones in spermatozoa in infertile men. Int J Androl. 1992;15(4):330–7.
114. Hofmann N, Hilscher B. Use of aniline blue to assess chromatin condensation in morphologically normal spermatozoa in normal and infertile men. Hum Reprod. 1991;6(7):979–82.
115. Terquem A, Dadoune J. Aniline bule staining of human spermatozoa chromatin: evaluation of nuclear maturation. The Hague: Martinus Nijhoff; 1983.
116. van Roijen HJ, Ooms MP, Spaargaren MC, et al. Immunoexpression of testis-specific histone 2B in human spermatozoa and testis tissue. Hum Reprod. 1998;13(6):1559–66.
117. Zhang X, SanGabriel M, Zini A. Sperm nuclear histone to protamine ratio in fertile and infertile men: evidence of heterogeneous subpopulations of spermatozoa in the ejaculate. J Androl. 2006;27(3):414–20.
118. Aoki VW, Liu L, Carrell DT. Identification and evaluation of a novel sperm protamine abnormality in a population of infertile males. Hum Reprod. 2005;20(5):1298–306.
119. Balhorn R, Reed S, Tanphaichitr N. Aberrant protamine 1/protamine 2 ratios in sperm of infertile human males. Experientia. 1988;44(1):52–5.
120. Belokopytova IA, Kostyleva EI, Tomilin AN, Vorobev VI. Human male infertility may be due to a decrease of the protamine-P2 content in sperm chromatin. Mol Reprod Dev. 1993;34(1):53–7.
121. Carrell DT, Emery BR, Hammoud S. Altered protamine expression and diminished spermatogenesis: what is the link? Hum Reprod Update. 2007;13(3):313–27.
122. Carrell DT, Liu L. Altered protamine 2 expression is uncommon in donors of known fertility, but common among men with poor fertilizing capacity, and may reflect other abnormalities of spermiogenesis. J Androl. 2001;22(4):604–10.
123. Chevaillier P, Mauro N, Feneux D, Jouannet P, David G. Anomalous protein complement of sperm nuclei in some infertile men. Lancet. 1987;2(8562):806–7.
124. Oliva R. Protamines and male infertility. Hum Reprod Update. 2006;12(4):417–35.
125. Aoki VW, Christensen GL, Atkins JF, Carrell DT. Identification of novel polymorphisms in the nuclear protein genes and their relationship with human sperm protamine deficiency and severe male infertility. Fertil Steril. 2006;86(5):1416–22.
126. Aoki VW, Emery BR, Liu L, Carrell DT. Protamine levels vary between individual sperm cells of infertile human males and correlate with viability and DNA integrity. J Androl. 2006;27(6):890–8.
127. Aoki VW, Liu L, Jones KP, et al. Sperm protamine 1/protamine 2 ratios are related to in vitro fertilization pregnancy rates and predictive of fertilization ability. Fertil Steril. 2006;86(5):1408–15.
128. Cho C, Jung-Ha H, Willis WD, et al. Protamine 2 deficiency leads to sperm DNA damage and embryo death in mice. Biol Reprod. 2003;69(1):211–7.
129. Depa-Martynow M, Kempisty B, Lianeri M, Jagodzinski PP, Jedrzejczak P. Association between fertilin beta, protamines 1 and 2 and spermatid-specific linker histone H1-like protein mRNA levels, fertilization ability of human spermatozoa, and quality of preimplantation embryos. Folia Histochem Cytobiol. 2007;45 Suppl 1:S79–85.
130. Mengual L, Ballesca JL, Ascaso C, Oliva R. Marked differences in protamine content and P1/P2 ratios in sperm cells from percoll fractions between patients and controls. J Androl. 2003;24(3):438–47.
131. Bedford JM, Calvin HI. The occurrence and possible functional significance of -S-S-crosslinks in sperm heads, with particular reference to eutherian mammals. J Exp Zool. 1974;188(2):137–55.

132. Calvin HI, Bedford JM. Formation of disulphide bonds in the nucleus and accessory structures of mammalian spermatozoa during maturation in the epididymis. J Reprod Fertil Suppl. 1971;13 Suppl 13:65–75.

133. Calvin HI, Yu CC, Bedford JM. Effects of epididymal maturation, zinc (II) and copper (II) on the reactive sulfhydryl content of structural elements in rat spermatozoa. Exp Cell Res. 1973;81(2):333–41.

134. Saowaros W, Panyim S. The formation of disulfide bonds in human protamines during sperm maturation. Experientia. 1979;35(2):191–2.

135. Sega GA, Generoso EE. Measurement of DNA breakage in spermiogenic germ-cell stages of mice exposed to ethylene oxide, using an alkaline elution procedure. Mutat Res. 1988;197(1):93–9.

136. Sega GA, Owens JG. Methylation of DNA and protamine by methyl methanesulfonate in the germ cells of male mice. Mutat Res. 1983;111(2):227–44.

137. Sega GA, Owens JG. Binding of ethylene oxide in spermiogenic germ cell stages of the mouse after low-level inhalation exposure. Environ Mol Mutagen. 1987;10(2):119–27.

138. Bjorndahl L, Kvist U. Human sperm chromatin stabilization: a proposed model including zinc bridges. Mol Hum Reprod. 2010;16(1):23–9.

139. Bench G, Corzett MH, Kramer CE, Grant PG, Balhorn R. Zinc is sufficiently abundant within mammalian sperm nuclei to bind stoichiometrically with protamine 2. Mol Reprod Dev. 2000;56(4):512–9.

140. Bianchi F, Rousseaux-Prevost R, Sautiere P, Rousseaux J. P2 protamines from human sperm are zinc -finger proteins with one CYS2/HIS2 motif. Biochem Biophys Res Commun. 1992; 182(2):540–7.

141. Gatewood JM, Schroth GP, Schmid CW, Bradbury EM. Zinc-induced secondary structure transitions in human sperm protamines. J Biol Chem. 1990;265(33):20667–72.

142. Hernandez-Ochoa I, Sanchez-Gutierrez M, Solis-Heredia MJ, Quintanilla-Vega B. Spermatozoa nucleus takes up lead during the epididymal maturation altering chromatin condensation. Reprod Toxicol. 2006;21(2):171–8.

143. Johansson L, Pellicciari CE. Lead-induced changes in the stabilization of the mouse sperm chromatin. Toxicology. 1988;51(1):11–24.

# Chapter 2
# Spermatogenesis: An Overview

**Rakesh Sharma and Ashok Agarwal**

## Neurological Pathways

Spermatogenesis is initiated through hormonal controls in the hypothalamus (Fig. 2.1). The hypothalamus secretes gonadotropin-releasing hormone (GnRH), triggering the release of luteinizing hormone (LH) and follicle-stimulating hormone (FSH) from the adenohypophysis or anterior lobe of the pituitary. LH assists with steroidogenesis by stimulating the Leydig cells of the interstitium, and FSH stimulates the Sertoli cells to aid with the proliferative and developmental stages of spermatogenesis. In addition to LH and FSH, the adenohypophysis also secretes adrenocorticotropic hormone, prolactin, growth hormone, and thyroid-stimulating hormone – all of these hormones play important roles throughout spermatogenesis. The primary hormones are responsible for initiating spermatogenesis inside the testes, which is the central organ of the reproductive axis. GnRH stimulations are regulated through three types of rhythmicity: (1) seasonal – peak GnRH production occurs during the spring (2) circadian – daily regulator with the highest output during the early morning and (3) pulsatile – highest output occurring on average every 90–120 min.

R. Sharma, PhD
Andrology Laboratory and Center for Reproductive Medicine,
Glickman Urological and Kidney Institute, OB-GYN
and Women's Health Institute, Cleveland Clinic,
Cleveland, OH, USA

A. Agarwal, PhD, HCLD (ABB) (✉)
Director, Center for Reproductive Medicine,
Glickman Urological and Kidney Institute,
Cleveland Clinic, 9500 Euclid Avenue, Desk A19.1,
Cleveland, OH 44195, USA
e-mail: agarwaa@ccf.org

A. Zini, A. Agarwal (eds.), *Sperm Chromatin for the Clinician*,
© Springer Science+Business Media New York 2013

23

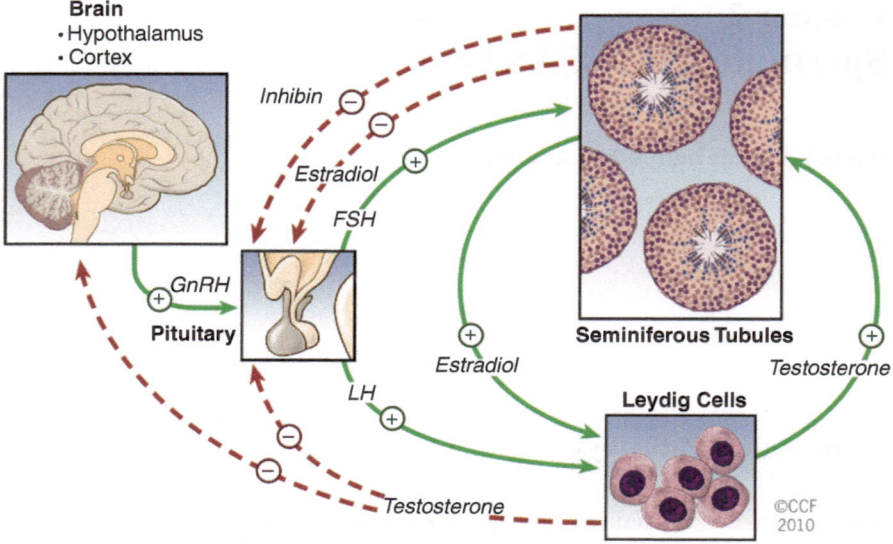

**Fig. 2.1** Schematic representation of the hypothalamic pituitary axis and the hormonal feedback system (reprinted with permission, Cleveland Clinic Center for Medical Art & Photography © 2010. All Rights Reserved)

## Steroid Hormone Interaction and Neurological Axis

Androgens are an integral part of spermatogenesis. Dihydrotestosterone is formed by metabolizing testosterone with 5 alpha-reductase. Both testosterone and dihydrotestosterone regulate various genes and the various developmental stages during gestation [1]. Estrogen is necessary for proper spermatogenesis [2, 3]. During Sertoli cell differentiation, estrogen levels drop to minimum levels. During the prepubescent years, estrogen shuts off androgen production by the Leydig cells. When puberty begins, estrogen levels fall to enable androgen production by Leydig cells and initiate spermatogenesis. Thyroid hormones play a key role in spermatogenesis involving Sertoli cell proliferation and development. All of these hormones interact with one another in the testicular axis in both the interstitial region and the Sertoli cells to enable spermatogenesis. In addition to the hormones, growth factors secreted directly by the Sertoli cells also play an important role in spermatogenesis. Transforming growth factor (alpha and beta), insulin-like growth factor, and beta fibroblast growth factor facilitate germ cell migration during embryonic development, proliferation, and regulation of meiosis and cellular differentiation.

## Organization of the Testis

The testes are ellipsoid in shape, measuring of 4.5–5.1 cm in length [4, 5], 2.5 × 4 cm in width [6] and have a volume of 15–25 mL [7]. They are engulfed by a strong connective tissues capsule (tunica albuginea) [6] and are the only

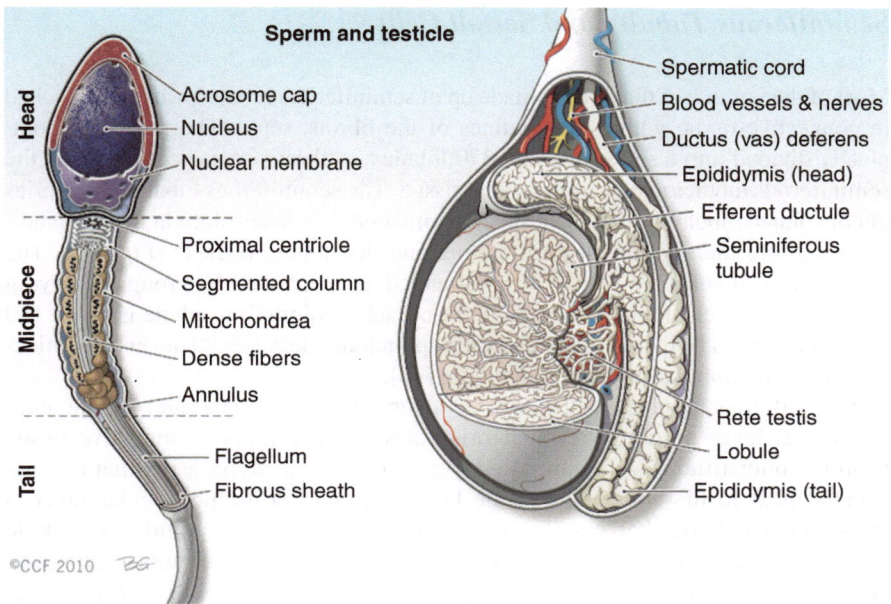

**Fig. 2.2** The human testis and the epididymis. The testis shows the tunica vaginalis and tunica albuginea, seminiferous tubule septae, rete testis, and the overlying head, body, and tail of the epididymis. To the *left* is a diagrammatic representation of a fully mature spermatozoon (reprinted with permission, Cleveland Clinic Center for Medical Art & Photography © 2010. All Rights Reserved)

organs in humans that are located outside the body. Spermatogenesis occurs at temperatures that are optimally 2–4° lower than that the temperature of main body [8]. The testis is loosely connected along its posterior border to the epididymis, which gives rise to the vas deferens at its lower pole [9]. The testis has two main functions: to produce hormones, in particular testosterone, and to produce male gametes – the spermatozoa (Fig. 2.2).

## Supporting Cells: Leydig Cells

The Leydig cells are irregularly shaped cells that have granular cytoplasm present individually or more often in groups within the connective tissue. They contribute to about 5–12% of the testicular volume [10–12]. Leydig cells are the prime source of the male sex hormone testosterone [13–15]. LH acts on Leydig cells to stimulate the production of testosterone. This acts as a negative "feedback" on the pituitary to suppress or modulate further LH secretion [15]. The intratesticular concentration of testosterone is significantly higher than the concentration in the blood. Some of the key functions of testosterone are as follows: (1) Activation of the hypophyseal-testicular axis, (2) Masculation of the brain and sexual behaviors, (3) Initiation and maintenance of spermatogenesis, (4) Differentiation of the male genital organs, and (5) Acquisition of secondary sex characteristics.

## Seminiferous Tubules and Sertoli Cells

Most of the volume of the testis is made up of seminiferous tubules, which are packed in connective tissue within the confines of the fibrous septa. The testis is incompletely divided into a series of about 370 lobules or fibrous septae consisting of the seminiferous tubules and the intertubular tissue. The seminiferous tubules are a series of convoluted tubules within the testes. Spermatogenesis takes place in these tubules, scattered into many different proliferating and developing pockets (Fig. 2.3). The seminiferous tubules are looped or blind-ended and separated by groups of Leydig cells, blood vessels, lymphatics, and nerves. Each seminiferous tubule is about 180 μm in diameter. The height of the germinal epithelium measures 80 μm and the thickness of the peritubular tissue is about 8 μm [16].

Seminiferous tubules consist of three layers of peritubular tissue: (1) the outer adventitial layer of fibrocytes that originates from primitive connective tissue from the interstitium, (2) the middle layer composed of myoid cells that are distributed next to the connective tissue lamellae, and (3) the peritubular layer, a thick, inner lamella that mainly consists of collagen. The seminiferous tubule space is divided into basal (basement membrane) and adluminal (lumen) compartments by strong intercellular junctional complexes called "tight junctions." The seminiferous tubules are lined with highly specialized Sertoli cells that rest on the tubular basement membrane and extend into the lumen with a complex ramification of cytoplasm. They encourage Sertoli cell proliferation and development during the gestational period. Both ends of the seminiferous tubules open into the spaces of the rete testis [17]. The fluid secreted by the seminiferous tubules is collected in the rete testis and delivered into the excurrent ductal system of the epididymis.

Approximately 40% of the seminiferous tubules consist of Sertoli cells, and roughly 40% of the Sertoli cells are occupied with elongated spermatids [18, 19]. Sertoli cells have larger nuclei than most cells, ranging from 250 to 850 cm$^3$ [18]. Each Sertoli cell makes contact with five other Sertoli cells and about 40–50 germ cells at various stages of development and differentiation. The Sertoli cells provide structural, functional, and metabolic support to germ cells. Functionally and endocrinologically competent Sertoli cells are necessary for optimal spermatogenesis. During spermatogenesis, the earlier germinal cells rest toward the epithelium region of the seminiferous tubules in order to develop and mature while the more developed germinal cells move toward the lumen of the seminiferous tubules in order to exit the seminiferous tubule system and continue with the final phases of spermatogenesis.

Sertoli cells function as "nurse" cells for spermatogenesis, nourishing germ cells as they develop and participating in germ cell phagocytosis. Multiple sites of communication exist between Sertoli cells and developing germ cells for the maintenance of spermatogenesis within an appropriate hormonal milieu. FSH binds to the high-affinity FSH receptors found on Sertoli cells, signaling the secretion of androgen-binding protein (ABP). ABP allows androgens such as testosterone and dihydrotestosterone to bind and increase their concentrations to initiate and/or

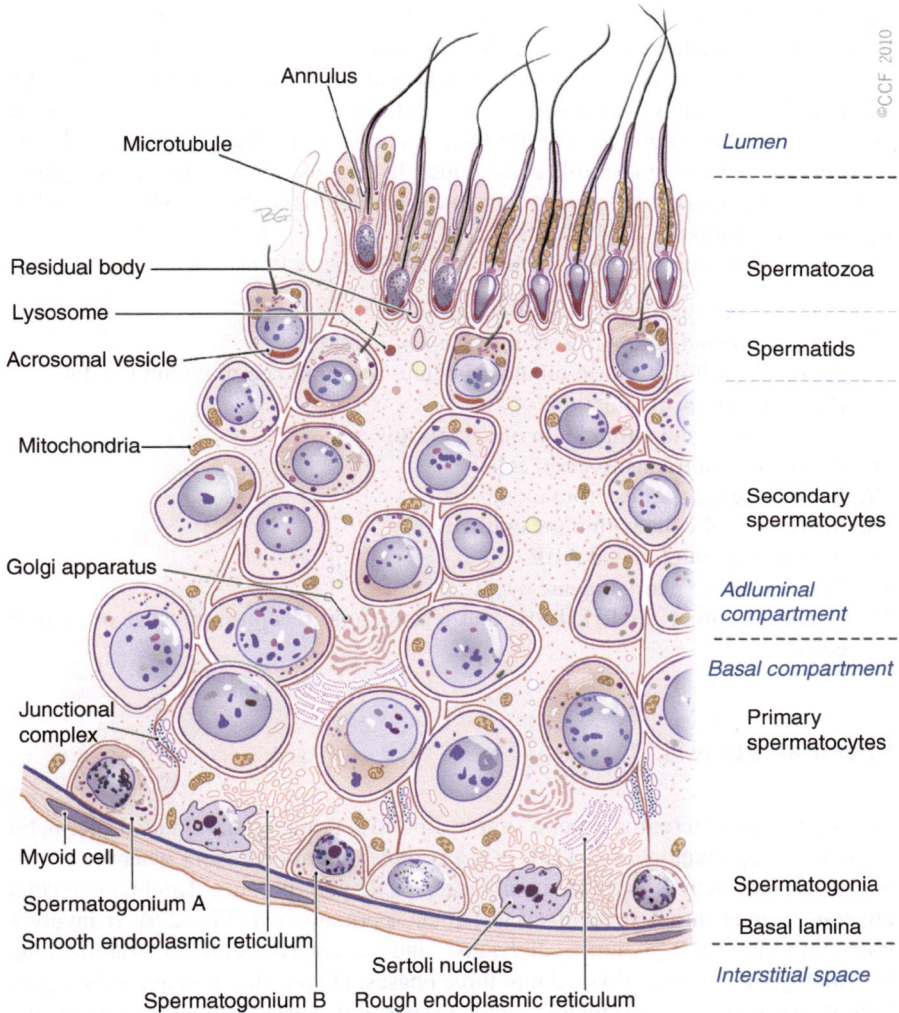

**Fig. 2.3** Section of the germinal epithelium in the seminiferous tubule. Sertoli cells divide the germinal epithelium into a basal and adluminal compartment, via the Sertoli cell. Spermatozoa are released into the lumen (reprinted with permission, Cleveland Clinic Center for Medical Art & Photography © 2010. All Rights Reserved)

continue the process of spermatogenesis. Sertoli cells also release anti-Müllerian hormone that allows for the embryonic development of the male by reducing the growth of the Müllerian ducts [20, 21]. Sertoli cells also secrete inhibin – a key macromolecule participating in pituitary FSH regulation.

Spermatozoa are produced at puberty but are not recognized by the immune system that develops during the first year of life. The blood–testis barrier provides a microenvironment for spermatogenesis to occur in an immunologically privileged site. The blood–testis barrier is divided into two regions: a basal region located near the seminiferous epithelium and an adluminal region that is positioned toward the lumen region of the seminiferous tubules. The basal region is the spermatogenic site for spermatogonial and primary spermatocyte development, while the adluminal region serves as the site for secondary spermatocyte and spermatid development. The blood–testis barrier has three different levels: (1) tight junctions between Sertoli cells, which helps separate premeiotic spermatogonia from the rest of the germ cells, (2) the endothelial cells in both the capillaries and (3) peritubular myoid cells.

Some of the main functions of the Sertoli cells are as follows:

1. Maintenance of integrity of seminiferous epithelium
2. Compartmentalization of seminiferous epithelium
3. Secretion of fluid to form tubular lumen to transport sperm within the duct
4. Participation in spermiation
5. Phagocytosis and elimination of cytoplasm
6. Delivery of nutrients to germ cells
7. Steroidogenesis and steroid metabolism
8. Movement of cells within the epithelium
9. Secretion of inhibin and ABP
10. Regulation of spermatogenic cycle
11. Provide a target for LH, FSH, and testosterone receptors present on Sertoli cells

## Spermatogenesis

The process of differentiation of a simple diploid spermatogonium into a spermatid is known as spermatogenesis [17]. It is a complex, temporal event whereby primitive, totipotent stem cells divide to either renew them or produce daughter cells that are transformed into a specialized testicular spermatozoon (Fig. 2.4). It involves both mitotic and meiotic divisions and extensive cellular remodeling. Spermatogenesis can be divided into three phases: (1) proliferation and differentiation of spermatogonia, (2) meiosis, and (3) spermiogenesis, a complex process that transforms round spermatids after meiosis into a complex structure called the spermatozoon. In humans, the process of spermatogenesis starts at puberty and continues throughout the entire life span of the individual. Once the gonocytes have differentiated into fetal spermatogonia, an active process of mitotic replication begins very early in the embryonic development.

Within the seminiferous tubule, germ cells are arranged in a highly ordered sequence from the basement membrane to the lumen. Spermatogonia lie directly on the basement membrane, followed by primary spermatocytes, secondary spermatocytes, and spermatids as they progress toward the tubule lumen. The tight junction barrier supports spermatogonia and early spermatocytes within the basal compartment and all subsequent germ cells within the adluminal compartment.

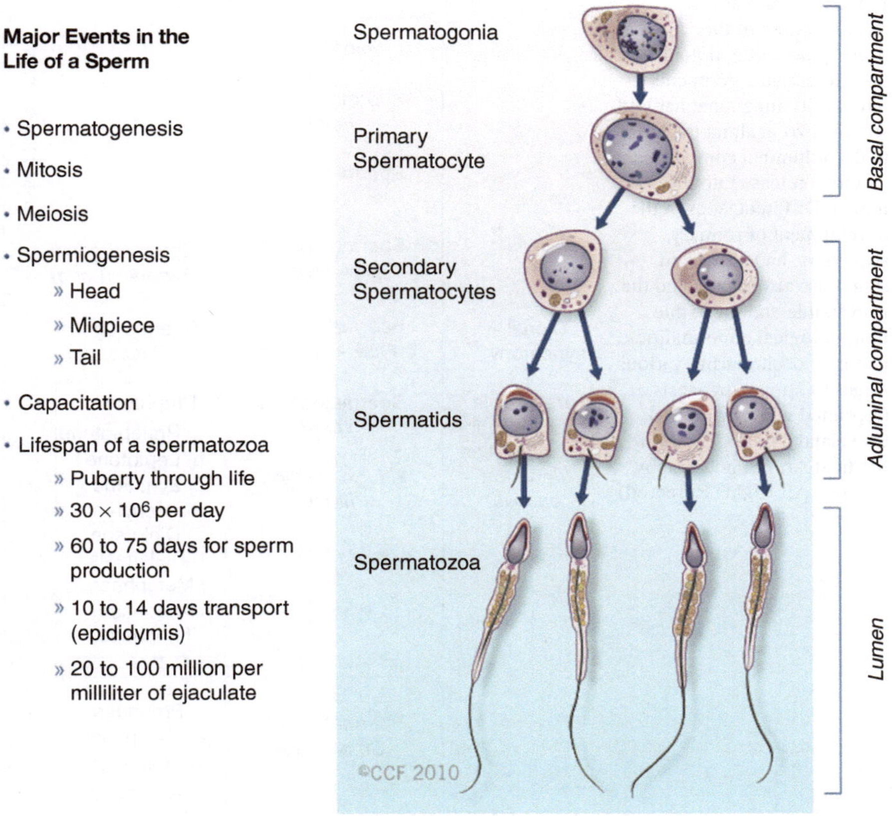

**Major Events in the Life of a Sperm**

- Spermatogenesis
- Mitosis
- Meiosis
- Spermiogenesis
  - » Head
  - » Midpiece
  - » Tail
- Capacitation
- Lifespan of a spermatozoa
  - » Puberty through life
  - » $30 \times 10^6$ per day
  - » 60 to 75 days for sperm production
  - » 10 to 14 days transport (epididymis)
  - » 20 to 100 million per milliliter of ejaculate

Spermatogonia

Primary Spermatocyte

Secondary Spermatocytes

Spermatids

Spermatozoa

Basal compartment

Adluminal compartment

Lumen

©CCF 2010

**Fig. 2.4** A diagrammatic representation of major events in the life of a sperm involving spermatogenesis, spermiogenesis, and spermiation during which the developing germ cells undergo mitotic and meiotic division to reduce the chromosome content (reprinted with permission, Cleveland Clinic Center for Medical Art & Photography © 2010. All Rights Reserved)

## Types of Spermatogonia

Fetal spermatogonia become transitional spermatogonia and later spermatogonia type Ad (dark). Spermatogonial stem cells undergo proliferative events and produce a population of cells that have distinct nuclear appearance that can be seen with hematoxylin and eosin staining. Spermatogonia can be categorized into three types: (1) Dark Type A, (2) Pale type A, and (3) Type B spermatogonia (Fig. 2.5).

Dark type A spermatogonia are stem cells of the seminiferous tubules that have an intensely stained dark ovoid nucleus containing fine granular chromatin. These cells divide by mitosis to generate Dark Type A and Pale Type A spermatogonia. Pale Type A spermatogonia have pale staining and fine granular chromatin in the ovoid

**Fig. 2.5** Schematic representation of the development of a diploid undifferentiated germ cell into a fully functional haploid spermatozoon along the basal to the adluminal compartment and final release into the lumen. Different steps in the development of primary, secondary, and spermatid stages are also shown and the irreversible and reversible morphological abnormalities that may occur during various stages of spermatogenesis (reprinted with permission, Cleveland Clinic Center for Medical Art & Photography © 2010. All Rights Reserved)

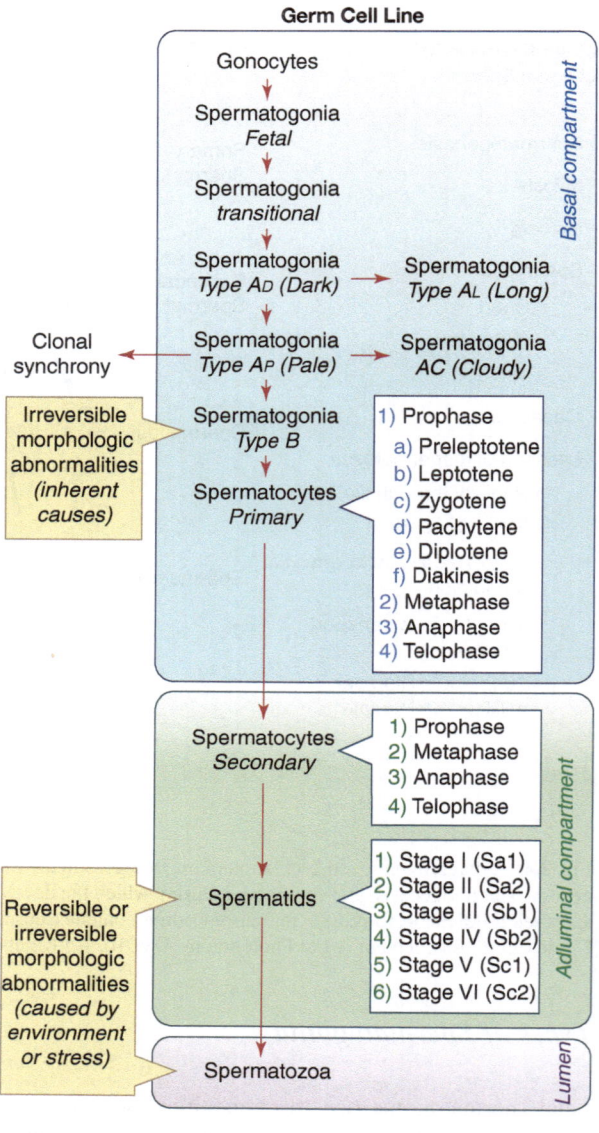

nucleus. Other proliferative spermatogonia include $A_{paired}$ ($A_{pr}$), resulting from dividing $A_{isolated}$, and subsequently dividing to form $A_{aligned}$ ($A_{al}$). Further differentiation of spermatogonia includes Type A1, A2, A3, A4, Intermediate, and Type B, each a result of the cellular division of the previous type. In humans, four spermatogonial cell types have been identified: $A_{long}$, $A_{dark}$, $A_{pale}$, and Type B [22–24]. In the rat, Type $A_{isolated}$ ($A_{is}$) is believed to be the stem cell [25, 26], whereas in humans, it is unclear which Type A spermatogonia is the stem cell. Type B spermatogonia are characterized by large clumps of condensed chromatin under the nuclear membrane of an ovoid nucleus. Type B spermatogonia divide mitotically to produce primary

**Fig. 2.6** Differentiation of a human diploid germ cell into a fully functional spermatozoon (reprinted with permission, Cleveland Clinic Center for Medical Art & Photography © 2010. All Rights Reserved)

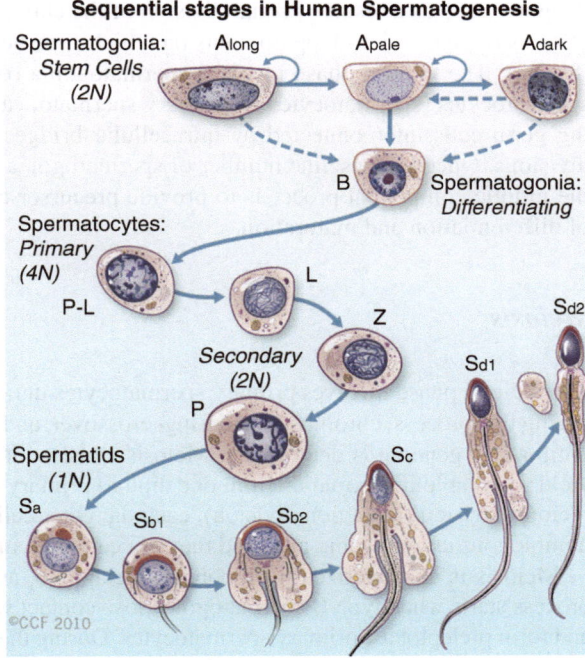

spermatocytes (preleptotene, leptotene, zygotene, and pachytene), secondary spermatocytes, and spermatids (Sa, Sb, Sc, $Sd_1$, and $Sd_2$), [22] (Fig. 2.6). Spermatogonia do not separate completely after meiosis but remain joined by intercellular bridges, which persist throughout all stages of spermatogenesis. This facilitates biochemical interactions and synchronizes germ cell maturation [27].

## Spermatocytogenesis

Spermatocytogenesis consists of the meiotic phase in which primary spermatocytes undergo meiosis I and meiosis II to give rise to haploid spermatids. This takes place in the basal compartment. Primary spermatocytes enter the first meiotic division to form secondary spermatocytes. The prophase of the first meiotic division is very long. Primary spermatocytes have the longest life span. Secondary spermatocytes undergo the second meiotic division to produce spermatids. Secondary spermatocytes are short-lived (1.1–1.7 days).

## *Mitosis*

Mitosis involves the proliferation and maintenance of spermatogonia. It is a precise, well-orchestrated sequence of events in which the genetic material (chromosomes) is duplicated, with breakdown of the nuclear envelope and formation of two daughter cells as a result of equal division of the chromosomes and cytoplasm [28] DNA is organized into loop domains on which specific regulatory proteins interact [29–33]. The mitotic phase involves spermatogonia (types A and B) and primary spermatocytes (spermatocytes I). Primary spermatocytes are produced by developing germ cells interconnected by intracellular bridges through a series of mitotic divisions. Once the baseline number of spermatogonia is established after puberty, the mitotic component proceeds to provide precursor cells and initiate the process of differentiation and maturation.

## Meiosis

The meiotic phase involves primary spermatocytes until spermatids are formed, and during this process, chromosome pairing, crossover, and genetic exchange take place until a new genome is determined. Meiosis consists of two successive divisions to yield four haploid spermatids from one diploid primary spermatocyte. After the first meiotic division (reduction division), each daughter cell contains one partner of the homologous chromosome pair, and they are called secondary spermatocytes (2n).

Meiosis is characterized by prophase, metaphase, anaphase, and telophase. The process starts when type B spermatogonia lose contact with the basement membrane and form preleptotene primary spermatocytes. During the leptotene stage of prophase, the chromosomes are arranged as long filaments. During the zygotene stage, the homologous chromosomes called tetrads are arranged linearly by a process known as synapsis and form synaptonemal complexes. Crossing over takes place during this phase, and the chromosomes shorten in the pachytene stage. The homologous chromosomes condense and separate from sites of crossing over during diakinesis. This random sorting is important to maintain genetic diversity in sperm. At the end of prophase, the nuclear envelope breaks down, and in metaphase, chromosomes are arranged in the equatorial plate. At anaphase, each chromosome consists of two chromatids migrating to opposite poles. In telophase, cell division occurs with the formation of secondary spermatocytes having half the number of chromosomes. Thus, each primary spermatocyte can theoretically yield four spermatids, although fewer actually result, as the complexity of meiosis is associated with a loss of some germ cells. The primary spermatocytes are the largest germ cells of the germinal epithelium.

The prophase of the second meiotic division is very short, and in this phase, the DNA content is reduced to half as the two chromatids of each chromosome separate and move to the opposite poles. At the end of telophase, the spermatids do not separate completely but remain interconnected by fine bridges for synchronous development. These spermatids are haploid with (22, X) or (22, Y) chromosome and undergo complete differentiation/morphogenesis known as spermiogenesis.

## Spermiogenesis

Spermiogenesis is the process of differentiation of the spermatids into spermatozoa with fully compacted chromatin. During this process, morphological changes occur once the process of meiosis is completed. In humans, six different stages have been described in the process of spermatid maturation; these are termed as $S_{a-1}$ and $S_{a-2}$, $S_{b-1}$ and $S_{b-2}$, and $S_{c-1}$ and $S_{c-2}$ (Fig. 2.6). Each stage can be identified by morphological characteristics. During the $S_{a-1}$ stage, both the Golgi complex and mitochondria are well developed and differentiated. In addition, the acrosomal vesicle appears, the chromatoid body develops in one pole of the cell opposite from the acrosomal vesicle, and proximal centriole and axial filament appear. During the $S_{b-1}$ and $S_{b-2}$ stages, acrosome formation is completed, the intermediate piece is formed and the tail develops. This process is completed during the Sc stages. During the postmeiotic phase, progressive condensation of the nucleus occurs with inactivation of the genome. The histones are converted into transitional proteins, and finally, protamines are converted into well-developed disulfide bonds.

## Spermiation

A mature spermatid frees itself from the Sertoli cell and enters the lumen of the tubule as a spermatozoon in a process called spermiation. Spermatids that originate from the same spermatogonia remain connected by bridges to facilitate the transport of cytoplasmic products. Sertoli cells actively participate in spermiation, which may also involve the actual movement of the cells as the spermatids advance toward the lumen of the seminiferous tubules [18]. The mature spermatids close their intracellular bridges, disconnect their contact with the germinal epithelium, and become free cells called spermatozoa. Portions of the cytoplasm in the Sertoli cell known as the cytoplasmic droplet are completely eliminated, or at times, they may be retained in the immature spermatozoon during the process of spermiation [34].

## The Cycle or Wave of Seminiferous Epithelium

A cycle of spermatogenesis involves the division of primitive spermatogonial stem cells into subsequent germ cell types through the process of meiosis. Type A spermatogonial divisions occur at a shorter time interval than the entire process of spermatogenesis. Therefore, at any given time, several cycles of spermatogenesis coexist within the germinal epithelium. Spermatogenesis is not a random but well orchestrated series of well-defined events in the seminiferous epithelium. Germ cells are localized in spatial units referred as stages. Each stage is recognized by development of the acrosome; meiotic divisions and shape of the nucleus and release of the sperm into lumen of the seminiferous tubule. A stage is designated by Roman numerals. Each cell type of the stage is morphologically integrated with the others in its development process. Each stage has a defined morphological entity of spermatid development called a step, which is designated by an Arabic number. Several steps occur together to form a stage, and several stages are necessary to form a mature sperm from immature stem cells [35, 36]. In rodent spermatogenesis, only one stage can be found in a cross section of seminiferous tubule.

Within any given cross section of the seminiferous tubule, there are four to five layers of germ cells. Cells in each layer comprise a generation or a cohort of cells that develop as a synchronous group. Each group has a similar appearance and function. Stages I–III have four generations comprising Type A spermatogonia, two primary spermatocytes, and an immature spermatid. Stages IV–VIII have five generations: Type A spermatogonia, one generation of primary spermatocyte, one generation of secondary spermatocytes, and one generation of spermatids. Thus, a position in the tubule that is occupied by cells comprising stage I will become stage II, followed by stage III, until the cycle repeats. The cycle of spermatogenesis can be identified for each species, but the duration of the cycle varies for each species [22].

The stages of spermatogenesis are sequentially arranged along the length of the tubule in such a way that it results in a "wave of spermatogenesis." Although it appears that the spatial organization is lacking or is poor in the human seminiferous tubule, these stages are tightly organized in an intricate helicine pattern [37]. In addition to the steps being organized spatially within the seminiferous tubule, the stages are organized in time. Spermatozoa are released only in certain cross sections along the length of the seminiferous tubule. In rat, all stages are involved in spermatogenesis, but spermatozoa are released only in stage VIII. In humans, this wave appears to be a spiral cellular arrangement as they progress down the tubule. This spatial arrangement probably exists to ensure that sperm production is a continuous and not a pulsatile process. The spermatocyte takes 25.3 days to mature. Spermiogenesis occurs in 21.6 days, and the duration of the cycle is 16 days. The progression from spermatogonia to spermatozoa or spermatogenesis is 74 days or 4½ cycles of the seminiferous cycle.

## Chromatin Remodeling/Alterations During Sperm Differentiation

Mammalian sperm chromatin is unique in that it is highly organized, condensed, and compacted. This feature protects the paternal genome during transport through the male and the female reproductive tracts and helps ensure that it is delivered to the ova in good condition. Mammalian sperm DNA is the most tightly compacted eukaryotic DNA [38]. This feature is in sharp contrast to the DNA structure in somatic cell nuclei. Somatic cell nuclear DNA is wrapped around an octamer of histones and packaged into a solenoid structure [39]. This type of packaging adds histones, which increase the chromatin volume. The sperm nucleus does not have this type of packaging, and the volume is highly compacted. Chromatin changes occur in the testis during meiosis in which copies of the genome are partitioned into haploid spermatid cells and during spermiogenesis in which spermatids elongate to form sperm with fully compacted chromatin. These events are largely controlled by posttranslational events for transcription. Translation greatly subsides as DNA becomes compacted and the cytoplasm is jettisoned during spermiogenesis [40, 41]. After meiosis, sperm DNA experiences extreme chromosome compaction during spermiogenesis.

Chromatin modeling is accompanied by changes in the nuclear shape, conversion of negatively supercoiled nucleosomal DNA into a nonsupercoiled state [42], induction of transient DNA breaks [43], and chromatin condensation. It is mediated by drastic changes at the most fundamental level of DNA packaging where a nucleosomal architecture shifts to a toroidal structure [44]. This change is implemented by sperm nuclear basic proteins (SNBs) that include variants of histone subunits, transition proteins, and protamine proteins [45, 46]. Chromatin proteins do not act exclusively to compact sperm DNA. This transition occurs in a stepwise manner, replacing somatic histones with testis-expressed histone variants, transition proteins, and finally protamines [47]. Histone localization and posttranslational modification of histones encode epigenetic information that may regulate transcription important for sperm development [48]. They may also serve to mark the heterochromatin state of specific regions of the genome that may be important after fertilization, when somatic histones are incorporated back into paternal chromatin or during subsequent zygotic development [49]. Male infertility can result from deficits of SNBs [50–52].

## Histone and Basic Nuclear Protein Transitions in Spermatogenesis

During spermatogenesis, histone proteins in developing sperm are replaced by testis-specific histone variants that are important for fertility [53]. The cells depend on posttranslational modifications to implement subsequent stages of sperm formation, maturation, and activation as de novo transcription in postmeiotic sperm is largely silenced [54]. During spermiogenesis, sperm chromatin undergoes a series of modifications in which histones are lost and replaced with transition proteins and subsequently with protamines [54–56]. Approximately 15% of the histones are retained in human sperm chromatin, subsequently making chromatin less tightly compacted [57, 58]. Chromatin remodeling is facilitated by the coordinated loosening of the chromatin by histone hyperacetylation and by the DNA topoisomerase II (topo II), which produce temporary nicks in the sperm DNA to relieve torsional stress that results from supercoiling [43, 59–61]. The same enzyme Topo II normally repairs these temporary nicks prior to completion of spermiogenesis and ejaculation. However, if these nicks are not repaired, DNA fragmented sperm may be present in the ejaculate [62].

## Role of Transition Proteins

The histone-to-protamine transition is important in the formation of spermatozoa [63]. This occurs in two steps in mammals: replacement of histones by transition nuclear proteins (TPs) – TP1 and TP2 – and replacement of TPs by protamines (protamine 1 and protamine 2). TPs are required for normal chromatin

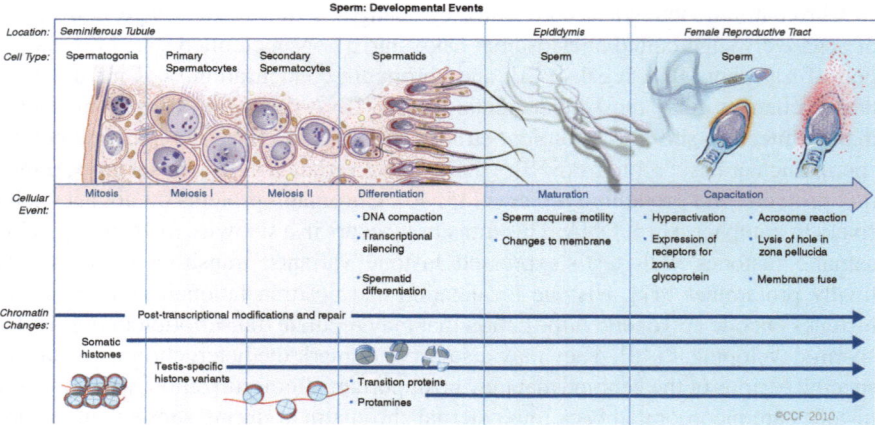

**Fig. 2.7** Diagrammatic representation of the series of cellular and chromatin changes during the development of the germ cell into a spermatozoon and its subsequent release and storage into the epididymis and its journey into the female reproductive tract (reprinted with permission, Cleveland Clinic Center for Medical Art & Photography © 2010. All Rights Reserved)

condensation, for reducing the number of DNA breaks and for preventing the formation of secondary defects in spermatozoa and the eventual loss of genomic integrity and sterility. TP1 is a 6.2-kDa, highly basic (about 20% each of arginine and lysine) protein with evenly distributed basic residues [64, 65], whereas TP2 is a 13-kDa basic (10% each of arginine and lysine) protein with distinct structural domains. The only similarity between the two is their high basicity, exon–intron genomic patterns, and developmental expression [66].

The transition nuclear proteins are localized exclusively to the nuclei of elongating and condensing spermatids [67] and were first detected in step 10–11 spermatids [68, 69] (Figs. 2.7 and 2.8). The maximum levels of TPs are acquired during steps 12–13, during which they constitute 90% of the chromatin basic protein, with the levels of TP1 being about 2.5 times those of TP2 [51]. They are not detected in the nucleus after the early part of step 15 [68, 69].

Some of the possible roles of TPs are as follows:

1. TP1 can destabilize nucleosomes and prevent binding of the DNA, both of which could contribute to displacement of histones [70, 71]
2. The zinc fingers of TP2 selectively bind to CpG sites and may be responsible for global expression of RNA synthesis [72]
3. Both TPs may play a role as alignment factors for DNA strand breaks, and TP1 is involved in the repair of strand breaks [73, 74]
4. Both TP1 and TP2 can condense DNA, and TP2 is more effective [70, 71, 75]. TP2 is not a critical factor for shaping of the sperm nucleus, histone displacement, initiation of chromatin condensation, binding of protamines to DNA, or fertility, but it is necessary for maintaining the normal processing of P2 and consequently the completion of chromatin condensation [52]

**Fig. 2.8** Diagrammatic representation of the steps where the histones are replaced with the transition proteins and protamines in the round spermatid progresses into a condensed spermatid just before it is released into the lumen (reprinted with permission, Cleveland Clinic Center for Medical Art & Photography © 2010. All Rights Reserved)

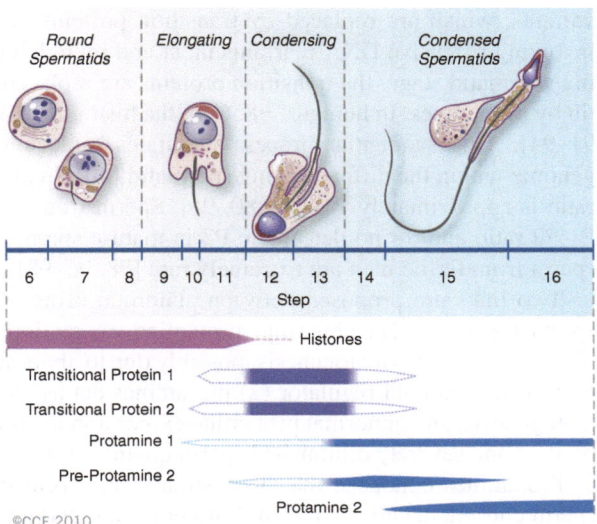

Mice lacking either TP1 or TP2 alone had normal numbers of sperm with only minor abnormalities and were fertile, indicating either that the TPs were not essential or that the individual TPs complement each other [51, 52, 76]. Protamine 2 processing defects do not inhibit postfertilization processes because late spermatids containing unprocessed protamine 2 are able to initiate normal development [77]. Defective protamine 2 processing is correlated with infertility in humans [78] and mouse mutants [51, 52] and could be due solely to the secondary cytoplasmic effects on sperm development resulting in a reduced ability to penetrate the egg.

## Protamines as Checkpoints of Spermatogenesis

Human sperm chromatin undergoes a complex transition during the elongating spermatid stage of spermiogenesis, in which histones are extensively replaced by protamines. Humans express equal quantities of two protamines: protamine 1 and protamine 2 [79–81]. Protamines are approximately half the size of histones [82]. They are highly basic sperm-specific nuclear proteins that are characterized by an arginine-rich core and cysteine residues [83, 84]. The high level of arginine causes a net positive charge, thereby facilitating strong DNA binding [85]. Cysteine residues facilitate the formation of multiple inter- and intraprotamine disulfide bonds essential for high-order chromatin packaging, which is necessary for normal sperm function [86–90]. P2 protamines contain fewer cysteine groups and thus contain fewer disulfide cross links [81]. This, theoretically, leaves the DNA more susceptible to damage. Altered P2 expression is common in men with infertility [77].

During spermiogenesis, protamines progressively replace somatic histones in a stepwise manner [83]. First, somatic histones are replaced by testis-specific histone variants, which are replaced by transition proteins (TP1a and TP2) in a process involving extensive DNA rearrangement and remodeling [42]. During the elongating spermatid stage, the transition proteins are replaced in the condensing chromatin by protamines. In humans, ~85% of the histones are replaced by protamines [54, 91–94]. This sequential process facilitates molecular remodeling of the male genome within the differentiating spermatid [40]. In human sperm, the mean P1/P2 ratio is approximately 1.0 [77, 80, 95]. Sperm from infertile men show an altered P1/P2 ratio and/ or no detectable P2 in mature sperm. Protamine abnormalities in sperm from fertile men are extremely rare [78, 95–98].

Two links are proposed between abnormal protamine expression and aberrant spermatogenesis: (1) abnormal protamine expression is indicative of a general abnormality of spermatogenesis, possibly due to abnormal function of the transcription or translational regulator (2) protamines act as checkpoint regulators of spermatogenesis, and abnormal protamine expression leads to induction of an apoptotic process and severely diminished sperm quality [99].

Protamines condense the DNA strands and form the basic packaging unit of sperm chromatin called a toroid. Intramolecular and intermolecular disulfide crosslinks between cysteine residues present in protamines result in further compaction of the toroids [100]. Protamines confer a higher order of DNA packaging in sperm than that found in somatic cells. All of these levels of compaction and organization help protect sperm chromatin during transport through the male and female reproductive tract. This also ensures delivery of the paternal genome in a form that allows developing embryo to accurately express genetic information [58, 75, 80, 101]. Protamine replacement may also be necessary for silencing the paternal genome and reprogramming the imprinting pattern of the gamete [102]. Abnormal protamine expression is associated with low sperm count, decreased sperm motility and morphology, diminished fertilization ability, and increased sperm chromatin damage [77, 98, 103]. Infertile men are reported to have a higher histone-to-protamine ratio in their sperm chromatin [95, 104].

## DNA Methylation During Spermatogenesis

Nucleohistones are present in human and rat sperm and are absent in mouse sperm. About ~15% of the histones are retained in the mature human spermatozoa [58]. The distribution of these histones within the sperm nucleus may have an important function. Chromatin associated with histones corresponds to specific sequences [58], suggesting that heterogeneity in the sperm nucleus may be the basis for male genetic information [105–107]. There are widespread differences in methylation of specific sequences during oogenesis and spermatogenesis. Maintenance methylases can stably preserve DNA methylation at cytosine residues through rounds of replication [108] and may have a role in gene regulation [109]. Methylation can also provide a mechanism for imprinting the maternal and paternal genomes as seen by the gametic differences in DNA methylation. This results in differential regulation of the paternal genomes during early development [110].The sequences that are highly methylated in pachytene spermatocytes are also highly methylated in spermatids and epididymal sperm, indicating that this state persists throughout spermatogenesis [111].

DNA methylation may be involved in genomic imprinting in mammals and is one of the major epigenetic marks established during spermatogenesis [112]. Mature sperms show a more unique DNA methylation profile than somatic cells [113]. The level of DNA methylation does not correlate with fertilization but with pregnancy rate after IVF [114].

## Sperm Nuclear DNA Strand Breaks

Mammalian spermiogenesis involves important changes in the cytoarchitecture and dramatic remodeling of the somatic chromatin; most of the nucleosomal DNA supercoiling is eliminated [115, 116]. This modification in chromatin structure occurs in elongating spermatids and is an important contributor to the nuclear integrity and acquisition of full fertilization potential of the male gamete [117]. DNA damage involves (1) abortive apoptosis initiated post meiotically when the ability to drive this process to completion is in decline (2) unresolved strand breaks created during spermiogenesis to relieve torsional stress associated with chromatin remodeling and (3) oxidative stress as a result of reactive oxygen species. Three major mechanisms for the creation of DNA damage in the male germ line have been proposed: chromatin remodeling by topoisomerase, oxidative stress, and abortive apoptosis. DNA damage could arise due to a combination of all the three mechanisms. Furthermore, a two-step hypothesis has been proposed [117, 118]. According to this hypothesis, the first step in the DNA damage cascade has its origin in spermiogenesis during which DNA is remodeled prior to condensation. Defects in the chromatin remodeling process result in the production of spermatozoa that are characterized by reduction in the efficiency of protamination, abnormal protamine 1 to protamine 2 ratio, and relatively high nucleohistone content [101, 119, 120]. These defects in chromatin modeling create a state of vulnerability whereby spermatozoa become increasingly susceptible to oxidative damage. In the second step of this DNA cascade, reactive oxygen species attack chromatin.

One of the first hypothesis concerning the origins of DNA damage in the male germ line focused on the physiological strand breaks created by topoisomerase during spermiogenesis as a means of relieving the torsional stresses created as DNA is condensed and packaged into the sperm head [60, 101]. Normally, these strand breaks are marked by a histone phosphorylation event and are fully resolved by topoisomerase before spermatozoa are released from germinal epithelium during spermiogenesis [121].

Sperm chromatin compaction is believed to play an important role in protecting the male genome from insult. This specific chromatin structure of the sperm essential for proper fertility and is in part due to the proteins that are bound to the DNA, including the protamines, histones, and components of the nuclear matrix [122, 123]. The cascade of events leading to DNA damage involves an error in chromatin remodeling during spermiogenesis. This leads to generation of spermatozoa with poorly protaminated nuclear DNA that is increasingly susceptible to oxidative attack [118].

Efficiency of chromatin remodeling during spermiogenesis has been studied employing DNA sensitive fluorochrome chromomycin (CM3). Chromomycin competes with the nucleoproteins for binding sites in the minor groove of GC-rich DNA and serves as a marker for the efficiency of DNA protamination during spermiogenesis. Staining with this probe is positively related to the presence of nuclear histones [124] and poor chromatin compaction [125] and negatively related with presence of protamines [126]. Impaired chromatin remodeling during spermiogenesis is a consistent feature of defective human spermatozoa possessing fragmented DNA [127–131]. DNA damage depends on fundamental errors that occur during spermatogenesis and may explain the correlation of pathology with sperm count [132].

## Sperm Apoptosis

Apoptosis in sperm is different from somatic apoptosis in many ways: (1) spermatozoa are transcriptionally and translationally silent, and therefore, cannot undergo programmed cell death or "regulated cell death," (2) sperm chromatin has a reduced nucleosome content due to extensive protamination and, therefore, lacks the characteristic DNA laddering seen in somatic cells, and (3) endonucleases that are activated in the cytoplasm or released from the mitochondria are prevented from physically accessing the DNA due to the inherent physical architecture of the spermatozoa. However, spermatozoa do exhibit some of the hallmarks of apoptosis including caspase activation and phosphatidylserine exposure on the surface of the cells [133].

Sertoli cells can support only a limited number of germ cells in the testis. In the testis, apoptosis normally occurs to prevent the overproduction of germ cells and to selectively remove injured germ cells [134]. Clonal expansion of the germ cells in the testis occurs at very high levels, and thus, apoptosis is necessary to limit the size of the germ cell population to one which the Sertoli cell is able to support [135]. Fas Ligand (FasL) is secreted by Sertoli cells. Fas is a protein located on the germ cell surface. Evidence of germ cell apoptosis has been demonstrated in FasL-defective mice [136]. Men with poor seminal parameters often display a large percentage of Fas-expressing sperm in their ejaculate [101]. Some of these sperms with DNA damage and Fas expression may have undergone "abortive apoptosis" in which they started but subsequently escaped the apoptotic pathway [137]. However, other studies have failed to find a correlation between DNA damage and Fas expression and other markers of apoptosis [62]. Recent studies examining loss of function have indicated that DNA damage checkpoints occur during spermatogenesis and may also involve excision repair genes, mismatch repair genes, and p53 [138].

## Oxidative Stress in the Testis

Sertoli cells provide nutritional support to the differentiating germ cells in the testis. They are protected from oxidative stress as these cells pass through meiosis and emerge as haploid cells known as round spermatids. At this stage of development, these cells are transcriptionally silent. Even in the absence of any regulated gene transcription, they are able to undergo cellular transformation into fully differentiated, highly specialized cells – the spermatozoa. This is accomplished through a highly orchestrated differential translation of preexisting mRNA species through a process called spermiogenesis. Cells are sensitive to oxidative stress during spermiogenesis. Throughout this phase, they are highly dependent on the nurturing Sertoli cells, which possess antioxidants such as superoxide dismutase, glutathione reductase, transferase, and peroxidase [139]. Isolated spermatozoa have a limited capacity for DNA repair [140].

## Spermiogenesis and Etiology of DNA Damage

Spermiogenesis, the process by which haploid round spermatids differentiate into spermatozoa, is a key event in the etiology of DNA damage in the male germ line. During spermiogenesis, the chromatin undergoes extensive remodeling, which enables the entire haploid genome to be compacted into a sperm head measuring $5 \times 2.5$ μm. This occurs as physiological DNA strand breaks are introduced by topoisomerase to relieve the torsional stresses involved in DNA packaging during sperm differentiation. These strand breaks are corrected by a complex process involving H2Ax expression, formation of poly(ADP-ribose) by nuclear poly (ADP-ribose) polymersases (PARP) and topoisomerase [141]. If the spermiogenesis process is disrupted for any reason, restoration of the cleavage sites is impaired, and defective spermatozoa with unresolved physiological strand breaks are released from the germinal epithelium. The "transition" proteins play a key role in maintaining DNA integrity during spermiogenesis as they move into the sperm nucleus between the removal of histones and the entry of protamines. Functional deletion of these proteins results in the production of spermatozoa with poor fertilizing ability, poor chromatin compaction, and high levels of DNA fragmentation [63]. DNA damage in human spermatozoa is associated with the disruption and poor chromatin remodeling during spermiogenesis [120, 128].

The efficiency of spermatogenesis is reflected by conventional semen characteristics such as sperm count and morphology and the correlation with DNA damage [132, 142]. Poor protamination results in spermatozoa that possess nucleohistone-rich regions of chromatin, which are vulnerable to oxidative attack [117]. Oxidative stress is a major determinant of the quality of spermiogenesis. When this process is disrupted, spermatozoa are produced that are vulnerable to oxidative stress, 8OHdg formation, and ultimately DNA fragmentation as a consequence of apoptosis [120, 143, 144].

## Efficiency of Spermatogenesis

The efficiency of spermatogenesis varies between different species; it appears to be relatively constant in man. The time needed for a spermatogonium to differentiate into a mature spermatid is estimated to be 70 ± 4 days [145]. In comparison to animals, the spermatogenetic efficiency in man is poor, and the daily rate of spermatozoa production is about 3–4 million/g of testicular tissue [146]. Although a much higher sperm count should be expected in the ejaculate than the 20 million/mL described by WHO manual [147], this is not the case. This is largely because most developed cells (>75%) are eliminated as a result of apoptosis. In the remaining cells, more than half are abnormal. Therefore, only about 12% of the spermatogenetic potential is available for reproduction [148]. Furthermore, daily sperm production in men also declines with age; this is associated with a loss of Sertoli cells, an increase in germ cell degeneration during prophase of meiosis, or loss of primary spermatocytes along with a reduction in the number of Leydig cells, non-Leydig interstitial cells, and myoid cells.

## Postspermiation Events

The process of spermiation and the journey of a sperm through the excurrent duct of the testis to a site where it can be included in the ejaculate take an additional 10–14 days. The nucleus progressively elongates as its chromatin condenses; the head is characterized by a flattened and pointed paddle shape, which is specific to each species, and involves the Golgi phase where the centrioles migrate from the cytoplasm to the base of the nucleus and proximal centriole becomes the implantation apparatus to anchor flagellum to the nucleus and distal centriole becomes the axoneme. In the cap phase, the acrosome forms a distinct cap over the nucleus covering about 30–50% of the nuclear surface [149]. The acrosome contains the hydrolytic enzymes necessary for fertilization. The manchette is formed, and the spermatids are embedded in Sertoli cells. During the maturation phase, mitochondria migrate toward the segment of the growing tail to form the mitochondrial sheath and dense outer fibers. A fibrous sheath is formed to complete the assembly of the tail. Most of the spermatid cytoplasm is discarded as a residual body, and the spermatid moves toward the lumen of the seminiferous tubule. Once elongation of the spermatid is complete, Sertoli cell cytoplasm retracts around the developing sperm, and all unnecessary cytoplasm is stripped. The spermatozoon is finally released it into the tubule lumen. The mature spermatozoon is an elaborate, highly specialized cell produced in large numbers – about 300 per gram of testis per second.

## Spermatozoa

Spermatozoa are highly specialized and condensed cells that do not grow or divide. A spermatozoon consists of a head containing the paternal material (DNA) and the tail, which provides motility. The spermatozoon is endowed with a large nucleus but lacks a large cytoplasm, which is characteristic of most body cells. The heterogeneity of the ejaculate is a characteristic feature in men [150–152].

## Head

The head is oval in shape, measuring about 4.0–5.5 μm in length and 2.5–3.5 μm in width. The normal length-to-width ratio is about 1.50–1.70 [153]. Under bright-field illumination, the most commonly observed aberrations include head shape/size defects (including large, small, tapering, pyriform, amorphous, and vacuolated (>20% of the head surface occupied by unstained vacuolar areas)) and double heads, or any combination thereof [154].

## Acrosome

The acrosome is represented by the Golgi complex and covers about two thirds or about 70% of the anterior head area [151, 152]. When observed under the scanning electron microscope, the sperm head is unequally divided into the acrosomal and postacrosomal regions. Under the electron microscope, the sperm head is a flattened ovoid structure consisting primarily of the nucleus. The acrosome contains several hydrolytic enzymes, including hyaluronidase and proacrosin, which are necessary for fertilization [150]. During fertilization of the egg, the fusion of the outer acrosomal membrane with the plasma membrane at multiple sites releases the acrosomal enzymes at the time of acrosome reaction. The anterior half of the head is covered only by the inner acrosomal membrane, while the posterior region of the sperm head is covered by a single membrane called the postnuclear cap. The overlap of the acrosome and the postnuclear cap results in an equatorial segment. The equatorial segment does not participate in the acrosome reaction. The nucleus comprises 65% of the head and is composed of DNA conjugated with protein. The chromatin is tightly packaged, and no distinct chromosomes are visible. The genetic information, including the sex determining X or Y chromosome, is "coded" and stored in the DNA [150].

## Neck

This forms a junction between the head and tail. It is fragile, and a common abnormality is the presence of a decapitated spermatozoon.

## Tail

The sperm tail arises at the spermatid stage. During spermatogenesis, the centriole is differentiated into midpiece, principal piece, and endpiece. The mitochondria reorganize around the midpiece. An axial core composed of two central fibrils surrounded by a concentric ring of nine double fibrils continues to the end of the tail. An additional outer ring is composed of nine coarse fibrils. The main piece is comprised of 9 coarse outer fibrils that diminish in thickness until only the inner 11 fibrils of the axial core surrounded by a fibrous sheath remain. The mitochondrial sheath of the midpiece is relatively short but slightly longer than the combined length of the head and neck [150].

## Endpiece

The endpiece is not distinctly visible by light microscopy. Both the tail sheath and coarse filaments are absent. The tail, which contains all the motility apparatus, is 40–50 μm long and arises from the spermatid centriole. It propels the sperm body via waves generated in the neck region. These waves pass distally along like a whiplash.

Under bright-field illumination, common neck and midpiece defects include bent tails, distended or irregular/bent midpieces, abnormally thin midpieces (no mitochondrial sheath), the absence of the neck or midpiece, or any of these combinations [154]. Tail defects include short, multiple hairpin broken tails, irregular widths, coiled tails with terminal droplets, or a combinations of these defects [154]. Cytoplasmic droplets greater than one third the area of a normal sperm head are considered abnormal. They are usually located in the neck/midpiece region of the tail [152].

Under scanning electron microscopy, the tail can be subdivided into three distinct parts, i.e., midpiece, principal piece, and endpiece. In the midpiece, the mitochondrial spirals can be clearly visualized. The midpiece narrows toward the posterior end. The short endpiece has a small diameter due to the absence of the outer fibers [150]. Under transmission electron microscopy, the midpiece possesses a cytoplasmic portion and a lipid-rich mitochondrial sheath that consists of several spiral mitochondria surrounding the axial filament in a helical fashion. The midpiece provides the sperm with the energy necessary for motility. An additional outer ring of 9 coarser fibrils surrounds the central core of 11 fibrils. Individual mitochondria are wrapped around these fibrils in a spiral manner to form the mitochondrial sheath, which contains the enzymes needed in the oxidative metabolism of the sperm. The mitochondrial sheath of the midpiece is relatively short and slightly longer than the combined length of the head and neck [150].

The principal or mainpiece is the longest part of the tail, and it provides most of the propellant machinery. The coarse nine fibrils of the outer ring diminish in thickness and finally disappear, leaving only the inner fibrils in the axial core for most of the length of the principal piece [155]. The tail terminates in the endpiece with a length of 4–10 μm and a diameter of <1 μm due to the absence of the outer fibrous sheath and distal fading of the microtubules.

# Regulation of Spermatogenesis

Both intrinsic and extrinsic regulations influence spermatogenic process.

## *Intrinsic Regulation*

Testosterone, neurotransmitters (neuroendocrine substances), and growth factors are secreted by Leydig cells to neighboring Leydig cells, blood vessels, the lamina propria of the seminiferous tubules and Sertoli cells [12, 148, 156] Leydig cells help maintain the nutrition of the Sertoli cells, and the cells of the peritubular tissue influence the contractility of myofibroblasts and regulate the peristaltic movements of seminiferous tubules and transportation of the spermatozoa. Leydig cells also help regulate blood flow in the intertubular microvasculature [6]. Sertoli cells deliver different growth factors, and various germ cells participate in the development and regulation of germ cells. These factors represent an independent intratesticular regulation of spermatogenesis.

## *Extrinsic Influences*

The hypothalamus and hypophysis control local regulation of spermatogenesis by pulsatile secretion of GnRH and release of LH. Leydig cells produce testosterone, which influences spermatogenesis and provides feedback to the hypophysis, which regulates the secretory activity of Leydig cells. FSH action on the Sertoli cells is necessary for maturation of the germ cells. Both FSH and LH are necessary for complete spermatogenesis. Testicular function is determined by interaction between the endocrine and paracrine mechanisms [157–159]. Sertoli cells secrete inhibin, which functions in the feedback mechanism directed to the hypophysis. Thus, both growth and differentiation of testicular germ cells involve a series of complex interactions between somatic and germinal elements [157–159].

# Immune Status of the Testis

The spermatozoa, late pachytene spermatocytes, and spermatids express unique antigens that are not formed until puberty, and therefore, immune tolerance is not developed. The blood–testis barrier develops as these autoantigens develop. The testis is considered to be an immune privileged site, i.e., transplanted foreign tissue can survive for a period of time without immunological rejection. An immune surveillance is present in the testis and the epididymis, which shows an active immunoregulation to prevent autoimmune disease [160, 161].

## Disturbances of Spermatogenesis

Disturbances in both proliferation and differentiation of the male germ cells and the intratesticular and extratesticular mechanisms regulating spermatogenesis can occur as a result of environmental influences or as a result of diseases that directly or indirectly affect spermatogenesis [162, 163]. In addition, nutrition, therapeutic drugs, hormones and their metabolites, increased scrotal temperature, toxic substances, and radiation can reduce or completely inhibit spermatogenesis.

## Sperm Transport in the Epididymis, Storage, and Capacitation

The epididymis lies along the dorsolateral border of each testis. It comprises the vasa efferentia, which emanates from the rete testis and the epididymal ducts. The primary function of the epididymis is posttesticular maturation and storage of spermatozoa during their passage from the testis to the vas deferens. The epididymal epithelium is androgen-dependent and has both absorptive and secretory functions. The epididymis is divided into three functionally distinct regions: the head, body, and tail, otherwise known as the caput epididymis, corpus epididymis, and cauda epididymis, respectively. Much of the testicular fluid that transports spermatozoa from the seminiferous tubules is reabsorbed in the caput, thereby increasing the concentration of the spermatozoa by 10- to 100-fold. As the newly developed spermatozoa pass through these regions of the epididymis, many changes occur including alterations in net surface charge, membrane protein composition, immunoreactivity, phospholipid and fatty acid content, and adenylate cyclase activity.

### Epididymal Sperm Storage

As many as half of the spermatozoa released from the testis die and disintegrate within the epididymis and are reabsorbed by the epididymal epithelium. The remaining mature spermatozoa are stored in the cauda epididymis, and this provides a capacity for repetitive fertile ejaculations. The capacity for sperm storage decreases distally, and the spermatozoa in the vas deferens may only be motile for a few days. After prolonged sexual activity, caudal spermatozoa first lose their fertilizing ability, followed by their motility and then their vitality. They ultimately disintegrate. Older, senescent spermatozoa must be eliminated from the male tract at regular intervals. Otherwise, their relative contribution to the next ejaculate(s) increases, reducing semen quality, even though such ejaculates do have a high sperm concentration. The vas deferens is not a physiological site of sperm storage and contains only about 2% of the total spermatozoa in the male tract. Sperms transit through the fine tubules of the epididymis in approximately 10–15 days in humans.

Sperms mature outside the testis. The spermatozoa within the testis have very limited motility, or none at all, and are incapable of fertilizing an egg. Both epididymal maturation and capacitation are necessary before fertilization. Capacitation – the final step required for fertilization – may be an evolutionary consequence of the development of a storage system for inactive sperm in the caudal epididymis. Preservation of optimal sperm function during this period of storage requires adequate testosterone levels in the circulation.

## Sperm Entry into Cervical Mucus

At the moment of ejaculation, spermatozoa from the cauda epididymis are mixed with secretions of the various accessory glands in a specific sequence and deposited around the external cervical os and in the posterior fornix of the vagina. The spermatozoa in the first fraction of the ejaculate have significantly better motility and survival than the later fractions. Most of the spermatozoa penetrate the cervical mucus within 15–20 min of ejaculation [164, 165]. Spermatozoa enter the uterine cavity from the internal "cervical os" by virtue of their own motility [166]. From here, the spermatozoa traverse to the site of fertilization in the ampulla of the Fallopian tube or the oviduct.

## Capacitation and Acrosome Reaction

Capacitation is a series of cellular or physiological changes that spermatozoa must undergo in order to fertilize an egg [167, 168]. It is characterized by the ability to undergo the acrosome reaction, bind to the zona pellucida, and acquire hypermotility. Capacitation per se does not involve any morphological changes, even at the ultrastructural level. It does, however, represent a change in the molecular organization of the intact sperm plasmalemma, which gives spermatozoa the ability to undergo the acrosome reaction in response to the induction of the stimulus. During capacitation, the seminal plasma factors that coat the surface of the sperm are removed, and the surface charge is modified along with the sperm membrane, sterols, lipids, and glycoproteins, and the outer acrosomal membrane lying immediately under it. Levels of intracellular free calcium also increase [169, 170].

The acrosome reaction enables sperm to penetrate the zona pellucida and also spurs the fusogenic state in the plasmalemma overlying the nonreactive equatorial segment, which is needed for interaction with the oolemma. The changes termed as "acrosome reaction" prepare the sperm to fuse with the egg membrane. The removal of cholesterol from the surface membrane prepares the sperm membrane for the acrosome reaction [171, 172]. In addition, D-mannose binding lectins are also involved in the binding of human sperm to the zona pellucida [173, 174]. Thus, all these series of changes are necessary to transform the stem cells into fully mature, functional spermatozoa equipped to fertilize an egg (Fig. 2.7).

## Conclusion

The testis is an immune privileged site. The blood–testis barrier provides a micro-environment for spermatogenesis to occur. The seminiferous tubules are the site of sperm production. The process of differentiation of a spermatogonium into a spermatid is known as spermatogenesis. It involves both mitotic and meiotic proliferation as well as extensive cell remodeling. In humans, the process of spermatogenesis starts at puberty and continues throughout life. Spermatogenesis produces genetic material necessary for the replication of the species. Meiosis assures genetic diversity. Along the length of the seminiferous tubule, there are only certain cross sections where spermatozoa are released. Sperm production is a continuous and not a pulsatile process. Spermatozoa are highly specialized cells that do not grow or divide. The spermatogenic process is maintained by different intrinsic and extrinsic influences. Spermatozoa have to undergo a series of cellular or physiological changes such as capacitation and acrosome reaction before they can fertilize. The epididymis is limited to a storage role. Nutrition, therapeutic drugs, hormones and their metabolites, increased scrotal temperature, toxic substances, or radiation can reduce or entirely inhibit spermatogenesis.

## References

1. Wilson JD. Syndromes of androgen resistance. Biol Reprod. 1992;46:168–73.
2. Lubahn DB, Moyer JS, Golding TS, Couse JF, Korach KS, Smithies O. Alteration of reproductive function but not prenatal sexual development after insertional disruption of the mouse estrogen receptor gene. Proc Natl Acad Sci USA. 1993;90:11162–6.
3. Smith EP, Boyd J, Frank GR, Takahashi H, Cohen RM, Specker B, et al. Estrogen resistance caused by a mutation in the estrogen-receptor gene in a man. N Engl J Med. 1994;331:1056–61.
4. Tishler PV. Diameter of testicles. N Engl J Med. 1971;285:1489.
5. Winter JS, Faiman C. Pituitary-gonadal relations in male children and adolescents. Pediatr Res. 1972;6:126–35.
6. Middendorff R, Müller D, Mewe M, Mukhopadhyay AK, Holstein AF, Davidoff MS. The tunica albuginea of the human testis is characterized by complex contraction and relaxation activities regulated by cyclic GMP. J Clin Endocrinol Metab. 2002;87:3486–99.
7. Prader A. Testicular size: assessment and clinical importance. Triangle. 1966;7:240–3.
8. Agger P. Scrotal and testicular temperature: its relation to sperm count before and after operation for varicocele. Fertil Steril. 1971;22:286–97.
9. de Kretser DM, Temple-Smith PD, Kerr JB. Anatomical and functional aspects of the male reproductive organs. In: Bandhauer K, Fricks J, editors. Handbook of urology, vol. XVI. Berlin: Springer; 1982. p. 1–131.

10. Christensen AK. Leydig cells. In: Hamilton DW, Greep RO, editors. Handbook of physiology. Baltimore: Williams and Wilkins; 1975. p. 57–94.
11. Kaler LW, Neaves WB. Attrition of the human Leydig cell population with advancing age. Anat Rec. 1978;192:513–8.
12. DeKretser DM, Kerr JB. The cytology of the testis. In: Knobill E, Neil JD, editors. The physiology of reproduction. New York: Raven; 1994. p. 1177–290.
13. Payne AH, Wong KL, Vega MM. Differential effects of single and repeated administrations of gonadotropins on luteinizing hormone receptors and testosterone synthesis in two populations of Leydig cells. J Biol Chem. 1980;255:7118–22.
14. Glover TD, Barratt CLR, Tyler JJP, Hennessey JF. Human male fertility. London: Academic; 1980. p. 247.
15. Ewing LL, Keeney DS. Leydig cells: structure and function. In: Desjardins C, Ewin LL, editors. Cell and molecular biology of the testis. New York: Oxford University Press; 1993.
16. Davidoff MS, Breucker H, Holstein AF, Seidel K. Cellular architecture of the lamina propria of human tubules. Cell Tissue Res. 1990;262:253–61.
17. Roosen-Runge EC, Holstein A. The human rete testis. Cell Tissue Res. 1978;189:409–33.
18. Russell LD, Griswold MD, editors. The Sertoli cell. Clearwater: Cache Press; 1993.
19. de França LR, Ghosh S, Ye SJ, Russell LD. Surface and surface-to-volume relationships of the Sertoli cell during the cycle of the seminiferous epithelium in the rat. Biol Reprod. 1993;49:1215–28.
20. Behringer RR. The müllerian inhibitor and mammalian sexual development. Philos Trans R Soc Lond B Biol Sci. 1995;350:285–8.
21. Josso N, di Clemente N, Gouédard L. Anti-Müllerian hormone and its receptors. Mol Cell Endocrinol. 2001;179:25–32.
22. Clermont Y. Kinetics of spermatogenesis in mammals: seminiferous epithelium cycle and spermatogonial renewal. Physiol Rev. 1972;52:198–236.
23. Clermont Y. The cycle of the seminiferous epithelium in man. Am J Anat. 1963;112:35–51.
24. Schulze C. Morphological characteristics of the spermatogonial stem cells in man. Cell Tissue Res. 1974;198:191–9.
25. Clermont Y, Bustos-Obregon E. Re-examination of spermatogonial renewal in the rat by means of seminiferous tubules mounted "in toto". Am J Anat. 1968;122:237–47.
26. Huckins C. The spermatogonial stem cell population in adult rats. I. Their morphology, proliferation and maturation. Anat Rec. 1971;169:533–57.
27. Dym M, Fawcett DW. Further observations on the numbers of spermatogonia, spermatocytes, and spermatids connected by intercellular bridges in the mammalian testis. Biol Reprod. 1971;4:195–215.
28. Berezney R, Coffey DS. Nuclear matrix. Isolation and characterization of a framework structure from rat liver nuclei. J Cell Biol. 1977;73:616–37.
29. Mirkovitch J, Mirault ME, Laemmli UK. Organization of the higher-order chromatin loop: specific DNA attachment sites on nuclear scaffold. Cell. 1984;39:223–32.
30. Gasse S. Studies on scaffold attachment sites and their relation to genome function. Int Rev Cytol. 1989;119:57.
31. Izaurralde E, Kas E, Laemmli UK. Highly preferential nucleation of histone H1 assembly on scaffold-associated regions. J Mol Biol. 1989;210:573–85.
32. Adachi Y, Kas E, Laemmli UK. Preferential cooperative binding of DNA topoisomerase II to scaffold-associated regions. EMBO J. 1989;13:3997.
33. Dickinson LA, Joh T, Kohwi Y, Kohwi-Shigematsu T. A tissue-specific MAR/SAR DNA-binding protein with unusual binding site recognition. Cell. 1992;70:631–45.
34. Breucker H, Schäfer E, Holstein AF. Morphogenesis and fate of the residual body in human spermiogenesis. Cell Tissue Res. 1985;240:303–9.
35. Leblond CP, Clermont Y. Definition of the stages of the cycle of the seminiferous epithelium in the rat. Ann N Y Acad Sci. 1952;55:548–73.
36. Clermont Y, Perey B. The stages of the cycle of the seminiferous epithelium of the rat: practical definitions in PA-Schiff-hematoxylin and hematoxylin-eosin stained sections. Rev Can Biol. 1957;16:451–62.

37. Schulze W, Rehder U. Organization and morphogenesis of the human seminiferous epithelium. Cell Tissue Res. 1984;237:395–407.
38. Ward WS, Coffey DS. DNA packaging and organization in mammalian spermatozoa: comparison with somatic cells. Biol Reprod. 1991;44:569–74.
39. McGhee JD, Felsenfeld G, Eisenberg H. Nucleosome structure and conformational changes. Biophys J. 1980;32:261–70.
40. Sassone-Corsi P. Unique chromatin remodeling and transcriptional regulation in spermatogenesis. Science. 2002;296:2176–8.
41. Dadoune JP, Siffroi JP, Alfonsi MF. Transcription in haploid male germ cells. Int Rev Cytol. 2004;237:1–56.
42. Ward WS, Partin AW, Coffey DS. DNA loop domains in mammalian spermatozoa. Chromosoma. 1989;98:153–9.
43. McPherson S, Longo FJ. Chromatin structure-function alterations during mammalian spermatogenesis: DNA nicking and repair in elongating spermatids. Eur J Histochem. 1993; 37:109–28.
44. Allen MJ, Lee C, Lee IV JD, Pogany GC, Balooch M, Siekhaus WJ, et al. Atomic force microscopy of mammalian sperm chromatin. Chromosoma. 1993;102:623–30.
45. Lewis JD, Abbott DW, Ausió J. A haploid affair: core histone transitions during spermatogenesis. Biochem Cell Biol. 2003;81:131–40.
46. Lewis JD, Song Y, de Jong ME, Bagha SM, Ausió J. A walk though vertebrate and invertebrate protamines. Chromosoma. 2003;111:473–82.
47. Braun RE. Packaging paternal chromosomes with protamine. Nat Genet. 2001;28:10–2.
48. Wu TF, Chu DS. Sperm chromatin: fertile grounds for proteomic discovery of clinical tools. Mol Cell Proteomics. 2008;7:1876–86.
49. Ooi SL, Henikoff S. Germline histone dynamics and epigenetics. Curr Opin Cell Biol. 2007;19:257–65.
50. Cho C, Willis WD, Goulding EH, Jung-Ha H, Choi YC, Hecht NB, et al. Haploinsufficiency of protamine-1 or -2 causes infertility in mice. Nat Genet. 2001;28:82–6.
51. Yu YE, Zhang Y, Unni E, Shirley CR, Deng JM, Russell LD, et al. Abnormal spermatogenesis and reduced fertility in transition nuclear protein 1-deficient mice. Proc Natl Acad Sci USA. 2000;97:4683–8.
52. Zhao M, Shirley CR, Yu YE, Mohapatra B, Zhang Y, Unni E, et al. Targeted disruption of the transition protein 2 gene affects sperm chromatin structure and reduces fertility in mice. Mol Cell Biol. 2001;21:7243–55.
53. Churikov D, Zalenskaya IA, Zalensky AO. Male germline-specific histones in mouse and man. Cytogenet Genome Res. 2004;105:203–14.
54. Dadoune JP. The nuclear status of human sperm cells. Micron. 1995;26:323–45.
55. Kierszenbaum AL. Transition nuclear proteins during spermiogenesis: unrepaired DNA breaks not allowed. Mol Reprod Dev. 2001;58:357–8.
56. Lee CH, Cho YH. Aspects of mammalian spermatogenesis: electrophoretical analysis of protamines in mammalian species. Mol Cells. 1999;9:556–9.
57. Bench GS, Friz AM, Corzett MH, Morse DH, Balhorn R. DNA and total protamine masses in individual sperm from fertile mammalian subjects. Cytometry. 1996;23:263–71.
58. Gatewood JM, Cook GR, Balhorn R, Bradbury EM, Schmid CW. Sequence-specific packaging of DNA in human sperm chromatin. Science. 1987;236:962–4.
59. Laberge RM, Boissonneault G. On the nature and origin of DNA strand breaks in elongating spermatids. Biol Reprod. 2005;73:289–96.
60. Marcon L, Boissonneault G. Transient DNA strand breaks during mouse and human spermiogenesis new insights in stage specificity and link to chromatin remodeling. Biol Reprod. 2004;70:910–8.
61. McPherson SM, Longo FJ. Nicking of rat spermatid and spermatozoa DNA: possible involvement of DNA topoisomerase II. Dev Biol. 1993;158:122–30.
62. Muratori M, Marchiani S, Maggi M, Forti G, Baldi E. Origin and biological significance of DNA fragmentation in human spermatozoa. Front Biosci. 2006;11:1491–9.

63. Zhao M, Shirley CR, Mounsey S, Meistrich ML. Nucleoprotein transitions during spermiogenesis in mice with transition nuclear protein Tnp1 and Tnp2 mutations. Biol Reprod. 2004;71:1016–25.
64. Kistler WS, Noyes C, Hsu R, Heinrikson RL. The amino acid sequence of a testis-specific basic protein that is associated with spermatogenesis. J Biol Chem. 1975;250:1847–53.
65. Kleene KC, Borzorgzadeh A, Flynn JF, Yelick PC, Hecht NB. Nucleotide sequence of a cDNA clone encoding mouse transition protein 1. Biochim Biophys Acta. 1988;950:215–20.
66. Schlüter G, Celik A, Obata R, Schlicker M, Hofferbert S, Schlung A, et al. Sequence analysis of the conserved protamine gene cluster shows that it contains a fourth expressed gene. Mol Reprod Dev. 1996;43:1–6.
67. Meistrich ML. Calculation of the incidence of infertility in human populations from sperm measures using the two-distribution model. Prog Clin Biol Res. 1989;302:275–85.
68. Alfonso PJ, Kistler WS. Immunohistochemical localization of spermatid nuclear transition protein 2 in the testes of rats and mice. Biol Reprod. 1993;48:522–9.
69. Heidaran MA, Showman RM, Kistler WS. A cytochemical study of the transcriptional and translational regulation of nuclear transition protein 1 (TP1), a major chromosomal protein of mammalian spermatids. J Cell Biol. 1988;106:1427–33.
70. Baskaran R, Rao MR. Interaction of spermatid-specific protein TP2 with nucleic acids, in vitro. A comparative study with TP1. J Biol Chem. 1990;265:21039–47.
71. Lévesque D, Veilleux S, Caron N, Boissonneault G. Architectural DNA-binding properties of the spermatidal transition proteins 1 and 2. Biochem Biophys Res Commun. 1998;252: 602–9.
72. Kundu TK, Rao MR. Zinc dependent recognition of a human CpG island sequence by the mammalian spermatidal protein TP2. Biochemistry. 1996;35:15626–32.
73. Boissonneault G. Chromatin remodeling during spermiogenesis: a possible role for the transition proteins in DNA strand break repair. FEBS Lett. 2002;514:111–4.
74. Caron N, Veilleux S, Boissonneault G. Stimulation of DNA repair by the spermatidal TP1 protein. Mol Reprod Dev. 2001;58:437–43.
75. Brewer L, Corzett M, Balhorn R. Condensation of DNA by spermatid basic nuclear proteins. J Biol Chem. 2002;277:38895–900.
76. Adham IM, Nayernia K, Burkhardt-Göttges E, Topaloglu O, Dixkens C, Holstein AF, et al. Teratozoospermia in mice lacking the transition protein 2 (Tnp2). Mol Hum Reprod. 2001;7: 513–20.
77. Carrell DT, Liu L. Altered protamine 2 expression is uncommon in donors of known fertility, but common among men with poor fertilizing capacity, and may reflect other abnormalities of spermiogenesis. J Androl. 2001;22:604–10.
78. de Yebra L, Ballescá JL, Vanrell JA, Corzett M, Balhorn R, Oliva R. Detection of P2 precursors in the sperm cells of infertile patients who have reduced protamine P2 levels. Fertil Steril. 1998;69:755–9.
79. Balhorn R, Corzett M, Mazrimas JA. Formation of intraprotamine disulfides in vitro. Arch Biochem Biophys. 1992;296:384–93.
80. Balhorn R, Cosman M, Thornton K, Krishnan VV, Corzett M, Bench G, et al. Protamine-mediated condensation of DNA in mammalian sperm. In: Gagnon C, editor. The male gamete: from basic science to clinical applications. Vienna: Cache River Press; 1999.
81. Corzett M, Mazrimas J, Balhorn R. Protamine 1: protamine 2 stoichiometry in the sperm of eutherian mammals. Mol Reprod Dev. 2002;61:519–27.
82. Fuentes-Mascorro G, Serrano H, Rosado A. Sperm chromatin. Arch Androl. 2000;45: 215–25.
83. Dixon GH, Aiken JM, Jankowski JM, McKenzie D, Moir R, States JC, et al. Organization and evolution of protamine gene of salmoind fishes. In: Reeck GR, Goodwin GH, Puigdomenech P, editors. Chromosomal proteins and gene expression. New York: Plenum; 1986.
84. Krawetz SA, Dixon GH. Sequence similarities of the protamine genes: implications for regulation and evolution. J Mol Evol. 1988;27:291–7.
85. Balhorn R, Brewer L, Corzett M. DNA condensation by protamine and arginine-rich peptides: analysis of toroid stability using single DNA molecules. Mol Reprod Dev. 2000;56:230–4.

86. Courtens JL, Loir M. Ultrastructural detection of basic nucleoproteins: alcoholic phospho-tungstic acid does not bind to arginine residues. J Ultrastruct Res. 1981;74:322–6.
87. Loir M, Lanneau M. Structural function of the basic nuclear proteins in ram spermatids. J Ultrastruct Res. 1984;86:262–72.
88. Singh J, Rao MR. Interaction of rat testis protein, TP, with nucleosome core particle. Biochem Int. 1988;17:701–10.
89. Le Lannic G, Arkhis A, Vendrely E, Chevaillier P, Dadoune JP. Production, characterization, and immunocytochemical applications of monoclonal antibodies to human sperm prot-amines. Mol Reprod Dev. 1993;36:106–12.
90. Szczygiel MA, Ward WS. Combination of dithiothreitol and detergent treatment of sperma-tozoa causes paternal chromosomal damage. Biol Reprod. 2002;67:1532–7.
91. Hecht NB. Post-meiotic gene expression during spermatogenesis. Prog Clin Biol Res. 1988;267:291–313.
92. Hecht NB. Regulation of 'haploid expressed genes' in male germ cells. J Reprod Fertil. 1990;88:679–93.
93. Oliva R, Dixon GH. Vertebrate protamine gene evolution I. Sequence alignments and gene structure. J Mol Evol. 1990;30:333–46.
94. Steger K. Transcriptional and translational regulation of gene expression in haploid sperma-tids. Anat Embryol (Berl). 1999;199:471–87.
95. Oliva R. Protamines and male infertility. Hum Reprod Update. 2006;12:417–35.
96. Chevaillier P, Mauro N, Feneux D, Jouannet P, David G. Anomalous protein complement of sperm nuclei in some infertile men. Lancet. 1987;2:806–7.
97. Balhorn R, Reed S, Tanphaichitr N. Aberrant protamine 1/protamine 2 ratios in sperm of infertile human males. Experientia. 1988;44:52–5.
98. Aoki VW, Moskovtsev SI, Willis J, Liu L, Mullen JB, Carrell DT. DNA integrity is compro-mised in protamine-deficient human sperm. J Androl. 2005;26:741–8.
99. Carrell DT, Emery BR, Hammoud S. Altered protamine expression and diminished sper-matogenesis: what is the link? Hum Reprod Update. 2007;13:313–27.
100. Kosower NS, Katayose H, Yanagimachi R. Thiol-disulfide status and acridine orange fluores-cence of mammalian sperm nuclei. J Androl. 1992;13:342–8.
101. Sakkas D, Mariethoz E, Manicardi G, et al. Origin of DNA damage in ejaculated human spermatozoa. Rev Reprod. 1999;4:31–7.
102. Aoki VW, Carrell DT. Human protamines and the developing spermatid: their structure, func-tion, expression and relationship with male infertility. Asian J Androl. 2003;5:315–24.
103. Mengual L, Ballescá JL, Ascaso C, Oliva R. Marked differences in protamine content and P1/P2 ratios in sperm cells from percoll fractions between patients and controls. J Androl. 2003;24:438–47.
104. Steger K, Pauls K, Klonisch T, Franke FE, Bergmann M. Expression of protamine-1 and -2 mRNA during human spermiogenesis. Mol Hum Reprod. 2000;6:219–25.
105. Rousseaux S, Caron C, Govin J, Lestrat C, Faure AK, Khochbin S. Establishment of male-specific epigenetic information. Gene. 2005;345:139–53.
106. Arpanahi A, Brinkworth M, Iles D, Krawetz SA, Paradowska A, Platts AE, et al. Endonuclease-sensitive regions of human spermatozoal chromatin are highly enriched in promoter and CTCF binding sequences. Genome Res. 2009;19:1338–49.
107. Hammoud SS, Purwar J, Pflueger C, Cairns BR, Carrell DT. Alterations in sperm DNA meth-ylation patterns at imprinted loci in two classes of infertility. Fertil Steril. 2010;94:1728–33.
108. Razin A, Riggs AD. DNA methylation and gene function. Science. 1980;210:604–10.
109. Cedar H. DNA methylation and gene expression. In: Razin A, Cedar H, Riggs AD, editors. DNA methylation: biochemistry and biological significance. New York: Springer; 1985.
110. Sanford JP, Clark HJ, Chapman VM, Rossant J. Differences in DNA methylation during oogenesis and spermatogenesis and their persistence during early embryogenesis in the mouse. Genes Dev. 1987;1:1039–46.
111. Rahe B, Erickson RP, Quinto M. Methylation of unique sequence DNA during spermatogen-esis in mice. Nucleic Acids Res. 1983;11:7947–59.

112. Trasler JM. Epigenetics in spermatogenesis. Mol Cell Endocrinol. 2009;306:33–6.
113. Oakes CC, La Salle S, Smiraglia DJ, Robaire B, Trasler JM. Developmental acquisition of genome-wide DNA methylation occurs prior to meiosis in male germ cells. Dev Biol. 2007;307:368–79.
114. Benchaib M, Braun V, Lornage J, et al. Sperm DNA fragmentation decreases the pregnancy rate in an assisted reproductive technique. Hum Reprod. 2003;18:1023–8.
115. Ward WS. The structure of the sleeping genome: implications of sperm DNA organization for somatic cells. J Cell Biochem. 1994;55:77–82.
116. Risley MS, Einheber S, Bumcrot DA. Changes in DNA topology during spermatogenesis. Chromosoma. 1986;94:217–27.
117. Aitken RJ, De Iuliis GN. On the possible origins of DNA damage in human spermatozoa. Mol Hum Reprod. 2010;16:3–13.
118. Aitken RJ, De Iuliis GN, McLachlan RI. Biological and clinical significance of DNA damage in the male germ line. Int J Androl. 2009;32:46–56.
119. Carrell DT, Emery BR, Hammoud S. The aetiology of sperm protamine abnormalities and their potential impact on the sperm epigenome. Int J Androl. 2008;31:537–45.
120. De Iuliis GN, Thomson LK, Mitchell LA, Finnie JM, Koppers AJ, Hedges A, et al. DNA damage in human spermatozoa is highly correlated with the efficiency of chromatin remodeling and the formation of 8-hydroxy-2´, -deoxyguanosine, a marker of oxidative stress. Biol Reprod. 2009;81:517–24.
121. Leduc F, Maquennehan V, Nkoma GB, Boissonneault G. DNA damage response during chromatin remodeling in elongating spermatids of mice. Biol Reprod. 2008;78:324–32.
122. Kramer JA, Krawetz SA. Nuclear matrix interactions within the sperm genome. J Biol Chem. 1996;271:11619–22.
123. Ward WS, Kimura Y, Yanagimachi R. An intact sperm nuclear matrix may be necessary for the mouse paternal genome to participate in embryonic development. Biol Reprod. 1999;60:702–6.
124. Singleton S, Zalensky A, Doncel GF, Morshedi M, Zalenskaya IA. Testis/sperm-specific histone 2B in the sperm of donors and subfertile patients: variability and relation to chromatin packaging. Hum Reprod. 2007;22:743–50.
125. Iranpour FG, Nasr-Esfahani MH, Valojerdi MR, al-Taraihi TM. Chromomycin A3 staining as a useful tool for evaluation of male fertility. J Assist Reprod Genet. 2000;17:60–6.
126. Bizzaro D, Manicardi GC, Bianchi PG, Bianchi U, Mariethoz E, Sakkas D. In-situ competition between protamine and fluorochromes for sperm DNA. Mol Hum Reprod. 1998;4:127–32.
127. Manicardi GC, Bianchi PG, Pantano S, Azzoni P, Bizzaro D, Bianchi U, et al. Presence of endogenous nicks in DNA of ejaculated human spermatozoa and its relationship to chromomycin A3 accessibility. Biol Reprod. 1995;52:864–7.
128. Bianchi PG, Manicardi GC, Bizzaro D, Bianchi U, Sakkas D. Effect of deoxyribonucleic acid protamination on fluorochrome staining and in situ nick-translation of murine and human mature spermatozoa. Biol Reprod. 1993;49:1083–8.
129. Zini A, Gabriel MS, Zhang X. The histone to protamine ratio in human spermatozoa: comparative study of whole and processed semen. Fertil Steril. 2007;87:217–9.
130. Aoki VW, Emery BR, Liu L, Carrell DT. Protamine levels vary between individual sperm cells of infertile human males and correlate with viability and DNA integrity. J Androl. 2006;27:890–8.
131. Carrell DT, De Jonge C, Lamb DJ. The genetics of male infertility: a field of study whose time is now. Arch Androl. 2006;52:269–74.
132. Irvine DS, Twigg JP, Gordon EL, Fulton N, Milne PA, Aitken RJ. DNA integrity in human spermatozoa: relationships with semen quality. J Androl. 2000;21:33–44.
133. Weng SL, Taylor SL, Morshedi M, Schuffner A, Duran EH, Beebe S, et al. Caspase activity and apoptotic markers in ejaculated human sperm. Mol Hum Reprod. 2002;8:984–91.
134. Sinha Hikim AP, Swerdloff RS. Hormonal and genetic control of germ cell apoptosis in the testis. Rev Reprod. 1999;4:38–47.
135. Rodriguez I, Ody C, Araki K, Garcia I, Vassalli P. An early and massive wave of germinal cell apoptosis is required for the development of functional spermatogenesis. EMBO J. 1997;16:2262–70.

136. Hikim AP, Lue Y, Yamamoto CM, Vera Y, Rodriguez S, Yen PH, et al. Key apoptotic pathways for heat-induced programmed germ cell death in the testis. Endocrinology. 2003;144: 3167–75.

137. Sakkas D, Seli E, Bizzaro D, Tarozzi N, Manicardi GC. Abnormal spermatozoa in the ejaculate: abortive apoptosis and faulty nuclear remodelling during spermatogenesis. Reprod Biomed Online. 2003;7:428–32.

138. Paul C, Povey JE, Lawrence NJ, Selfridge J, Melton DW, Saunders PT. Deletion of genes implicated in protecting the integrity of male germ cells has differential effects on the incidence of DNA breaks and germ cell loss. PLoS One. 2007;3:e989.

139. Bauché F, Fouchard MH, Jégou B. Antioxidant system in rat testicular cells. FEBS Lett. 1994;349:392–6.

140. Fraga CG, Motchnik PA, Wyrobek AJ, Rempel DM, Ames BN. Smoking and low antioxidant levels increase oxidative damage to sperm DNA. Mutat Res. 1996;351:199–203.

141. Meyer-Ficca ML, Lonchar J, Credidio C, Ihara M, Li Y, Wang ZQ, et al. Disruption of poly(ADP-ribose) homeostasis affects spermiogenesis and sperm chromatin integrity in mice. Biol Reprod. 2009;81:46–55.

142. Aitken RJ, Gordon E, Harkiss D, Twigg JP, Milne P, Jennings Z, et al. Relative impact of oxidative stress on the functional competence and genomic integrity of human spermatozoa. Biol Reprod. 1998;59:1037–46.

143. Piña-Guzmán B, Solís-Heredia MJ, Rojas-García AE, Urióstegui-Acosta M, Quintanilla-Vega B. Genetic damage caused by methyl-parathion in mouse spermatozoa is related to oxidative stress. Toxicol Appl Pharmacol. 2006;216:216–24.

144. Zubkova EV, Robaire B. Effects of ageing on spermatozoal chromatin and its sensitivity to in vivo and in vitro oxidative challenge in the Brown Norway rat. Hum Reprod. 2006;11: 2901–10.

145. Heller C, Clermont Y. Kinetics of the germinal epithelium in man. Recent Prog Horm Res. 1964;20:545–75.

146. Sculze W, Salzbrunn A. Spatial and quantitative aspects of spermatogenetic tissue in primates. In: Neischlag E, Habenicht U, editors. Spermatogenesis-fertilization-contraception. Berlin: Springer; 1992. p. 267–83.

147. Rowe PJ, Comhaire F, Hargreave TB, Mellows HJ, editors. WHO manual for the standardized investigation and diagnosis of the infertile couple. Cambridge: Cambridge University Press; 1993.

148. Sharpe RM. Regulation of spermatogenesis. In: Knobill E, Neil JD, editors. The physiology of reproduction. New York: Raven; 1994. p. 1363–434.

149. De Kretser DM. Ultrastructural features of human spermiogenesis. Z Zellforsch Mikrosk Anat. 1969;98:477–505.

150. Hafez ES. The human semen and fertility regulation in the male. J Reprod Med. 1976;16: 91–6.

151. Kruger TF, Menkveld R, Stander FS, Lombard CJ, Van der Merwe JP, van Zyl JA, et al. Sperm morphologic features as a prognostic factor in in vitro fertilization. Fertil Steril. 1986;46:1118–23.

152. Menkveld R, Stander FS, Kotze TJ, Kruger TF, van Zyl JA. The evaluation of morphological characteristics of human spermatozoa according to stricter criteria. Hum Reprod. 1990;5:586–92.

153. Katz DF, Overstreet JW, Samuels SJ, Niswander PW, Bloom TD, Lewis EL. Morphometric analysis of spermatozoa in the assessment of human male fertility. J Androl. 1986;7:203–10.

154. World Health Organization. World Health Organization laboratory manual for the examination of human semen and sperm-cervical mucus interaction. 4th ed. Cambridge: Cambridge University Press; 1999.

155. White IG. Mammalian sperm. In: Hafez ESE, editor. Reproduction of farm animals. Philadelphia: Lea & Febiger; 1974.

156. Jegou B. The Sertoli cell. Baillières Clin Endocrinol Metab. 1992;6:273–311.

157. Bellve AR, Zheng W. Growth factors as autocrine and paracrine modulators of male gonadal functions. J Reprod Fertil. 1989;85:771–93.
158. Sharpe T. Intratesticular control of steroidogenesis. Clin Endocrinol. 1990;33:787–807.
159. Sharpe RM. Monitoring of spermatogenesis in man-measurement of Sertoli cell- or germ cell-secreted proteins in semen or blood. Int J Androl. 1992;15:201–10.
160. Mahi-Brown CA, Yule TD, Tung KS. Evidence for active immunological regulation in prevention of testicular autoimmune disease independent of the blood-testis barrier. Am J Reprod Immunol Microbiol. 1988;16:165–70.
161. Barratt CL, Bolton AE, Cooke ID. Functional significance of white blood cells in the male and female reproductive tract. Hum Reprod. 1990;5:639–48.
162. Holstein AF, Schulze W, Breucker H. Histopathology of human testicular and epididymal tissue. In: Hargreave TB, editor. Male infertility. London: Springer; 1994. p. 105–48.
163. Nieschlag E, Behre H. Andrology. Male reproductive health and dysfunction. Berlin: Springer; 2001.
164. Tredway DR, Settlage DS, Nakamura RM, Motoshima M, Umezaki CU, Mishell Jr DR. Significance of timing for the postcoital evaluation of cervical mucus. Am J Obstet Gynecol. 1975;121:387–93.
165. Tredway DR, Buchanan GC, Drake TS. Comparison of the fractional postcoital test and semen analysis. Am J Obstet Gynecol. 1978;130:647–52.
166. Settlage DSF, Motoshima M, Tredway DR. Sperm transport from the external cervical os to the fallopian tubes in women: a time and quantitation study. In: Hafez ESE, Thibault CG, editors. Sperm transport, survival and fertilizing ability in vertebrates, vol. 26. Paris: INSERM; 1974. p. 201–17.
167. Eddy EM, O'Brien DA. The spermatozoon. In: Knobill EO, NO'Nneill JD, editors. The physiology of reproduction. New York: Raven; 1994.
168. Yanagamachi R. Mammalian fertilization. In: Knobill E, O'Brien NJ, editors. The physiology of reproduction. New York: Raven; 1994.
169. Mahanes MS, Ochs DL, Eng LA. Cell calcium of ejaculated rabbit spermatozoa before and following in vitro capacitation. Biochem Biophys Res Commun. 1986;134:664–70.
170. Thomas P, Meizel S. Phosphatidylinositol 4,5-bisphosphate hydrolysis in human sperm stimulated with follicular fluid or progesterone is dependent upon $Ca^{2+}$ influx. Biochem J. 1989; 264:539–46.
171. Parks JE, Ehrenwalt E. Cholesterol efflux from mammalian sperm and its potential role in capacitation. In: Bavister BD, Cummins J, Raldon E, editors. Fertilization in mammals. Norwell: Serono Symposia; 1990.
172. Ravnik SE, Zarutskie PW, Muller CH. Purification and characterization of a human follicular fluid lipid transfer protein that stimulates human sperm capacitation. Biol Reprod. 1992;47: 1126–33.
173. Benoff S, Cooper GW, Hurley I, Mandel FS, Rosenfeld DL. Antisperm antibody binding to human sperm inhibits capacitation induced changes in the levels of plasma membrane sterols. Am J Reprod Immunol. 1993;30:113–30.
174. Benoff S, Hurley I, Cooper GW, Mandel FS, Hershlag A, Scholl GM, et al. Fertilization potential in vitro is correlated with head-specific mannose-ligand receptor expression, acrosome status and membrane cholesterol content. Hum Reprod. 1993;8:2155–66.

# Chapter 3
# Role of Oxidative Stress in the Etiology of Sperm DNA Damage

R. John Aitken and Geoffry N. De Iuliis

Male infertility is the single largest defined cause of human infertility and, along with maternal age, is the major reason why patients are referred for assisted conception therapy. Maternal age is a significant factor in the etiology of human infertility because it affects the quality of the oocytes and their capacity to support normal embryonic development. Importantly, the fertilizability of such oocytes is not impaired by advances in maternal age. As a consequence, even when conception is facilitated in such patients using assisted reproductive technologies (ARTs) such as in vitro fertilization (IVF) or intracytoplasmic sperm injection (ICSI), the live birth rate declines with maternal age much as it does in the natural population [1]. The fact is that an old oocyte cannot be rescued by facilitating contact with a spermatozoon because achieving fertilization is not the limiting issue with such patients; it is the establishment of normal embryonic development. As a result, the use of ART to treat age-related infecundity is of questionable utility. On the other hand, ART is a perfectly rational treatment for male infertility, which generally involves defects in the fertilizing potential of the spermatozoa that can be effectively remedied by facilitating contact with an egg, even if that treatment involves bypassing the entire physiology of fertilization by physically injecting a spermatozoon into the ooplasm.

R.J. Aitken, PhD, Dsc, FRSE (✉)
Discipline of Biological Sciences,
School of Environmental and Life Sciences,
University of Newcastle, University Drive, Callaghan, NSW 2308, Australia

ARC Centre of Excellence in Biotechnology and Development,
Priority Research Centre in Reproductive Science,
University of Newcastle, Callaghan, NSW 2308, Australia
e-mail: john.aitken@newcastle.edu.au

G.N. De Iuliis, PhD, BSc
Department of Biological Sciences,
ARC Centre of Excellence in Biotechnology and Development,
Priority Research Centre in Reproductive Science,
University of Newcastle, Newcastle, NSW, Australia

A. Zini, A. Agarwal (eds.), *Sperm Chromatin for the Clinician*,
© Springer Science+Business Media New York 2013

Even though defective sperm function is recognized as the largest single defined cause of human infertility [2], relatively little is known about the etiology of this condition. A majority of infertile men produce spermatozoa in sufficient numbers to fertilize the egg; however, in this subpopulation of individuals, the fertilizing potential of these cells has been compromised for reasons that are still not fully elucidated. The only major breakthrough we have seen in the past half-century is the awareness that one of the major causes of defective sperm function is oxidative stress [3, 4]. Analysis of the impact of oxidative stress on the male gamete initially focused on the impaired fertilizing potential of these cells as a consequence of lipid peroxidation in the plasma membrane [5–7]. Spermatozoa are particularly vulnerable to lipid peroxidation because they possess a high cellular content of unsaturated fatty acids, particularly arachidonic and decosahexaenoic acids [5, 8]. As a consequence of free radical attack and the initiation of a lipid peroxidation cascade, the sperm plasma membrane loses its fluidity and hence its capacity for engaging in the membrane fusion events associated with fertilization including acrosomal exocytosis and the act of sperm–oocyte fusion itself [9]. This association between oxidative stress and male infertility has been established in a large number of independent studies [10–12], and as a result, we can now safely conclude that the fertilizing potential of human spermatozoa is frequently impaired by the excessive generation of reactive oxygen species (ROS) and peroxidative damage. However, this is not the whole story.

The initial emphasis on lipid peroxidation and lost fertilizing potential has recently given way to the realization that polyunsaturated fatty acids are not the only target for free radical attack. A second vulnerable substrate for free radical attack in spermatozoa is the DNA in the sperm nucleus and mitochondria [13–15]. Sperm DNA damage is now recognized as a major attribute of the human condition, which is significantly elevated in the spermatozoa of subfertile males and highly correlated with a number of adverse clinical outcomes including poor fertilization rates, poor development of the preimplantation embryo, high rates of miscarriage, and an increased incidence of disease in offspring [12, 16–19]. The consequences of DNA damage in the paternal genome for the F1 generation are many and varied but include cancer and complex neurological conditions such as autism, spontaneous schizophrenia, bipolar disease, and epilepsy [17]. The existence of these correlations has served to broaden our concept of what constitutes a normal fertile male. Normal reproductive function is not just about producing spermatozoa that will fertilize the egg. It is also about producing spermatozoa that will support normal embryonic development and the birth of normal, healthy children.

Since sperm DNA damage is highly represented in the subfertile population and since DNA integrity cannot be determined in the spermatozoon that achieves fertilization in vitro, there is a high probability that DNA-damaged spermatozoa are being used in ART. Such involvement of DNA-damaged spermatozoa in assisted conception may explain the increased risk of abnormalities in the offspring conceived by such methods. Thus, we already know that the incidence of birth defects following assisted conception is double that seen in the naturally conceived population [20] and that imprinting disorders, notably the Beckwith–Wiedemann and Angelman syndromes, appear to be increased in such children [21]. Infants produced by ART are also significantly more likely to be admitted to a neonatal intensive care unit, to be hospitalized, and to stay in hospital longer than their naturally conceived counterparts [22]. Recent studies using record linkage have also shown an increase in the hospitalization of ART offspring in infancy and early childhood compared with spontaneously conceived children [23–25]. Additional independent investigations have also revealed abnormal retinal vascularization in such children, while another study has uncovered an eightfold increase in the incidence of undescended testicles in boys conceived by ICSI [26, 27].

In light of this information, it is clearly important that we understand the etiology of DNA damage in spermatozoa and take steps to reduce its incidence. At present the factors contributing to this damage are poorly understood, although paternal age certainly plays a major role, as does infection, lifestyle (e.g., smoking), and exposure to environmental pollutants. A common denominator that cuts across all of the factors thought to contribute to DNA damage in the male germ line is that they are all capable of generating a state of oxidative stress. In keeping with this assertion is the recent observation that DNA fragmentation in human spermatozoa is highly correlated with oxidative DNA damage as reflected by the presence of 8-hydroxy 2' deoxyguanosine (8OHdG), a marker of oxidative stress. Indeed, this correlation is so high that we have been forced to conclude that oxidative stress is the major cause of DNA damage in the male germ line [28, 29]. This finding raises a number of questions about the detection, cause, prevention, and treatment of DNA damage in the germ line that are addressed in this review. Before these biological issues are discussed, we first examine the fundamental chemistry of free radicals and consider how they precipitate a state of oxidative stress.

## The Chemistry of Oxidative Stress

### Reactive Oxygen Species

The term reactive oxygen species (ROS) covers a wide range of metabolites derived from the reduction of molecular oxygen, including free radicals, such as the superoxide anion ($O_2^{-\bullet}$) and powerful oxidants such as hydrogen peroxide ($H_2O_2$). The term also covers molecules derived from the reaction of carbon-centered radicals with oxygen including peroxyl radicals ($ROO^{\bullet}$), alkoxyl radicals ($RO^{\bullet}$), and organic hydroperoxides ($ROOH$). It may also refer to other powerful oxidants such as peroxynitrite ($ONOO^-$) or hypochlorous acid ($HOCl$), as well as the highly biologically active free radical, nitric oxide ($NO^{\bullet}$).

The specific term "free radicals" refers to any atom or molecule containing one or more unpaired electrons. As unpaired electrons are highly energetic and seek out other electrons with which to pair, they confer upon free radicals considerable reactivity. Thus, free radicals and related "reactive species" have the ability to react with, and modify the structure of, many different kinds of biomolecules including proteins, lipids, and nucleic acids. The wide range of targets that can be attacked by ROS is a critical aspect of their chemistry that contributes significantly to the pathological significance of these metabolites. In this context, it is important to emphasize that ROS are not discrete single entities but, by virtue of their very reactivity, react with one another to generate complex mixtures of reactive metabolites, classic examples being the dismutation (reaction with itself) of $O_2^{-\bullet}$ to generate $H_2O_2$ or the reaction of $NO^{\bullet}$ and $O_2^{-\bullet}$ to generate $ONOO^-$. One of the most important such processes is the reaction of $O_2^{-\bullet}$ with $H_2O_2$ in the presence of transition metals to generate the hydroxyl radical ($OH^{\bullet}$). The latter is extremely reactive and a major factor in the initiation of oxidative damage to vulnerable substrates including polyunsaturated fatty acids and DNA.

## Lipid Peroxidation

Since most biological molecules only have paired electrons, free radicals are also likely to be involved in chain reactions that can propagate the damage induced by ROS. A classic example of such a chain reaction is the peroxidation of lipids in biological membranes. In this process, a ROS-mediated attack on unsaturated fatty acids generates peroxyl ($ROO^{\bullet}$) and alkoxyl ($RO^{\bullet}$) radicals that, in order to stabilize, abstract a hydrogen atom from an adjacent carbon, generating the corresponding acid (ROOH) or alcohol (ROH). The abstraction of a hydrogen atom from an adjacent lipid creates a carbon-centered radical that combines with molecular oxygen to re-create another lipid peroxide. In order to stabilize, the latter must again abstract a hydrogen atom from a nearby lipid, creating another carbon radical that combines with molecular oxygen to create yet another lipid peroxide. In this manner, a chain reaction is created that, if unchecked, would propagate the peroxidative damage throughout the plasma membrane, leading to a rapid loss of membrane-dependent functions.

Such chain reactions are promoted by the presence of transition metals such as iron and copper that can vary their valency states by gaining or losing electrons. Significantly, there is sufficient free iron and copper in human seminal plasma to promote lipid peroxidation once this process has been initiated [30]. When iron sulfate and ascorbate (added as a reductant to maintain the iron in a reduced state) are added to suspensions of human spermatozoa, large amounts of lipid peroxide are generated. A majority of these peroxides arise from the iron-catalyzed propagation, rather than de novo initiation, of lipid peroxidation cascades [31], according to the following equations:

$$\underset{\text{lipid hydroperoxide}}{ROOH} + Fe^{2+} \rightarrow \underset{\text{alkoxyl radical}}{RO^{\bullet}} + OH^- + Fe^{3+}$$

$$\underset{\text{lipid hydroperoxide}}{ROOH} + Fe^{3+} \rightarrow \underset{\text{peroxyl radical}}{ROO^{\bullet}} + H^+ + Fe^{2+}$$

Thus, the amounts of lipid peroxide generated on addition of transition metals, such as iron, to human sperm suspensions will reflect the amount of lipid peroxide present in these cells at the moment the catalyst was added. The lipid peroxide content of these cells will, in turn, reflect differences in the amount of oxidative stress the spermatozoa have suffered during their life history. As a result, transition metals such as iron have been used to promote lipid peroxidation cascades in human spermatozoa in order to generate sufficient reaction product (e.g., malondialdehyde or 4-hydroxyalkenals) to monitor for diagnostic purposes. Such measurements of the "lipoperoxidative potential" of human spermatozoa have been shown to have clear diagnostic value [32, 33].

## Oxidative DNA Damage

DNA fragmentation can be induced enzymatically, as that occurs during apoptosis, or be initiated by free radical attack. Like lipid peroxidation, the latter can also be catalyzed by transition metals, which serve to localize these reactions at the DNA molecule, vastly increasing the efficiency of the generated OH˙ to attack DNA. As in the case of lipid peroxidation, such attacks create carbon radicals that, in the presence of oxygen, form peroxyl radicals. The initiating radical, OH˙, can attack sugars, purines, and pyrimidines, generating a wide variety of oxidatively damaged DNA metabolites. One of the most important metabolites from a diagnostic perspective is 8OHdG, formed by the ability of OH˙ to add to the C-8 carbon in the purine ring of guanine. One of the eventual consequences of free radical attack on bases such as guanine is to labilize the glycosyl bond that attaches the base to the ribose unit with the resultant generation of an abasic site. Abasic sites have a strong destabilizing effect on the DNA backbone and can subsequently result in strand breaks. Strand breaks can also occur through free-radical-mediated attacks of the DNA sugar moiety.

## Antioxidant Protection

Protection against oxidative stress includes membrane-associated antioxidants epitomized by α-tocopherol, a hydrophobic vitamin that is capable of intercepting alkoxyl and peroxyl radicals and terminating the peroxidation chain reaction. Significantly, this vitamin has been shown to significantly improve the fertility of males selected on the basis of high levels of lipid peroxidation in their spermatozoa [34]. Moreover, this vitamin has been known since the 1940s to be essential for male reproduction. Of the small molecular mass scavengers involved in the protection of human spermatozoa while they are suspended in seminal plasma, the most important are vitamin C, uric acid, tryptophan, and taurine [35, 36]. In terms of antioxidant enzymes, spermatozoa possess both the mitochondrial and cytosolic forms of superoxide dismutase (SOD) and the enzymes of the glutathione cycle, but little catalase.

SOD catalyzes the dismutation of $O_2^{-\bullet}$ to generate $H_2O_2$. Such dismutation can occur spontaneously without SOD; however, the reaction proceeds much more slowly in the absence of this enzyme. There is sufficient SOD activity in the mitochondria and cytosol of human spermatozoa to account for most, if not all, of the $H_2O_2$ produced by these cells [2]. Although SOD is usually thought of in antioxidant terms, this is only true if this enzyme is tightly coupled with additional enzymes that can metabolize the $H_2O_2$ generated as a consequence of $O_2^{-\bullet}$ dismutation. In isolation, SOD converts a short-lived, rather inert, membrane-impermeable free radical $(O_2^{-\bullet})$ into a powerful, membrane-permeable oxidant, $H_2O_2$. Although the latter is not a free radical, it is, nevertheless, a potentially pernicious molecule. If not rapidly metabolized, it has the potential to both initiate lipid peroxidation in the sperm plasma membrane and, in the presence of transition metals, trigger DNA damage to both the nuclear and mitochondrial genomes of these cells.

Some insight into the relative importance of $O_2^{-\bullet}$ and $H_2O_2$ in the initiation of peroxidative damage in human spermatozoa has come from studies employing xanthine oxidase to generate an extracellular mixture of ROS in vitro [37]. In the presence of this ROS-generating system, human spermatozoa rapidly lose their motility as a consequence of the initiation and propagation of peroxidative damage. If SOD is added to the medium to remove $O_2^{-\bullet}$, motility loss still occurs. However, if catalase is added to the incubation mixture to remove the $H_2O_2$, then lipid peroxidation is suppressed and sperm motility is fully maintained. The implication of such experiments is that $H_2O_2$ is the major cytotoxic species of ROS as far as spermatozoa are concerned. This conclusion has been confirmed by experiments in which the direct addition of this oxidant has been shown to disrupt the movement of human spermatozoa, their competence for oocyte fusion, and the integrity of their DNA [38, 39].

Given the damaging nature of $H_2O_2$, it is obviously important that this oxidant is rapidly removed from spermatozoa before it can initiate lipid peroxidation or DNA damage. The enzymes of the glutathione cycle (glutathione peroxidase and reductase) are responsible for peroxide metabolism in these cells. Under normal circumstances, sufficient nicotinamide adenine dinucleotide phosphate (NADPH) is generated by the oxidation of glucose through the hexose monophosphate shunt to fuel glutathione reductase and maintain an adequate pool of reduced glutathione (GSH) to counteract the $H_2O_2$ and lipid peroxides generated as a consequence of sperm metabolism [40]. It should also be noted that the detoxification of lipid peroxides by glutathione peroxidase requires the concerted action of an additional enzyme in the form of phospholipase A2. This enzyme is required to cleave the lipid peroxide away from the parent phospholipid so that it becomes available for the detoxifying action of glutathione peroxidase.

In addition to these intracellular antioxidants, spermatozoa are also protected by highly specialized extracellular antioxidant enzymes secreted by the male reproductive tract. These enzymes include glutathione peroxidase 5 (GPX5) as well as the extremely large amounts of extracellular SOD present in epididymal and seminal plasma [41, 42]. Indeed, seminal plasma contains more SOD than any other fluid in biology.

# Measurement of Oxidative Stress in Spermatozoa

## Assessment of Reactive Oxygen Species Generation

### Confounding Effect of Leukocyte Contamination

If oxidative stress is such a major factor in the etiology of human infertility, the measurement of free radical generation by human spermatozoa should feature in the routine diagnostic workup of male infertility patients. Unfortunately, this is much more difficult than it sounds. One of the major reasons for this is that most human sperm populations are contaminated by leukocytes, particularly neutrophils and macrophages. These phagocytes are much more powerful generators of ROS than spermatozoa, so only a small level of white cell contamination can overwhelm the signal generated by the spermatozoa and obfuscate the analysis. Although seminal leukocytes are clearly capable of generating ROS [43], the presence of these cells in subclinical concentrations ($<1 \times 10^6$/mL) does not appear to have any impact on sperm quality [44]. The reason for this is that under normal circumstances a majority of seminal phagocytes originate from the secondary sexual glands and only enter the seminal fluid and make contact with the spermatozoa at the moment of ejaculation. At this juncture, spermatozoa are protected from leukocyte-derived ROS by the powerful antioxidants present in seminal plasma. Once the seminal plasma has been removed, however, as occurs when spermatozoa are being prepared for assisted conception therapy, then the free radicals generated by the leukocyte population have unfettered access to the spermatozoa and are capable of inducing significant damage to these cells [45]. Thus, the use of a formyl peptide provocation test to examine the presence of leukocytes in sperm preparations used for assisted conception purposes has confirmed not only that such cells are present in these suspensions but also that their presence significantly disrupts fertilization [46]. Experimentally, the addition of activated leukocytes to human sperm suspensions has been found to suppress sperm function [47], while the physical removal of these cellular contaminants using magnetic beads or ferrofluids coated with a monoclonal antibody against the common leukocyte antigen significantly increases fertilization rates [48]. In addition, it has also been shown that the disruptive effect of leukocytes in vitro can be reversed by the addition of antioxidants to the medium including GSH, N-acetylcysteine, hypotaurine, and catalase [47].

There are important implications in these findings for the methods used to prepare spermatozoa for ART. In order to avoid a leukocyte-mediated free radical attack on spermatozoa, it is essential that the spermatozoa are separated from these cells while still protected by the antioxidants present in seminal plasma. Thus, separation of spermatozoa by discontinuous gradient centrifugation or swim-up from semen, are superior to swim-up from a washed pellet, where the spermatozoa would have no protection against attack by free-radical-generating leukocytes [45]. Importantly, preparation of human spermatozoa in the absence of seminal plasma has been found to significantly increase the levels of DNA damage sustained by the spermatozoa as well as their potential for fertilization [49]. Given the importance of sperm DNA damage to the ultimate health and well-being of the embryo, every precaution should be taken during assisted conception therapy to prevent such iatrogenically generated DNA damage from occurring.

## Chemiluminescence

One of the earliest techniques used to detect ROS generation by human sperm suspensions was chemiluminescence [3]. This technique involves the use of probes such as lucigenin or luminol, which ostensibly generate light in the presence of ROS. Luminol is often used in conjunction with horseradish peroxidase, in order to sensitize the assay for $H_2O_2$ [50], although lucigenin appears to be the more capable of identifying populations of defective spermatozoa [51]. Such assays are simple, convenient, sensitive, and cheap; however, there are major problems associated with their clinical application. To begin with, the precise redox activity measured by these probes is open to question. In the case of lucigenin, for example, we have demonstrated that the chemiluminescent signals generated in the presence of this probe do not reflect the generation of ROS. Rather, this probe detects the presence of oxidoreductases including cytochrome b5 reductase [52] and cytochrome P450 reductase [53] that are capable of effecting the one-electron reduction of lucigenin to generate the corresponding lucigenin radical ($LucH^{\bullet}+$). The latter will readily give up its electron to ground-state oxygen to generate $O_2^{-\bullet}$ and regenerate the parent lucigenin molecule ($Luc^{2+}$). $O_2^{-\bullet}$ will then react with another lucigenin radical ($LucH^{\bullet}+$) to create dioxetane that, in turn, decomposes with the generation of light (chemiluminescence). Similar issues apply to luminol when used in isolation as a probe for ROS. Thus, luminol chemiluminescence can also be activated by any one of a number of factors capable of inducing univalent oxidation of the probe, including ferricyanide, persulfate, hypochlorite, $ONOO^-$, and xanthine oxidase, as well as $H_2O_2$. It is therefore impossible to determine whether the intense chemiluminescence signals generated by populations of defective human spermatozoa represent the excessive generation of ROS or redox cycling of the probes [54].

A second problem with chemiluminescence is that it is impossible to accurately calibrate the output from conventional luminometers because the readout from the photomultipliers used in these machines is in relative units. Thus, the results generated by individual luminometers will differ in terms of sensitivity and number of counts recorded in accordance with the properties of the individual photomultiplier used in their construction. While brave attempts have been made to provide diagnostic thresholds for chemiluminescent assays, the numbers described in such publications are only relevant for the luminometer used in their calculation and do not have wider application.

Finally, because luminescence gives an integrated picture of redox activity in the entire sperm suspension, the results will be profoundly influenced by the presence of any leukocytes that are present in the same sperm suspension. Any

**Fig. 3.1** Superoxide anion generation by human spermatozoa. This sperm suspension was stained with dihydroethidium (DHE) and, as a vitality stain, Sytox green. In the presence of superoxide anion, DHE generates DNA-sensitive fluorochromes (ethidium and 2-hydroxyethidium) that stain the sperm nuclei red. The cells in this micrograph that have *red* nuclei, and no trace of *green* staining, are therefore, viable and generating superoxide anion. *Green* cells are nonviable. Magnification ×1,000

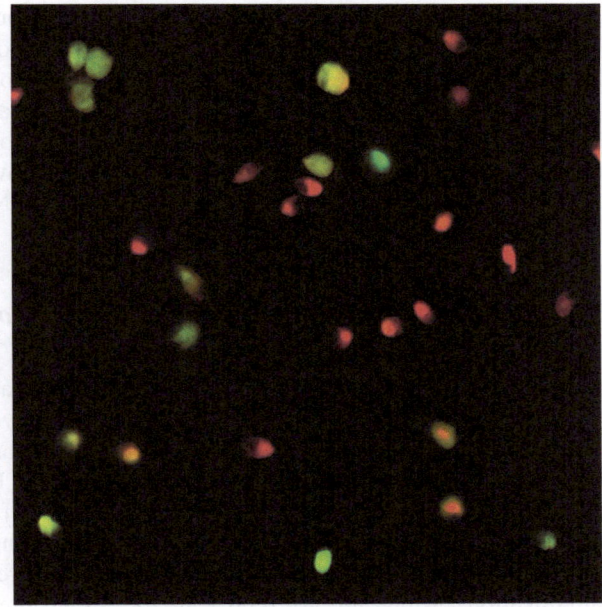

chemiluminescent studies of ROS production that have not rigorously removed all contaminating leukocytes beforehand cannot generate meaningful data on ROS generation by the spermatozoa. If it is the latter we are interested in, then techniques need to be used that focus on these cells to the exclusion of all others. In this context, flow cytometry is the technique of choice.

## DHE and Mitosox Red

Flow cytometers can be set up in such a way that only spermatozoa are analyzed by virtue of their unique size and light scattering characteristics. In this context, we have recently described and validated an improved assay for the generation of ROS by spermatozoa [55], which utilizes the fluorogenic probe, dihydroethidium (DHE). In the presence of ROS, DHE generates DNA-sensitive fluorochromes that stain the nuclei of free-radical-generating cells red (Fig. 3.1). Molecular analysis of the fluorescent products of DHE oxidation in the presence of spermatozoa revealed the generation of ethidium (the 2 electron oxidation product of DHE) and 2-hydroxyethidium. The latter is significant because it is a unique reaction product created by the interaction between DHE and $O_2^{-\bullet}$. Its presence is a conclusive proof that spermatozoa can generate ROS and, specifically, the $O_2^{-\bullet}$ [55].

A further refinement of the DHE method is to use a charged variant of this molecule, MitoSox red, to monitor free radical generation by the sperm mitochondria. We had originally thought that because $O_2^{-\bullet}$ production by human spermatozoa was insensitive to rotenone and the inhibition of mitochondrial membrane potential (MMP), the source must be nonmitochondrial [55]. However, subsequent studies demonstrated that the source is indeed largely mitochondrial but is unexpectedly impervious to changes in MMP and is actually stimulated by rotenone [56]. Our current hypothesis is that the mitochondria *are* the major source of free radicals in human spermatozoa and that mitochondrial ROS are involved in both the etiology of defective sperm function [56] and the induction of DNA damage [29].

## Measurement of DNA Damage in Spermatozoa

Analysis of sperm DNA damage in a majority of laboratories focuses on the measurement of DNA strand breaks. For this purpose, a wide variety of assays have been developed including sperm chromatin dispersion assays [57], sperm chromatin structure assays (SCSA) [58], comet [15, 59] and TUNEL (terminal deoxynucleotidyl transferase dUTP nick-end labeling) assays [13, 60]. The SCSA assay measures the existence of single-stranded DNA following denaturation of the chromatin under pH stress (around pH 1.2). Importantly, preexisting, acid-labile DNA modifications, which are not represented as strand breaks in the original sperm sample, will contribute to the DNA fragmentation index readout with this method. The comet assay exists in two forms, the neutral and the alkaline. The alkaline version, like the SCSA assay, yields information on strand breaks but also encompasses the presence of DNA adducts or abasic sites that transform into strand breaks at high pH and contribute to the overall DNA fragmentation readout. The TUNEL assay measures the existence of preexisting 3′-OH ends but cannot discriminate whether these are double- or single-strand breaks or provide information on the origins of the DNA damage. This assay is performed by adding to the spermatozoa a terminal nucleotidyl transferase and a fluorescently labeled UTP substrate. The transferase attaches the fluorescently tagged UTP to any accessible 3′-OH phosphate group and the resulting fluorescent signal intensity is monitored by microscopy or flow cytometry. The conventional version of this assay underestimates DNA damage because the terminal transferase cannot adequately penetrate the condensed chromatin in the sperm nucleus. However, a modified version of this assay, involving relaxation of the chromatin with a reducing agent (dithiothreitol) prior to performing the TUNEL assay, is able to detect DNA damage induced by clastogens such as $H_2O_2$ [60]. Furthermore, this version of the assay is readily able to distinguish between semen samples produced by donors or ART patients, detecting significantly higher levels of DNA damage in the latter [61]. The DNA fragmentation detected with this assay is also highly correlated with levels oxidative DNA damage in the form of 8OHdG expression [61]. Oxidative DNA adducts of this type are not only potentially mutagenic but also destabilize the nucleic acid structure, resulting in fragmentation of the DNA and leaving it more vulnerable to further attack. This type of DNA damage has been identified as being central to the initiation of cancer in other cell types [62].

## *Criteria for Diagnosing Oxidative DNA Damage in the Germ Line*

Given that oxidative stress appears to be a major cause of DNA damage in human spermatozoa, it is now important that we development robust criteria for assessing the incidence of this damage in the spermatozoa of male infertility patients, including the establishment of thresholds of normality for diagnostic purposes. This is more problematical than it seems because the distribution of DNA damage among human sperm donors is not bimodal, i.e., there is no easily identifiable subpopulation of males suffering from oxidative damage to their sperm DNA. In every ejaculate some spermatozoa are 8OHdG positive and in the population at large these data are normally distributed (Fig. 3.2). This raises the obvious question as to how much DNA damage is too much, and therefore, requiring some form of therapeutic intervention. In order to address this question, we have

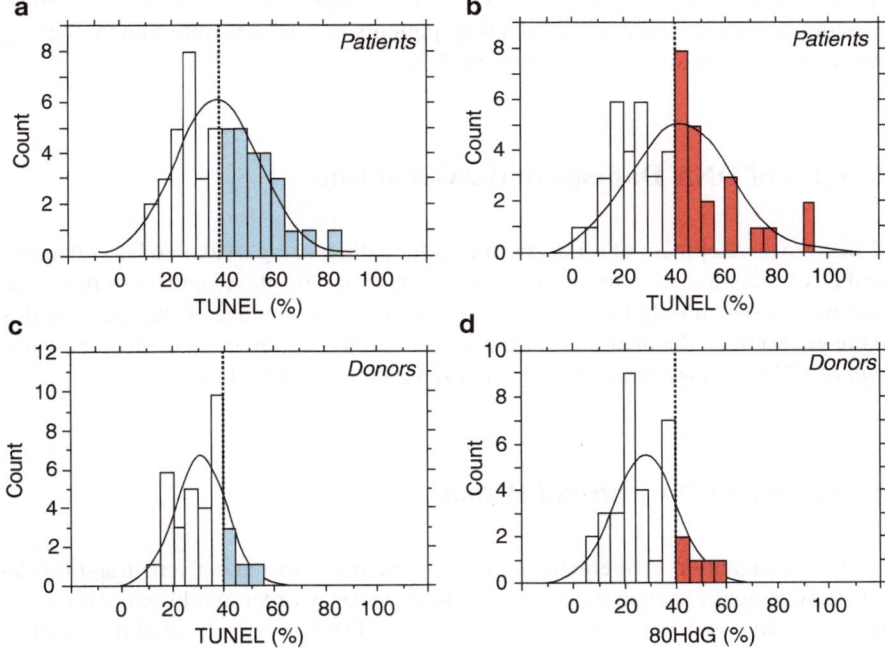

**Fig. 3.2** Frequency distribution data for 8-hydroxy, 2′-deoxyguanosine (8OHdG) expression and TUNEL positivity in the spermatozoa of assisted conception patients and semen donors. Panels (**a**, **b**), present the TUNEL data, while panels (**c**, **d**), focus on the 8OHdG results. *Dotted line* represents the diagnostic threshold of around 40% positivity for the optimal discrimination of patient and donors samples, as determined by Youden's J statistic following Receiver Operating Characteristic curve analysis. *Colored bars* represent those samples that would have been identified as abnormal. *Solid line* represents normal distribution. For both TUNEL and 8OHdG frequency distributions, the difference between patients and donors was highly significant ($P < 0.001$)

compared the frequency distribution of 8OHdG positivity in human spermatozoa recovered from normal donors and a random cross section of patients attending an assisted conception clinic. The assumption unpinning this analysis was that although the frequency distribution 8OHdG data in each of these populations would be normally distributed and overlapping (since fertile men would be present in both groups of subjects), the patient samples would be shifted to the right because this population would be enriched with samples exhibiting excessively high levels of oxidative DNA damage and DNA fragmentation. Using Receiver Operating Curve analyses, the frequency distribution of data for both the TUNEL and 8OHdG assays was indeed found to be extended to the right in the patient population, as anticipated (Fig. 3.2). Applying Youden's J statistic, we were able to determine those threshold values for the TUNEL and 8OHdG assays that optimally separated the patient and donor populations. The results of this analysis were consistent in recommending a diagnostic threshold of around 40% positive cells for both the TUNEL and 8OHdG assays in sperm suspensions prepared by repeated centrifugation in medium BWW. Using this threshold, populations of spermatozoa suffering from oxidative DNA damage could be readily identified, proving a rational means of selecting patients for whom antioxidant therapy would be rational and appropriate (Fig. 3.2).

## Origins of DNA Damage in the Germ Line

While the development of robust protocols for a diagnosing oxidative DNA damage and DNA fragmentation in spermatozoa is important, the development of preventative measures can only be achieved through an understanding of the cause of this damage. Some of the major theories that have been constructed to explain the etiology of DNA damage in human spermatozoa are presented below.

### *Physiological DNA Strand Breaks*

DNA fragmentation in spermatozoa may be the result of unresolved strand breaks created during the normal process of spermiogenesis in order to relieve the torsional stresses involved in packaging a large amount of DNA into the head of the smallest cell in the body. Normally, these "physiological" strand breaks are corrected by a complex process involving H2Ax phosphorylation and the subsequent activation of nuclear poly (ADP-ribose) polymerase and topoisomerase [63]. However, if spermiogenesis should be disrupted for some reason, then the restoration of these cleavage sites might be impaired, and the spermatozoa, lacking any capacity for DNA repair in their own right, would be released from the germinal epithelium still carrying their unresolved strand breaks.

## Antioxidant Depletion

A second possible cause of DNA damage is the creation of oxidative stress due to the poor availability of antioxidant protection. The spermatozoon is very vulnerable to a lack of antioxidants because, while it might possess some SOD and glutathione peroxidase activities, these enzymes are in short supply given the limited volume and restricted distribution of cytoplasm in these highly specialized cells. As a result, spermatozoa are very dependent on extracellular antioxidant protection, particularly while they are being matured and stored in the epididymis. Any disruption in the availability of these extrinsic antioxidants leads to a state of oxidative stress within the male reproductive tract and oxidative DNA damage to the spermatozoa. This chain of cause and effect has recently been demonstrated in the GPx5 knockout mouse. GPx5 is one of the major antioxidant enzymes present in the mammalian epididymis. Its functional deletion results in an age-related phenotype associated with a significant increase in the incidences of miscarriage and birth defects in the offspring as a consequence of high levels of oxidative DNA damage in the spermatozoa [64]. Clinically, systemic antioxidant depletion is observed in men who smoke heavily [65] and is correlated with high levels of oxidative DNA damage in their spermatozoa and the appearance of severe pathology in their offspring, including cancer [66]. Although there are many other examples in the literature supporting the notion that a loss of antioxidant protection leads to oxidative stress and male infertility, as in the GPx4 knockout mouse or the aging brown Norway rat [67, 68], very few clinical analyses have been performed on patients where idiopathic infertility is involved. The limited data available to date suggest that GPx4 deficiency in the spermatozoa of infertile patients could be involved in the etiology of their oxidative stress [69]. Whether oxidative DNA damage can result from such a deficiency has not yet been examined in clinical material. However, it has been shown experimentally that removal of seminal antioxidant protection through surgical ablation of the secondary sexual glands in an animal model leads to a state of oxidative stress characterized by high rates of DNA damage in the spermatozoa [70]. Some data are also available to suggest that the antioxidant status of human seminal plasma is inversely correlated with DNA damage in the spermatozoa [71]. More specifically, men with insufficient seminal ascorbic acid frequently possess high levels of sperm DNA damage [72]. Furthermore, the presence of varicocele has been linked with a loss of antioxidant protection from seminal plasma and the induction DNA damage in the spermatozoa, via mechanisms that can be reversed by varicocele ligation [73, 74].

Overall, the current literature suggests that DNA damage in the male germ line can, and occasionally is, induced as a consequence of systemic antioxidant depletion. Whether this is a major factor in the idiopathic DNA damage we encounter regularly in the patient population is still an open question. It is also debatable whether a patient's antioxidant status can be gleaned from an analysis of their seminal plasma for two major reasons. First, spermatozoa, especially those destined for fertilization, spend very little time in seminal plasma before colonizing the female reproductive tract. Second, although many authors have argued that oxidative stress in the ejaculate is generated by a decline in antioxidant protection, it is just as likely that the antioxidant status of human seminal plasma is a consequence of oxidative stress, not its cause. In other words, ROS production in the ejaculate rapidly consumes antioxidant equivalents from seminal plasma lowering the level of protection that can be afforded to the spermatozoa. In this context, the major culprits responsible for lowering the antioxidant capacity of human semen are not the spermatozoa, but infiltrating leucocytes.

## Leukocytic Infiltration

Since every human semen sample is contaminated with leukocytes and these cells are actively generating ROS, a relationship between DNA damage and leukocytic infiltration would seem rational. For reasons given above, subclinical seminal leukocyte contamination ($<1 \times 10^6$/mL) does not seem to have a profound effect on DNA damage in spermatozoa [75, 76], although some sperm samples may be more vulnerable to free radical attack than others [77]. However, when levels of leukocyte infiltration are high, as in cases of leukocytospermia, then the presence of these cellular contaminants appears to overwhelm the male tract's antioxidant defenses and induce significant levels of DNA damage in the spermatozoa [78]. This relationship could reflect a direct effect of leukocyte-derived ROS on sperm DNA integrity and/or the indirect creation of oxidative stress through the consumption of seminal antioxidants. However, we should also recognize the possibility that there may be no direct causal relationship between DNA damage and leukocytic infiltration. Rather, the leukocytes could be attracted into the seminal fluid by the presence of DNA damaged spermatozoa that are prematurely undergoing a program of regulated senescence, similar to apoptosis.

## Apoptosis

The role that apoptosis plays in the etiology of DNA damage in the germ line has been a subject of some confusion and controversy. It has been postulated that as spermatozoa enter the postmeiotic stages of differentiation, they lose the capacity to complete the process of apoptosis [79]. As a result, differentiating germ cells may enter the apoptotic pathway in response to stress within the germinal epithelium of the testes, and this process may then proceed to the point where endonucleases have been activated and the DNA has become cleaved. However, because the germ cell has lost some of the cellular machinery needed to effect cell death, it is proposed that spermiogenesis and spermiation continue normally with the result that viable spermatozoa are released from the germinal epithelium still carrying the DNA strand breaks left over from their abortive attempt at apoptosis-mediated suicide.

There can be no doubt that spermatozoa can exhibit many of the characteristics of apoptosis including activation of caspases 1, 3, 8, and 9, annexin-V binding, mitochondrial generation of ROS, and DNA fragmentation [56, 80–83]. Although many of the reagents that have been shown to induce apoptosis in somatic cells (staurosporine, lipopolysaccharide, 3-deoxy-D-manno-octulosonic acid, and genistein) are ineffective with human spermatozoa, these cells will default to the intrinsic apoptotic pathway in response to oxidative stress. Thus, exposure of human spermatozoa to $H_2O_2$ can readily trigger an apoptotic cascade characterized by the activation of caspase 3 and the appearance of annexin-V binding positivity [84]. Furthermore preexposure of human spermatozoa to antioxidants, such as melatonin or catalase, will prevent this apoptotic response to oxidative stress [85, 86]. Such an apoptotic cascade can also be precipitated by a variety of factors that induce oxidative stress in spermatozoa by triggering free radical generation, including exposure to radio-frequency electromagnetic radiation [87], unsaturated fatty acids [88] and exposure to the PI3 kinase inhibitor, wortmannin (A. Koppers and R.J. Aitken, unpublished observations).

Whether the activation of apoptosis is a cause or consequence of DNA cleavage in the germ line is a matter of debate. If it is a potential cause, then we might anticipate that apoptosis would have to be activated in the testes before chromatin remodeling and sperm morphogenesis has reached completion. In the mature gamete, it is physically unlikely that endonucleases activated in the cytosol or released from the mitochondria as a consequence of apoptosis could damage the DNA for two reasons. First, the spermatozoon is unique in that the mitochondria and surrounding cytoplasm are located in a different compartment of the cell, the midpiece, from the nucleus in the sperm head. As illustrated in Fig. 3.3, it is extremely difficult to imagine how endonucleases could move out of the midpiece and penetrate the sperm head to induce DNA cleavage. Second, the chromatin present in mature spermatozoa is so densely compacted that it would be difficult to imagine how an enzyme might penetrate into the heart of this structure and induce DNA fragmentation (Fig. 3.3). This problem would be solved if spermatozoa possessed a nuclease that was already integrated into the structure of the chromatin as described by Sotolongo et al. [89]. Such an enzyme could be activated when the spermatozoa are losing vitality in order to ensure the complete destruction of the DNA, as an aid to cell disposal.

The only other way in which apoptosis could induce DNA damage would be through an oxidative attack mediated by mitochondrial ROS generation. When apoptosis is induced in human spermatozoa, the mitochondria generate $O_2^{-\bullet}$, which then rapidly dismutates to $H_2O_2$. Such a mechanism fits comfortably with the fact that most DNA damage in human spermatozoa is oxidatively induced [29] and supports the apparent ameliorating effect of antioxidant treatment on DNA damage in the germ line [90].

## Impaired Spermiogenesis

A final piece of the DNA damage puzzle is the tight correlation that has been observed by several authors concerning the relationship between DNA damage in the male germ line and impaired chromatin remodeling during spermiogenesis, as measured with the chromomycin A3 (CMA) assay [29, 91]. The latter is a fluorescent probe

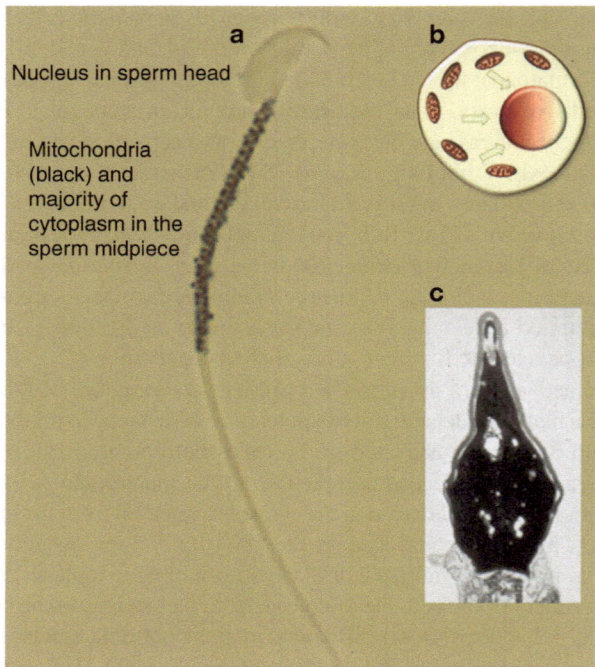

**Fig. 3.3** Apoptosis and DNA cleavage in spermatozoa. (**a**) High-power image of a mouse spermatozoon stained to reveal the location of the mitochondria (stained *black*) in the sperm midpiece,
emphasizing the separation of these organelles from the nucleus in the sperm head (magnification
×4,000). It is difficult to envisage how nucleases released from the mitochondria or activated in the
cytoplasm could make their way to the nucleus to induce DNA cleavage. (**b**) This situation con-
trasts with most somatic cells in which the nucleus is typically surrounded by cytoplasm and
mitochondria, and nuclease migration to the nucleus is a characteristic feature of apoptosis. (**c**) The
sperm chromatin is also so densely packed that nucleases would find it difficult to penetrate this
structure to induce DNA fragmentation (magnification ×12,000)

that competes with protamines for binding sites on the minor groove of DNA so that
cells with inadequately protaminated chromatin fluoresce brightly and can be readily
identified by flow cytometry. Such signals correlate extremely well with measures of
DNA damage [29]. This association between defective spermiogenesis and DNA
damage is further supported by the fact that several independent studies have recorded
correlations between DNA damage in human spermatozoa and elements of the conventional semen profile (specifically sperm count and morphology) that, in turn,
reflect the efficiency of the spermatogenic process [15, 92, 93].

That defective chromatin remodeling should be associated with DNA damage is
not surprising because the efficient protamination and compaction of DNA is known
to protect this material from oxidative attack [94]. DNA that is poorly protaminated
will possess domains that are relatively open and relaxed as a consequence of the
presence of residual histones, and are therefore vulnerable to free radical attack –
but why would such an attack occur? One possibility is that poorly differentiated

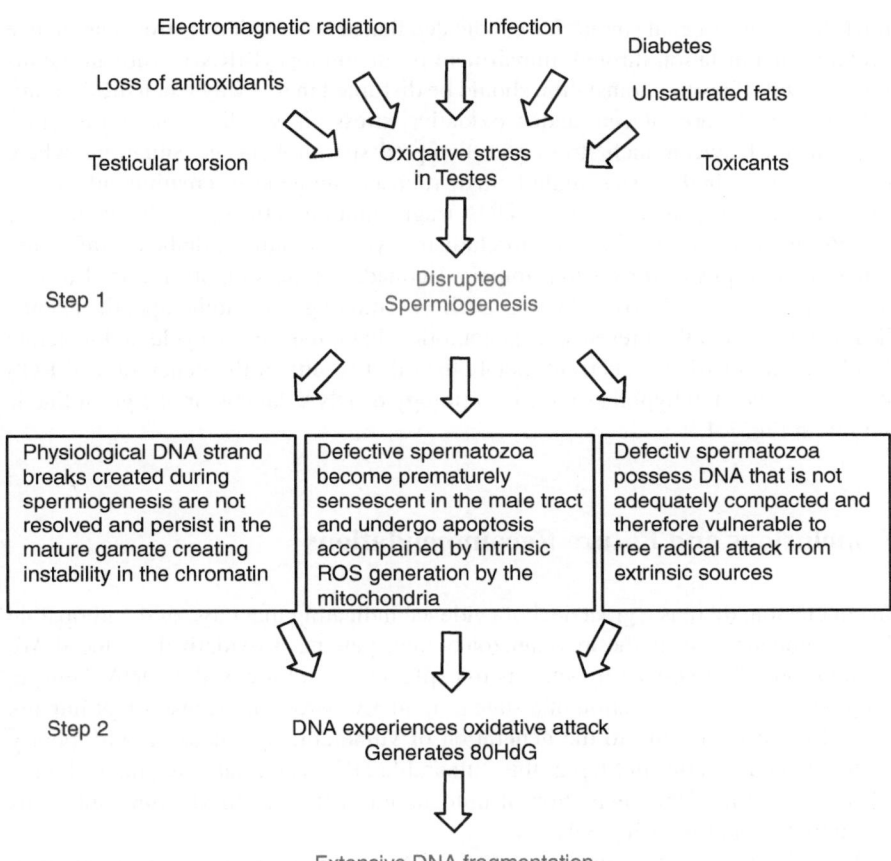

**Fig. 3.4** Hypothesis to explain the etiology of DNA fragmentation in the male germ line. The core of this concept is a two-step hypothesis: Step 1, the disruption of spermiogenesis as a consequence of oxidative stress within the testes created via a large array of lifestyle and environmental factors, as well as pathological conditions such as diabetes or testicular torsion. The result of this disrupted spermiogenic process is the production of spermatozoa with poorly remodeled chromatin that are themselves vulnerable to oxidative attack; Step 2 refers to this oxidative attack. It may involve the intrinsic generation of reactive oxygen species by the sperm mitochondria, as these defective cells default to the apoptotic pathway. Alternatively, the free radicals may come from extrinsic sources such as infiltrating leukocytes or redox-cycling xenobiotics

spermatozoa have a tendency to default to an apoptotic pathway that features the generation of mitochondrial ROS as discussed above (Fig. 3.4). A second possibility is that impaired spermatogenesis and DNA fragmentation share a common cause in the presence of oxidative stress within the testes. Spermiogenesis is highly susceptible to oxidative stress because isolated spermatids have a limited capacity for both DNA repair and glutathione replenishment [95]. It may also be significant that spermiogenesis is entirely dependent on the regulated translation of preexisting mRNA species. Recent studies have indicated that severe oxidative stress can induce protein mistranslation through impairment of an aminoacyl-tRNA synthetase editing site [96]. If protein translation should be disrupted in this way when differentiating spermatids are placed under oxidative stress, it would explain the close relationship between such stress and disrupted spermiogenesis. Situations where oxidative stress in the testes might both disrupt spermiogenesis, creating vulnerability in the gametes, and then trigger DNA fragmentation in the spermatozoa, include varicocele, testicular torsion, cryptorchidism, hyperthyroidism, diabetes, infection, inflammation, physical exertion, impaired gonadotrophic support, reduced testosterone production, lifestyle factors such as smoking, chemotherapeutic agents, heavy metals, and the presence of xenobiotics that either redox-cycle and generate ROS directly or trigger aberrant metabolism that results in the generation of ROS [97]. This two-step hypothesis for the etiology of DNA damage in the germ line is set out in Fig. 3.4.

## Conclusions and Future Recommendations

In conclusion, there is a great deal of evidence indicating that most of the idiopathic DNA damage we see in the spermatozoa of male patients is oxidatively induced. We have proposed a two-step hypothesis to explain the etiology of this DNA damage. Step 1 features the generation of a state of oxidative stress in the testes that impairs spermiogenesis, leading to the generation of vulnerable spermatozoa with poorly remodeled chromatin. In Step 2, this vulnerable DNA is oxidatively attacked, possibly as a result of the generation of mitochondrial ROS as these vulnerable cells succumb to apoptosis (Fig. 3.4).

If oxidative stress is a major cause of DNA damage in the male germ line, then antioxidants should be part of the cure. It is remarkable that despite the current awareness of the importance of oxidative stress in the etiology of male infertility, there have still been no definitive assessments of the therapeutic value of antioxidant therapy using a double-blind, placebo-controlled, crossover design. The field urgently needs such studies to be conducted.

**Acknowledgments** We gratefully acknowledge the support of the NHMRC and ARC Centre of Excellence in Biotechnology and Development.

## References

1. Jansen RP. The effect of female age on the likelihood of a live birth from one in-vitro fertilisation treatment. Med J Aust. 2003;178:258–61.
2. Hull MGR, Glazener CMA, Kelly NJ, Conway DI, Foster PA, Hunton RA, et al. Population study of causes, treatment and outcome of infertility. BMJ. 1985;291:1693–7.

3. Alvarez JG, Touchstone JC, Blasco L, Storey BT. Spontaneous lipid peroxidation and production of hydrogen peroxide and superoxide in human spermatozoa. J Androl. 1987;8: 338–48.
4. Aitken RJ, Clarkson JS. Cellular basis of defective sperm function and its association with the genesis of ROS by human spermatozoa. J Reprod Fertil. 1987;81:459–69.
5. Jones R, Mann T, Sherins RJ. Peroxidative breakdown of phospholipids in human spermatozoa: spermicidal effects of fatty acid peroxides and protective action of seminal plasma. Fertil Steril. 1979;31:531–7.
6. Aitken RJ, Harkiss D, Buckingham D. Relationship between iron-catalysed lipid peroxidation potential and human sperm function. J Reprod Fertil. 1993;98:257–65.
7. de Lamirande E, Gagnon C. Impact of reactive oxygen species on spermatozoa: a balancing between beneficial and detrimental effects. Hum Reprod. 1995;10:15–21.
8. Koppers AJ, Garg ML, Aitken RJ. Stimulation of mitochondrial reactive oxygen species production by unesterified, unsaturated fatty acids in defective human spermatozoa. Free Radic Biol Med. 2010;48:112–9.
9. Aitken RJ, Clarkson JS, Fishel S. Generation of reactive oxygen species, lipid peroxidation and human sperm function. Biol Reprod. 1989;41:183–7.
10. Tremellen K. Oxidative stress and male infertility – a clinical perspective. Hum Reprod Update. 2008;14:243–58.
11. Agarwal A, Sharma RK, Desai NR, Prabakaran S, Tavares A, Sabanegh E. Role of oxidative stress in pathogenesis of varicocele and infertility. Urology. 2009;73:461–9.
12. Aitken RJ, De Iuliis GN. On the possible origins of DNA damage in human spermatozoa. Mol Hum Reprod. 2010;16:3–13.
13. Sun JG, Jurisicova A, Casper RF. Detection of deoxyribonucleic acid fragmentation in human sperm: correlation with fertilization in vitro. Biol Reprod. 1997;56:602–7.
14. Sawyer DE, Roman SD, Aitken RJ. Relative susceptibilities of mitochondrial and nuclear DNA to damage induced by hydrogen peroxide in two mouse germ cell lines. Redox Rep. 2001;6:182–4.
15. Irvine DS, Twigg JP, Gordon EL, Fulton N, Milne PA, Aitken RJ. DNA integrity in human spermatozoa: relationships with semen quality. J Androl. 2000;21:33–44.
16. Aitken RJ, De Iuliis GN. Origins and consequences of DNA damage in male germ cells. Reprod Biomed Online. 2007;14:727–33.
17. Aitken RJ, De Iuliis GN, McLachlan RI. Biological and clinical significance of DNA damage in the male germ line. Int J Androl. 2009;32:46–56.
18. Zini A, Boman JM, Belzile E, Ciampi A. Sperm DNA damage is associated with an increased risk of pregnancy loss after IVF and ICSI: systematic review and meta-analysis. Hum Reprod. 2008;23:2663–8.
19. Zini A, Sigman M. Are tests of sperm DNA damage clinically useful? Pros and cons. J Androl. 2009;30:219–29.
20. Hansen M, Kurinczuk JJ, Bower C, Webb S. The risk of major birth defects after intracytoplasmic sperm injection and in vitro fertilization. N Engl J Med. 2002;346:725–30.
21. Shiota K, Yamada S. Intrauterine environment-genome interaction and children's development (3): assisted reproductive technologies and developmental disorders. J Toxicol Sci. 2009;34 Suppl 2:SP287–91.
22. Hansen M, Colvin L, Petterson B, Kurinczuk JJ, de Klerk N, Bower C. Admission to hospital of singleton children born following assisted reproductive technology (ART). Hum Reprod. 2008;23:297–1305.
23. Ericson A, Nygren KG, Olausson PO, Kallen B. Hospital care utilization of infants born after IVF. Hum Reprod. 2002;7:929–32.
24. Kallen B, Finnstrom O, Nygren KG, Olausson PO. In vitro fertilization in Sweden: child morbidity including cancer risk. Fertil Steril. 2005;84:605–10.
25. Klemetti R, Sevon T, Gissler M, Hemminki E. Health of children born as a result of in vitro fertilization. Pediatrics. 2006;118:1819–27.

26. Ludwig AK, Katalinic A, Thyen U, Sutcliffe AG, Diedrich K, Ludwig M. Physical health at 5.5 years of age of term-born singletons after intracytoplasmic sperm injection: results of a prospective, controlled, single-blinded study. Fertil Steril. 2009;91:115–24.

27. Wikstrand MH, Niklasson A, Strömland K, Hellström A. Abnormal vessel morphology in boys born after intracytoplasmic sperm injection. Acta Paediatr. 2008;97:1512–7.

28. Kodama H, Yamaguchi R, Fukuda J, Kasi H, Tanak T. Increased deoxyribonucleic acid damage in the spermatozoa of infertile male patients. Fertil Steril. 1997;65:519–24.

29. De Iuliis GN, Thomson LK, Mitchell LA, Finnie JM, Koppers AJ, Hedges A, et al. DNA damage in human spermatozoa is highly correlated with the efficiency of chromatin remodeling and the formation of 8-hydroxy-2′-deoxyguanosine, a marker of oxidative stress. Biol Reprod. 2009;81:517–24.

30. Kwenang A, Krous MJ, Koster JF, Van Eijk HG. Iron, ferritin and copper in seminal plasma. Hum Reprod. 1987;2:387–8.

31. Aitken RJ, Harkiss D, Buckingham DW. Analysis of lipid peroxidation mechanisms in human spermatozoa. Mol Reprod Dev. 1993;35:302–15.

32. Gomez E, Irvine DS, Aitken RJ. Evaluation of a spectrophotometric assay for the measurement of malondialdehyde and 4-hydroxyalkenals in human spermatozoa: relationships with semen quality and sperm function. Int J Androl. 1998;21:81–94.

33. Virji N, Eliasson R. LDH-C4 in human seminal plasma and testicular function. III. Relationship to other semen variables. Int J Androl. 1985;8:376–84.

34. Suleiman SA, Elamin Ali M, Zaki ZMS, El-Malik EMA, Nasr MA. Lipid peroxidation and human sperm motility: protective role of vitamin E. J Androl. 1996;7:530–7.

35. van Overveld FW, Haenen GR, Rhemrev J, Vermeiden JP, Bast A. Tyrosine as important contributor to the antioxidant capacity of seminal plasma. Chem Biol Interact. 2000;127:151–61.

36. Rhemrev JP, van Overveld FW, Haenen GR, Teerlink T, Bast A, Vermeiden JP. Quantification of the nonenzymatic fast and slow TRAP in a postaddition assay in human seminal plasma and the antioxidant contributions of various seminal compounds. J Androl. 2000;21:913–20.

37. Aitken RJ, Buckingham D, Harkiss D. Use of a xanthine oxidase free radical generating system to investigate the cytotoxic effects of reactive oxygen species on human spermatozoa. J Reprod Fertil. 1993; 97:441–50.

38. Aitken RJ, Gordon E, Harkiss D, Twigg JP, Milne P, Jennings Z, et al. Relative impact of oxidative stress on the functional competence and genomic integrity of human spermatozoa. Biol Reprod. 1998;59:1037–46.

39. Oehninger S, Blackmore P, Mahony M, Hodgen G. Effects of hydrogen peroxide on human spermatozoa. J Assist Reprod Genet. 1995;12:41–7.

40. Storey BT, Alvarez JG, Thompson KA. Human sperm glutathione reductase activity in situ reveals limitation in the glutathione antioxidant defense system due to supply of NADPH. Mol Reprod Dev. 1998;49:400–7.

41. Vernet P, Rigaudiére N, Ghyselinck N, Dufaure JP, Drevet JR. In vitro expression of a mouse tissue specific glutathione-peroxidase-like protein lacking the selenocysteine can protect stably transfected mammalian cells against oxidative damage. Biochem Cell Biol. 1996;74:125–31.

42. Mennella MRF, Jones R. Properties of spermatozoal superoxide dismutase and lack of involvement of superoxides in metal-ion-catalysed lipid-peroxidation reactions in semen. Biochem J. 1980;191:289–97.

43. Aitken RJ, West KM. Analysis of the relationship between reactive oxygen species production and leucocyte infiltration in fractions of human semen separated on Percoll gradients. Int J Androl. 1990; 13:433–51.

44. Aitken RJ, Buckingham DW, Brindle J, Gomez E, Baker HW, Irvine DS. Analysis of sperm movement in relation to the oxidative stress created by leukocytes in washed sperm preparations and seminal plasma. Hum Reprod. 1995;10:2061–71.

45. Aitken RJ, Clarkson JS. Significance of reactive oxygen species and antioxidants in defining the efficacy of sperm preparation techniques. J Androl. 1988;9:367–76.

46. Krausz C, Mills C, Rogers S, Tan SL, Aitken RJ. Stimulation of oxidant generation by human sperm suspensions using phorbol esters and formyl peptides: relationships with motility and fertilization in vitro. Fertil Steril. 1994;62:599–605.
47. Baker HW, Brindle J, Irvine DS, Aitken RJ. Protective effect of antioxidants on the impairment of sperm motility by activated polymorphonuclear leukocytes. Fertil Steril. 1996;65:411–9.
48. Aitken RJ, Buckingham DW, West K, Brindle J. On the use of paramagnetic beads and ferro-fluids to assess and eliminate the leukocytic contribution to oxygen radical generation by human sperm suspensions. Am J Reprod Immunol. 1996;35:541–51.
49. Twigg J, Irvine DS, Houston P, Fulton N, Michael L, Aitken RJ. Iatrogenic DNA damage induced in human spermatozoa during sperm preparation: protective significance of seminal plasma. Mol Hum Reprod. 1998;4:439–45.
50. Aitken RJ, Buckingham DW, West KM. Reactive oxygen species and human spermatozoa: analysis of the cellular mechanisms involved in luminol- and lucigenin-dependent chemilumi-nescence. J Cell Physiol. 1992;151:466–77.
51. Aitken RJ, Ryan AL, Curry BJ, Baker MA. Multiple forms of redox activity in populations of human spermatozoa. Mol Hum Reprod. 2003;9:645–61.
52. Baker MA, Krutskikh A, Curry BJ, Hetherington L, Aitken RJ. identification of cytochrome-b5 reductase as the enzyme responsible for NADH-dependent lucigenin chemiluminescence in human spermatozoa. Biol Reprod. 2005;73:334–42.
53. Baker MA, Krutskikh A, Curry BJ, McLaughlin EA, Aitken RJ. identification of cytochrome P450-reductase as the enzyme responsible for NADPH-dependent lucigenin and tetrazolium salt reduction in rat epididymal sperm preparations. Biol Reprod. 2004;71:307–18.
54. Aitken RJ, Baker MA, O'Bryan M. Shedding light on chemiluminescence: the application of chemiluminescence in diagnostic andrology. J Androl. 2004;25:455–65.
55. De Iuliis GN, Wingate JK, Koppers AJ, McLaughlin EA, Aitken RJ. Definitive evidence for the nonmitochondrial production of superoxide anion by human spermatozoa. J Clin Endocrinol Metab. 2006;91:1968–75.
56. Koppers AJ, De Iuliis GN, Finnie JM, McLaughlin EA, Aitken RJ. Significance of mitochon-drial reactive oxygen species in the generation of oxidative stress in spermatozoa. J Clin Endocrinol Metab. 2008; 93:3199–207.
57. Muriel L, Garrido N, Fernández JL, Remohí J, Pellicer A, de los Santos MJ, et al. Value of the sperm deoxyribonucleic acid fragmentation level, as measured by the sperm chromatin disper-sion test, in the outcome of in vitro fertilization and intracytoplasmic sperm injection. Fertil Steril. 2006;85:371–83.
58. Evenson DP, Kasperson K, Wixon RL. Analysis of sperm DNA fragmentation using flow cytometry and other techniques. Soc Reprod Fertil Suppl. 2007;65:93–113.
59. Lewis SE, Agbaje IM. Using the alkaline comet assay in prognostic tests for male infertility and assisted reproductive technology outcomes. Mutagenesis. 2008;23:163–70.
60. Mitchell LA, De Iuliis GN, Aitken RJ. The TUNEL assay consistently underestimates DNA damage in human spermatozoa and is influenced by DNA compaction and cell vitality: devel-opment of an improved methodology. Int J Androl. 2011;34(1):2–13.
61. Aitken RJ, De Iuliis GN, Finnie JM, Hedges A, McLachlan RI. Analysis of the relationships between oxidative stress, DNA damage and sperm vitality in a patient population: develop-ment of diagnostic criteria. Hum Reprod. 2010;25:2415–26.
62. Cavalieri EL, Rogan EG. A unifying mechanism in the initiation of cancer and other diseases by catechol quinones. Ann N Y Acad Sci. 2004;1028:247–57.
63. Meyer-Ficca ML, Lonchar J, Credidio C, Ihara M, Li Y, Wang ZQ, et al. Disruption of poly(ADP-ribose) homeostasis affects spermiogenesis and sperm chromatin integrity in mice. Biol Reprod. 2009;81:46–55.
64. Chabory E, Damon C, Lenoir A, Kauselmann G, Kern H, Zevnik B, et al. Epididymis seleno-independent glutathione peroxidase 5 maintains sperm DNA integrity in mice. J Clin Invest. 2009;119:2074–85.

65. Fraga CG, Motchnik PA, Wyrobek AJ, Rempel DM, Ames BN. Smoking and low antioxidant levels increase oxidative damage to DNA. Mutat Res. 1996;351:199–203.

66. Ji BT, Shu XO, Linet MS, Zheng W, Wacholder S, Gao YT, et al. Paternal cigarette smoking and the risk of childhood cancer among offspring of non-smoking mothers. J Natl Cancer Inst. 1997;89:238–44.

67. Imai H, Hakkaku N, Iwamoto R, Suzuki J, Suzuki T, Tajima Y, et al. Depletion of selenoprotein GPx4 in spermatocytes causes male infertility in mice. J Biol Chem. 2009;284:32522–32.

68. Zubkova EV, Robaire B. Effect of glutathione depletion on antioxidant enzymes in the epididymis, seminal vesicles, and liver and on spermatozoa motility in the aging brown Norway rat. Biol Reprod. 2004; 71:1002–8.

69. Imai H, Suzuki K, Ishizaka K, Ichinose S, Oshima H, Okayasu I, et al. Failure of the expression of phospholipid hydroperoxide glutathione peroxidase in the spermatozoa of human infertile males. Biol Reprod. 2001;64:674–83.

70. O WS, Chen H, Chow PH. Male genital tract antioxidant enzymes – their ability to preserve sperm DNA integrity. Mol Cell Endocrinol. 2006;250:80–3.

71. Shamsi MB, Venkatesh S, Tanwar M, Talwar P, Sharma RK, Dhawan A, et al. DNA integrity and semen quality in men with low seminal antioxidant levels. Mutat Res. 2009;665:29–36.

72. Song GJ, Norkus EP, Lewis V. Relationship between seminal ascorbic acid and sperm DNA integrity in infertile men. Int J Androl. 2006;29:569–75.

73. Abd-Elmoaty MA, Saleh R, Sharma R, Agarwal A. Increased levels of oxidants and reduced antioxidants in semen of infertile men with varicocele. Fertil Steril. 2010;94:1531–4.

74. Smith R, Kaune H, Parodi D, Madariaga M, Rios R, Morales I, et al. Increased sperm DNA damage in patients with varicocele: relationship with seminal oxidative stress. Hum Reprod. 2006;21:986–93.

75. Brackett NL, Ibrahim E, Grotas JA, Aballa TC, Lynne CM. Higher sperm DNA damage in semen from men with spinal cord injuries compared with controls. J Androl. 2008;29:93–9.

76. Moskovtsev SI, Willis J, White J, Mullen JB. Leukocytospermia: relationship to sperm deoxyribonucleic acid integrity in patients evaluated for male factor infertility. Fertil Steril. 2007;88:737–40.

77. Erenpreiss J, Hlevicka S, Zalkalns J, Erenpreisa J. Effect of leukocytospermia on sperm DNA integrity: a negative effect in abnormal semen samples. J Androl. 2002;23:717–23.

78. Fariello RM, Del Giudice PT, Spaine DM, Fraietta R, Bertolla RP, Cedenho AP. Effect of leukocytospermia and processing by discontinuous density gradient on sperm nuclear DNA fragmentation and mitochondrial activity. J Assist Reprod Genet. 2009; 26:151–7.

79. Sakkas D, Mariethoz E, St. John JC. Abnormal sperm parameters in humans are indicative of an abortive apoptotic mechanism linked to the Fas-mediated pathway. Exp Cell Res. 1999;251:350–5.

80. Gorczyca W, Traganos F, Jesionowska H, Darzynkiewicz Z. Presence of DNA strand breaks and increased sensitivity of DNA in situ to denaturation in abnormal human sperm cells: analogy to apoptosis of somatic cells. Exp Cell Res. 1993;207(1):202–5.

81. Barroso G, Morshedi M, Oehninger S. Analysis of DNA fragmentation, plasma membrane translocation of phosphatidylserine and oxidative stress in human spermatozoa. Hum Reprod. 2000;15:1338–44.

82. Paasch U, Grunewald S, Agarwal A, Glandera HJ. Activation pattern of caspases in human spermatozoa. Fertil Steril. 2004;81 Suppl 1:802–9.

83. Grunewald S, Sharma R, Paasch U, Glander HJ, Agarwal A. Impact of caspase activation in human spermatozoa. Microsc Res Tech. 2009;72:878–88.

84. Lozano GM, Bejarano I, Espino J, González D, Ortiz A, García JF, et al. Relationship between caspase activity and apoptotic markers in human sperm in response to hydrogen peroxide and progesterone. J Reprod Dev. 2009;55:615–21.

85. Libman J, Gabriel MS, Sairam MR, Zini A. Catalase can protect spermatozoa of FSH receptor knock-out mice against oxidant-induced DNA damage in vitro. Int J Androl. 2010;33: 818–22.

86. Espino J, Bejarano I, Ortiz A, Lozano GM, García JF, Pariente JA, et al. Melatonin as a potential tool against oxidative damage and apoptosis in ejaculated human spermatozoa. Fertil Steril. 2010;94:1915–7.
87. De Iuliis GN, Newey RJ, King BV, Aitken RJ. Mobile phone radiation induces reactive oxygen species production and DNA damage in human spermatozoa in vitro. PLoS One. 2009;4:e6446.
88. Aitken RJ, Wingate JK, De Iuliis GN, Koppers AJ, McLaughlin EA. Cis-unsaturated fatty acids stimulate reactive oxygen species generation and lipid peroxidation in human spermatozoa. J Clin Endocrinol Metab. 2006;91:4154–63.
89. Sotolongo B, Huang TT, Isenberger E, Ward WS. An endogenous nuclease in hamster, mouse, and human spermatozoa cleaves DNA into loop-sized fragments. J Androl. 2005;26:272–80.
90. Greco E, Romano S, Iacobelli M, Ferrero S, Baroni E, Minasi MG, et al. ICSI in cases of sperm DNA damage: beneficial effect of oral antioxidant treatment. Hum Reprod. 2005;20:2590–4.
91. Bianchi PG, Manicardi GC, Bizzaro D, Bianchi U, Sakkas D. Effect of deoxyribonucleic acid protamination on fluorochrome staining and in situ nick-translation of murine and human mature spermatozoa. Biol Reprod. 1993;49:1083–8.
92. Lolis D, Georgiou I, Syrrou M, Zikopoulos K, Konstantelli M, Messinis I. Chromomycin A3-staining as an indicator of protamine deficiency and fertilization. Int J Androl. 1996;19:23–7.
93. Iranpour FG, Nasr-Esfahani MH, Valojerdi MR, al-Taraihi TM. Chromomycin A3 staining as a useful tool for evaluation of male fertility. J Assist Reprod Genet. 2000;17:60–6.
94. Bennetts LE, Aitken RJ. A comparative study of oxidative DNA damage in mammalian spermatozoa. Mol Reprod Dev. 2005;71:77–87.
95. Den Boer PJ, Poot M, Verkerk A, Jansen R, Mackenbach P, Grootegoed JA. Glutathione-dependent defence mechanisms in isolated round spermatids from the rat. Int J Androl. 1990;13:26–38.
96. Ling J, Söll D. Severe oxidative stress induces protein mistranslation through impairment of an aminoacyl-tRNA synthetase editing site. Proc Natl Acad Sci USA. 2010;107:4028–33.
97. Aitken RJ, Roman SD. Antioxidant systems and oxidative stress in the testes. Adv Exp Med Biol. 2008;636:154–71.

# Chapter 4
# Abortive Apoptosis and Sperm Chromatin Damage

Hasan M. El-Fakahany and Denny Sakkas

The term *programmed cell death* was originally used to describe the coordinated series of events leading to cell demise during development. The term *apoptosis* refers to a morphologically distinct form of cell death that plays a major role during the normal development and homeostasis of multicellular organisms. This mode of cell death is a tightly regulated series of energy-dependent molecular and biochemical events orchestrated by a genetic program [1].

Apoptosis is either developmentally regulated (launched in response to specific stimuli, such as deprivation of survival factors, exposure to ionizing radiation and chemotherapeutic drugs, or activation by various death factors and their ligands) or induced in response to cell injury or stress. It is now widely accepted that apoptosis serves as a prominent force in sculpting body parts, in deleting unneeded structures, in maintaining tissue homeostasis, and it also serves as a defense mechanism to remove unwanted and potentially dangerous cells, such as self-reactive lymphocytes, virus-infected cells, and tumor cells. Apoptosis is also being recognized in the pathogenesis of many diverse human diseases including cancer, acquired immune deficiency syndrome, neurodegenerative disorders, atherosclerosis, and cardiomyopathy. Maintaining the homeostatic relationship between apoptosis and cell proliferation is important for tissue development and degeneration. Decreased apoptosis may lead to neoplasia, whereas increased apoptosis may lead to a dystrophic condition [1].

H.M. El-Fakahany, MD (✉)
Department of Dermatology, STD's and Andrology,
Al-Minya University, 61519, Al-Minya, Egypt
e-mail: fakahany@hotmail.com

D. Sakkas, PhD
Department of Obstetrics, Gynecology and Reproductive Sciences,
Yale University School of Medicine, New Haven, CT, USA

A. Zini, A. Agarwal (eds.), *Sperm Chromatin for the Clinician*,
© Springer Science+Business Media New York 2013

## Cellular Characteristics of Apoptosis Versus Necrosis

The process of apoptosis is associated with well-defined morphological and biochemical changes, including a reduction in cell volume, blebbing of the cell membrane, chromatin condensation and margination, and formation of apoptotic bodies. In contrast to physiological cell death or apoptosis, necrosis is a passive process that does not require energy expenditure by the cell and occurs in response to a wide variety of noxious agents. Necrosis does not occur in a developmental context, usually affects a group of contiguous cells, and is characterized by swelling of the cell and its organelles (as a result of ion pump failure) and results ultimately in membrane rupture and cell lysis [1].

A unique biochemical event in apoptosis is the activation of calcium–magnesium-dependent endonuclease activity, which specifically cleaves cellular DNA between regularly spaced nucleosomal units. Such fragments possess a characteristic DNA pattern, which is considered the hallmark of apoptosis. In necrosis, as opposed to apoptosis, the genomic DNA is degraded randomly by a host of cytosolic and lysosomal endonucleases, producing a continuous spectrum of sizes [2].

Another important distinguishing feature of apoptosis is the rapid clearance of dead cells by "professional" phagocytes (such as macrophages) before they can lyse, spill their noxious contents, and cause an inflammatory reaction. This clearance mechanism is efficient and rapid. By contrast, during the pathological or accidental cell death that results from overwhelming cellular injury, cells swell and lyse, releasing noxious contents that often trigger an inflammatory response. An additional change associated with cells during the early phases of apoptosis is the alteration of plasma membrane phosphatidylserine asymmetry. In normal cells, the phosphatidylserine is located on the cytoplasmic side or on the inner leaflet of the plasma membrane. Early in apoptosis, phosphatidylserine is translocated from the inner to the outer surface of the plasma membrane and, consequently, is exposed to the external cellular environment. Surface exposure of phosphatidylserine occurs along with chromatin condensation, and it precedes the increase in membrane permeability and constitutes one of the principal targets of phagocyte recognition [3].

A disruption in the mitochondrial transmembrane potential occurring before nuclear changes has been observed in many cells undergoing apoptosis. This permeability transition involves the opening of a large channel in the inner membrane of the mitochondrion that leads to the release of apoptosis-inducing factors (AIF) from mitochondria to the cytosol. In addition, permeability transition causes the mitochondrial generation of ROS, and rapid expression of phosphatidylserine residues in the outer plasma membrane leaflet [4].

Moreover, during apoptosis, mitochondrial inner membrane proteins, such as cytochrome c, leak out into the cytosol. At least two other cytosolic proteins, apoptotic protease activating factor 1 (Apaf-1) and Apaf-3, have been identified that collaborate with cytochrome c (also known as Apaf-2) to induce proteolytic processing and caspase activation and, in turn, kill cells by apoptosis [5–7].

# Programmed Cell Death Cascade

Broadly, the programmed cell death cascade can be divided into at least three to four phases: signal activation, control, execution, and structural alterations. Multiple signaling pathways lead from death-triggering extrinsic signals to a central control and execution stage [8].

Three major pathways are involved in the process of caspase activation and apoptosis in mammalian cells. The intrinsic pathway for apoptosis involves the release of cytochrome c into the cytosol where it binds to Apaf-1. Once activated by the cytochrome c, Apaf-1 then binds to procaspase 9, resulting in the activation of the initiator caspase 9 and the subsequent proteolytic activation of the executioner caspase 3, 6, and 7. The active executioners are then involved in the cleavage of a set of proteins as poly (ADP-ribose)polymerase (PARP) and cause morphological changes to the cell and nucleus typical of apoptosis. Members of the Bcl-2 family of proteins play a major role in governing this mitochondria-dependent apoptotic pathway, with proteins such as Bax functioning as inducers and proteins such as Bcl-2 as suppressors of cell death [5].

The extrinsic pathway for apoptosis involves ligation of a death receptor (e.g., Fas) to its ligand [e.g., Fas ligand (FasL)]. For the Fas pathway, binding of FasL to Fas activates Fas receptors, which recruit the Fas-associated death domain, which in turn binds to the initiator caspase 8 or 10 [9].

A third subcellular compartment, the endoplasmic reticulum, has also shown to be involved in apoptotic execution. Cross talk between these pathways does occur at numerous levels. In certain cells, caspase 8 through cleavage of Bid, a proapoptotic Bcl-2 family member, can induce cytochrome c release from mitochondria in Fas-mediated death signaling. All these pathways converge on caspase 3 and other executioner caspases and nucleases that drive the terminal events of programmed cell death [9].

## *Testicular Germ Cells Apoptosis in Normal Spermatogenesis*

Spermatogenesis is a dynamic process of germ cell proliferation and differentiation. Sertoli cells and germ cells, the only cell types within the seminiferous epithelium, are in close contact. Sertoli cells, lining the seminiferous epithelium, supervise spermatogenesis by providing structural and nutritional support to germ cells. The seminiferous epithelium of the testis is a rapidly proliferating tissue in which germ cells degenerate spontaneously. Up to 75% of the spermatogonia die in the process of programmed cell death before reaching maturity. The testes of normal men produce $10^8$ spermatozoa daily. This output depends on proliferative activity in the basal compartment of the seminiferous epithelium where the spermatogonial cells are found and differentiate toward the lumen where meiosis and spermatogenesis occur. During regular spermatogenesis testicular germ cells degenerate by an apoptotic process. The significance of regulating the cell population by apoptosis is more apparent when sperm production is halted. A number of factors can trigger regression of the epithelium and render the testis sterile [10].

In mammals, germ cell death is conspicuous during spermatogenesis and occurs spontaneously at various phases of germ cell development such that seminiferous epithelium yields fewer spermatozoa than might be anticipated from spermatogonial proliferations [11].

In normal newborns, apoptotic cells in the seminiferous cords were identified as being mostly spermatogonia, even though Sertoli cells were also detected. The extent of testicular cell proliferation during fetal and neonatal development determines the final adult testis size and potential for sperm output in the human with subsequent stabilization during the first years of prepuberty. Even though gonadotropins start to increase during the first month of life, it is remarkable that the peak of the activation of the gonadotropin testicular axis that takes place during the second and third month of life was not associated with a lower rate of apoptosis, or with increase in testis weight. Hormonal or growth factors present in the fetoplacental unit might influence testicular cell growth for a few weeks after birth. The newborn period is characterized by increased cell mass in the two compartments of the testis. This cell growth seems to be mainly mediated by decreased apoptosis. The main mechanism for modulation of cell number in the prepubertal testis is the regulation of apoptotic cell death relative to cell proliferation [12].

Apoptosis is the underlying mechanism of germ cell death during normal spermatogenesis in humans. Human testes exhibit spontaneous occurrence of germ cell apoptosis involving all three classes of germ cells, including spermatogonia, spermatocytes, and spermatids. The incidence of spontaneous germ cell apoptosis in humans varies with ethnic background. For example, the incidence of spermatogonial and spermatid apoptosis was higher in Chinese men than in Caucasian men. The triggering factors for spontaneous germ cell apoptosis during normal spermatogenesis are not known, and it is uncertain why there are ethnic differences in the inherent susceptibility of germ cells to programmed cell death. However, it should be noted that, in testes, as in many other tissues, the contribution of spontaneous germ cell apoptosis has been grossly underestimated due to the rapid and efficient clearance of apoptotic cells by professional phagocytes (Sertoli cells) [13].

The survival of conjoined spermatogonial cell progenies depends in part on maintaining structural and functional relationships with both neighboring Sertoli cells and with the basal lamina of the seminiferous tubular wall. Spermatocytes are less dependent on the basal lamina relationship and more dependent on Sertoli cell support. When apoptosis signaling is activated, caspases initiate a cell disassembling procedure, generating apoptotic bodies and leading to the final demise of entire spermatogonial and spermatocyte progenies [14].

During spermatogenesis, spermatogonia and round spermatids almost certainly die by apoptosis [15]. Peak germ cell loss has been observed during the stages of mitosis of type A spermatogonia, during meiotic division of spermatocytes, and during spermiogenesis [16]. Apoptotic germ cells are either sloughed into the tubule lumen or phagocytosed by Sertoli cells. Spermatozoa also demonstrate changes consistent with apoptosis. The percentage of germ cells undergoing apoptosis in

normal subjects is significantly lower than that seen in men with oligoasthenotera-
tozoospermia, Hodgkin's disease, and testicular cancer [17].

Five possible functional roles have been proposed in the literature for the presence of apoptosis during normal spermatogenesis:

1. *Maintenance of an optimal germ cell/Sertoli cell ratio.* It has been established
   that each Sertoli cell can support only a definite number of germ cells throughout
   their development into spermatozoa. Therefore, supraoptimal numbers of spermatogonia may undergo apoptosis to maintain an optimal ratio [18].
2. *Elimination of abnormal germ cells.* There may be a selective process in which
   abnormal germ cells, especially chromosomally abnormal germ cells, are eliminated from the population by apoptosis [11].
3. *The formation of the blood–testis barrier by tight junctions between Sertoli cells
   requires the elimination of excessive germ cells.* Suppression of germ cell apoptosis by means of inactivating Bax, an apoptosis-inducing gene, prevents the
   formation of these tight junctions [19].
4. *Creation of a prepubertal apoptotic wave facilitates the eventual functional
   development of mature spermatogenesis.* A massive wave of germ cell apoptosis
   normally takes place as mammalian species approach puberty. This wave serves
   as a regulator of the ratio between germinal cells in various stages and Sertoli
   cells. There is evidence that preventing this wave of apoptosis by expression of
   apoptosis-inhibitory proteins, such as Bcl-xL or Bcl-2, results in highly abnormal
   adult spermatogenesis accompanied by sterility [20].
5. *Selective removal of unneeded portions of sperm cytoplasm.* Apoptosis plays
   an important role in the spermatogenesis such as removing abnormal sperm.
   For example, spermatids display many of the histological and molecular fin-
   gerprints of apoptosis. Maturing spermatids form darkly staining basophilic
   bodies and express multiple caspases within these "residual bodies." In addition, these bodies contain proteins linked to the regulation of cell death such as
   Fas and p53. The cytoplasm of maturing spermatids is collected and removed
   by residual bodies. This is probably done by neighboring Sertoli cells, which
   recognize and phagocytose them as they are shed. All of this has led to the idea
   that developing spermatozoa use the apoptotic machinery to selectively dissi-
   pate unneeded portions of their cytoplasm. In this view, apoptotic factors are
   somehow segregated to the cytoplasm – away from the nucleus – and this segregation permits the emerging sperm to utilize the apoptotic machinery without dying [21].

## Regulators of Testicular Apoptosis

Apoptotic cell death seems to be strictly regulated by extrinsic and intrinsic factors
and can be triggered by a wide variety of stimuli. Examples of extrinsic stimuli
potentially important in testicular apoptosis are irradiation, trauma, viral infection,

toxin exposure, and the withdrawal of hormonal support. It has been widely assumed that certain hormones, growth factors, or cytokines are necessary for cell survival and cell cycle progression and that their absence leads to apoptosis of their target cells. Moreover, genetic control plays a prominent role in apoptosis through molecular regulatory factors, which act as intrinsic mediators [22].

## *Intrinsic Regulators*

### Genes Regulating Germ Cell Apoptosis

Disruption of a number of genes can result in infertility through accelerated germ cell apoptosis in mice. These findings give a first glimpse of the regulatory mechanisms involved in the regulation of germ cell apoptosis and may help in defining important genetic principles that may apply to genes important for human fertility. Male-mice deficient in Bax were infertile and displayed accumulation of premeiotic germ cells with complete loss of advanced spermatids. In addition, mice misexpressing Bcl-2 in spermatogonia displayed an accumulation of spermatogonia before puberty but during adulthood exhibited a loss of germ cells in the majority of the tubules [23].

*Fas-FasL.* The cell surface receptor Fas is a transmembrane glycoprotein that belongs to the tumor necrosis factor/nerve growth factor family. The Fas–FasL interaction triggers the death of cells expressing Fas. Expression of Fas and FasL is detected not only in Sertoli cells but also in germ cells and Leydig cells [24].

In testis, the Fas system has been implicated in maintaining immune privilege. According to this hypothesis, FasL-expressing Sertoli cells eliminate Fas-positive activated T-cells, providing general protection against rejection in the testicular environment. Moreover, if Sertoli cells are injured, they increase the expression of FasL to eliminate Fas-positive germ cells, which cannot be supported adequately. These findings strongly implicate the Sertoli cell in the paracrine control of germ cell output during spermatogenesis by a Fas-mediated pathway [25].

Although Fas may contribute to germ cell homeostasis, it is not essential. Mice with complete lack of Fas are fertile without any overt defects in germ cell apoptosis [26].

*Bcl-2 Family.* Bcl-2 is the first member identified of a growing family of genes that regulates cell death in either a positive or a negative fashion. The Bcl-2 family of proteins, which contains both proapoptotic (Bax, Bak, Bcl-xs, Bad) and anti-apoptotic (Bcl-2, Bcl-xL, Mcl, A1) proteins, constitutes a critical, intracellular checkpoint within a common cell-death pathway that determines the susceptibility of a cell to apoptosis. It is generally believed that the ratio of proapoptotic to anti-apoptotic Bcl-2 family proteins is the critical determinant of cell fate, with an excess of Bcl-2 resulting in cell survival but an excess of Bax resulting in cell death. Although these molecules compete, it has not been established firmly yet whether antiapoptotic or proapoptotic members are dominant in determining the key survival-promoting decision point. Paradoxically, a given family member may perform either function, depending on the cell systems used [8].

Bcl-2 protects cells from apoptosis by its capacity to reduce production of ROS. Other members of the Bcl-2 family, including Bax, Bak, and Bad, can block the ability of Bcl-2 to inhibit apoptosis and subsequently to promote cell death. Bax, for example, functions to increase the sensitivity of cells to apoptotic stimuli [27]. Disruption of Bax, an apoptosis-inducing gene, prevented the process of apoptosis in the testis and resulted in an accumulation of immature germ cells (mainly spermatocytes) in the tubules [19].

*p53.* p53 suppresses oncogenic transformation by promoting apoptosis. p53 is found in high concentration in the testis and plays a significant role in temperature-induced germ cell apoptosis. This cell-cycle regulator also seems to be required for radiation-induced apoptosis of spermatogonia, as evidenced by de novo induction of p53 expression in spermatogonia and degenerating giant cells in the testes following irradiation [22].

p53-induced testicular apoptosis involves the following:

1. Activation of redox-related genes also known as p53-induced genes.
2. Generation of ROS.
3. Oxidative degradation of mitochondrial components permitting the release of apoptosis-inducing factors, including AIF, cytochrome c, Apaf-1, Apaf-3, into the cytosol to activate the Caspases [28].

*Caspases.* Caspases are cystein proteases that promote apoptosis in mammals. Evidence for the role of caspases in cell death is based on findings that their inhibition can prevent apoptosis, whereas their overexpression and activation cause apoptosis. Caspases mediate apoptosis by cleaving selected intracellular proteins, including PARP, lamin and actin, and cause morphological changes to the cell and nuclei [29].

In vitro, apoptosis of human male germ cells can be prevented by caspase inhibition [30]. On the contrary, caspase activity could not be detected in human adult germ cells obtained from men with normal spermatogenesis and cultured in vitro under conditions that led to massive DNA fragmentation, suggesting the implication of an alternative, caspase-independent mechanism [31].

*c-Myc.* c-Myc is a nuclear phosphoprotein, encoded by a proto-oncogene, c-Myc. It plays a key role in the control of cell proliferation by acting as a transcription factor. Overexpression of the c-Myc gene in transgenic rats induces germ cell apoptosis at the meiotic prophase of primary spermatocytes. Depletion of sperm and seminiferous tubule atrophy, causing sterility, have been observed in the male transgenic rats [32].

*Cyclic adenosine monophosphate responsive element modulator (CREM).* The transcriptional activator, cyclic adenosine monophosphate (cAMP) responsive element modulator (CREM), which is highly expressed in postmeiotic cells, may be responsible for the activation of haploid germ-cell-specific genes involved in the structuring of the spermatozoa. CREM is responsive to the cAMP signal pathway and is required for expression of postmeiotic germ-cell-specific genes. Mice that are CREM-deficient are phenotypically normal but have a maturation arrest at the early spermatid stage associated with a marked increase in apoptosis [33].

CREM is expressed in the nuclei of round spermatids, but not in elongated spermatids. CREM may be important for spermatid development and as a stage-specific regulator of human spermatogenesis. Absence of CREM may play a causative role in testicular failure associated with various types of human male infertility [34].

*c-kit*. c-kit has been identified as a germ cell apoptosis preventing gene. Blockade or loss of the c-kit receptor results in the inability of the mature spermatozoa to undergo the acrosome reaction. Decreased expression of the c-kit receptor and its ligand, stem cell factor, may alter the balance between cell proliferation/differentiation and cell death, resulting in increased apoptosis in the testes [35].

In mice, c-kit is involved in the migration of primordial germ cells and is expressed early in spermatogenesis. It is expressed in type A, intermediate, and type B spermatogonia, and its ligand is expressed in Sertoli cells [36].

## Genetic Regulators of DNA Repair

DNA damage is one of the most potent triggers of apoptosis. DNA damage (e.g., chromosomal abnormalities, failure of DNA repair or genetic recombination, ionizing radiation, chemotherapy) leads to the elimination of damaged cells scattered within the epithelium via apoptosis [37].

PARP is a chromatin-associated enzyme with a presumptive role in DNA repair during replication and recovery from strand breaks caused by genotoxic agents. It is particularly active in the testis, where its expression varies according to the stage of germ cell differentiation. The degradation of PARP is also one of the classic indicators of apoptosis [38].

## Extrinsic Regulation (Hormonal Regulation)

Withdrawal of gonadotropins or testosterone can markedly accelerate germ cell apoptosis. In rodents, spermatogenesis and apoptosis have been shown to be hormonally dependent. As in other hormonally sensitive reproductive organs, such as the prostate, endometrium, and ovary, the withdrawal of hormonal stimulation results in the selective degeneration of specific cell types [22].

Assessing the relationship between hormonal deprivation and the induction of germ cell apoptosis in adult rats following the withdrawal of testosterone demonstrated a significant rise in testicular cells with a low DNA content in combination with a decrease in haploid cells after testosterone deprivation [39].

Glucocorticoids act at the level of the pituitary and testis to suppress testosterone secretion and as a result may generate testicular apoptosis. Also, administration of exogenous glucocorticoid resulted in testicular germ cell apoptosis in rats. Severe stress may provoke the release of endogenous glucocorticoids in men, resulting in decreased serum testosterone and possibly triggering apoptosis [40].

There is an increase in DNA fragmentation in seminiferous tubules after hypophysectomy, further supporting the concept that androgen deprivation increases programmed cell death in the seminiferous epithelium. GnRH antagonist-induced germ cell apoptosis is most prominent among meiotic spermatocytes. Administration of a

GnRH antagonist resulted in morphologic signs of germ cell degeneration in spermatocytes and spermatids [41].

Gonadotropin-dependent germ cell apoptosis seems to be age-related. A marked increase in apoptotic DNA fragmentation was seen in aging rats treated with a potent GnRH antagonist to suppress circulating levels of FSH, LH, and testosterone. Testicular apoptosis may, therefore, be enhanced in the aging male given the decline in free testosterone levels that occur with advancing age [42].

## Testicular Germ Cells Apoptosis During Testicular Dysfunction Conditions

### Aging

With aging, both potential daily sperm production and Leydig cell function decline. As for spermatogenesis, histopathological examination reveals that there is a significant decline in the number of Sertoli cells per seminiferous tubule and the number of spermatids and primary spermatocytes per Sertoli cell [43].

Germ cell loss associated with aging occurs by apoptosis, probably because of a combination of a primary testicular defect and secondary hypothalamic pituitary dysfunction. Reproductive aging in the rat is characterized by decreased Leydig cell steroidogenesis associated with seminiferous tubule dysfunction. Accelerated germ cell apoptosis involving spermatogonia, spermatocytes, and spermatids is greater in the testes of aging rats than in the testes of younger animals [44].

Downregulated apoptosis of spermatogonia was detected with aging. Diminished spermatogonial proliferation was also found concomitant with low spermatogonial apoptosis. The decline of spermatogonial apoptosis might reflect a compensatory role of apoptosis in spermatogonia for the diminished proliferation that occurred during aging. Accelerated apoptosis of primary spermatocytes was detected in the testis of elderly men. It was speculated that apoptosis of primary spermatocytes might be the most relevant cause of impaired spermatogenesis in the aged testis. Apoptotic rates of round spermatids and elongated spermatids showed no significant elevations, whereas quantitative analysis revealed a reduction in their number. Sertoli cells might already have digested many apoptotic spermatids at the time of the detection of DNA fragmentation because those cells are phagocytosed in the early phase of the apoptotic process in the rat testis [45].

### Varicocele

Several varicocele-associated factors, including heat stress, androgen deprivation, and exposure to toxic elements, may induce pathways, which result in apoptosis [46].

*Apoptosis in the ejaculate of men with varicocele.* Varicocele induces apoptosis, which is initiated in the testicular tissue and is then expressed in the semen. Up to 10%

of sperm cells in the ejaculate of men with a varicocele were apoptotic, as compared with 0.1% in fertile controls [47]. Saleh et al. [48] showed that infertile men with varicoceles had significantly greater DNA damage in spermatozoa than had normal men. Bertolla et al. [49] also evaluated DNA fragmentation in adolescents with clinically diagnosed varicoceles, and determined that these boys had a higher percentage of cells with DNA fragmentation than did adolescents with no varicocele.

The expression of Fas protein was upregulated in semen samples obtained from patients with varicocele when compared to a control group, whereas little or no changes in FasL expression were detected in both groups. The relationship between varicoceles and apoptosis was explored by monitoring the concentrations of the soluble form of Fas (s-Fas) in seminal plasma, to characterize the Fas signaling system with regard to hypospermatogenesis as a result of varicocele. By screening the seminal plasma of oligospermic men with varicoceles, oligospermic men with no varicocele, and normal controls, for the levels of s-Fas and the s-Fas ligand, s-Fas ligand was not detected in any of the cases, whereas s-Fas levels were specifically lower only in cases of varicocele. These reduced s-Fas levels were reversed by varicocelectomy. However, although higher temperatures may inhibit s-Fas production in patients with varicocele, the reason for this decrease in s-Fas levels remains unknown [50].

By contrast, Chen et al. [51] identified no relationship between semen quality and apoptosis. Although the varicocele patients had a significantly higher apoptotic index (AI) than fertile controls, semen quality and sperm motion characteristics were not significantly different between the groups.

Seminal ROS may result in sperm DNA damage in patients with varicoceles. At the molecular level, ROS affect DNA directly and alter the levels of intracellular $Ca^{+2}$, which is known to be one of the most effective means of inducing apoptosis. Morphological alterations in testicular tissues have been reported as "stress patterns" in patients with varicoceles. This stress pattern is reminiscent of, although not identical to, the cytomorphological changes in apoptosis [46].

High levels of seminal ROS and reduced total antioxidant capacity were detected in both fertile and infertile men with a clinical diagnosis of varicocele. Therefore, it was hypothesized that spermatozoal dysfunction in association with varicoceles may be related, at least in part, to elevated levels of sperm DNA damage induced by the high levels of ROS, which are common in such patients [52].

Infertile men with varicoceles had significant increase in spermatozoal DNA damage, which appeared to be associated with high ROS levels in the semen. This finding of high seminal ROS levels in patients with varicoceles might indicate that ROS plays a role in the pathogenesis of sperm DNA damage in such patients [48].

*Apoptosis in the testicular tissue in men with varicocele.* Simsek et al. [53] evaluated the presence of apoptosis in testicular tissue, using the TUNEL assay. Apoptosis was very rare in the testicular tissues of the control group compared to the varicocele group. The mean percentage of apoptotic cells per total germ cell was 2% in the control and 14.7% in the varicocele group.

Hurley et al. [54] also reported that there were far more apoptotic nuclei in the seminiferous tubules of men with varicocele than in normal controls. Recently, Benoff et al. [55] have reported that the percentage of apoptotic nuclei was noticeably higher in some men with varicoceles.

On the contrary, Fujisawa et al. [56] reported fewer apoptotic germ cells in testicular biopsy material obtained from subfertile men with varicoceles than in biopsies of normal men. There were also fewer apoptotic cells per Sertoli cell in the testes of men with varicocele than in those of normal men.

Although Bcl-2 was not expressed in the germ cells in infertile patients with varicocele, these cells expressed low levels of Bax, with no significant differences to the specimens from fertile men. In the testes from infertile patients with varicoceles stained for caspase 3, significantly fewer germ cells were detected than those in the testes of normal controls. It was suggested that apoptosis might be suppressed as the result of reduced expression of caspase 3 and that the mitochondrial pathway involving Bcl-2 and Bax may not be involved in apoptotic regulation in germ cells [57].

**Spermatogenesis Failure**

The causes of complete spermiogenesis failure are not completely known. These include the withdrawal of some developmentally important ligands, such as testosterone [58] or vitamin A [59], mutations of the receptors with which these ligands and their metabolites can act, such as the retinoic acid receptor A [60] or the retinoid X receptor B [61], alterations of molecules involved in signal transduction pathways, downstream of receptors, such as CREM protein [33], or mutations of components of cell DNA repair enzyme systems [62]. Such conditions are often associated with germ cell apoptosis [63].

Reduced expression of CREM was also detected in patients with predominant round spermatid maturation arrest in comparison with men with normal spermatogenesis or with mixed testicular atrophy [34], and increased apoptosis of testicular cells has been demonstrated in patients with abnormal spermatogenesis [64]. It can, thus, be postulated that the low efficacy of round spermatid sperm injection in cases of complete spermiogenesis failure is due to the activation of apoptosis-promoting mechanisms similar to those operating in the experimental models of spermiogenesis arrest [65].

Apoptosis is involved in the removal of arrested germ cells from the testis of patients with spermatogenic disorders. The degree of spermatocyte and spermatid DNA fragmentation in the group of patients with incomplete spermiogenesis failure appears higher as compared to men with normal spermatogenesis [13].

In addition to DNA fragmentation, apoptotic cells also undergo a rearrangement of plasma membrane lipids, leading to translocation of phosphatidylserine from the inner side of the plasma membrane to the outer layer, probably as a result of disintegration of plasma membrane cytoskeleton that, in healthy cells, stabilizes membrane structure by connecting plasma membrane components to the cellular interior. It was suggested that this plasma membrane modification may serve to mark apoptotic cells for subsequent recognition and removal by the phagocytotic machinery [66].

Tesarik et al. [67], using double labeling with TUNEL and Annexin-V, concluded that patients with complete spermiogenesis failure (round spermatids is the latest stage detected histolgically in the testicular biopsy in azoospermic patients) had significantly higher frequencies of primary spermatocytes and round spermatids carrying the apoptosis-specific DNA damage in comparison with patients with incomplete spermiogenesis failure (elongated spermatids is the latest stage detected histolgically in the testicular biopsy in azoospermic patients). Apoptosis-related phosphatidylserine externalization occurs rarely until the advanced stages of spermiogenesis. Since externalized phosphatidylserine is expected to be involved in the recognition of apoptotic cells by phagocytes, apoptotic spermatocytes and round spermatids may not be removed easily by phagocytosis. The high frequency of DNA damage in round spermatids from patients with complete spermiogenesis failure explains the low success rates of spermatid conception in these cases. They also recommended that the evaluation of apoptosis could help to predict success rates of spermatid conception.

Caspase activation and DNA fragmentation are frequent phenomena in germ cells from men with nonobstructive azoospermia, especially in cases of meiotic and postmeiotic maturation arrest. The incidence of Caspase activation and DNA fragmentation is somewhat lower in samples from patients with hypospermatogenesis, in which some germ cells achieve the late elongated spermatid stage [68].

## Obstructive Azoospermia

The mechanism inducing apoptosis after obstruction remains unknown. Since the obstruction of the vas deferens would also induce an increase of pressure in the seminal tract, it may cause apoptosis. Increased pressure occurring prior to testicular development might have a more adverse effect than that occurring in adulthood. The difference in apoptotic change between prepubertal and adult cases might, thus, relate to the susceptibility to pressure. However, these pressure increases also seem to be reduced by epididymal development [69].

Flickinger et al. [70] reported that obstruction of the seminal tract in immature rats caused epididymal granulomas, which might in turn have caused fairly high pressure to the seminal tract. In the case of prepubertal obstruction, when epididymis is not well developed, the increased pressure may directly affect the testes to cause increased germ cell apoptosis.

Patients with congenital absence of the vas deferens who generally have good spermatogenesis are somewhat different from acquired obstructions. They have life-long history of seminal tract obstruction; however, the increase or the fluctuation of the pressure may not occur. This could be supported by the report that the vasectomized men showed significantly greater seminiferous tubular wall thickness than the patients who had congenital absence of the vas deferens [71].

# References

1. Sinha HA, Swerdloff RS. Hormonal and genetic control of germ cell apoptosis in the testis. Rev Reprod. 1999;4(1):38–47.
2. Tilly J, Ratts V. Biological and clinical importance of ovarian cell death. Contemp Obstet Gynecol. 1996;41:49–86.
3. Kroemer G, Petit P, Zamzami N, Vayssiere J, Mignotte B. The biochemistry of programmed cell death. FASEB J. 1995;9:1277–87.
4. Kroemer G, Zamzami N, Susin SA. Mitochondrial control of apoptosis. Immunol Today. 1997;18:44–51.
5. Reed JC. Mechanisms of apoptosis. Am J Pathol. 2000;157(5):1415–30.
6. Reed JC. Double identity for proteins of the Bcl-2 family. Nature. 1997;387(6635):773–6.
7. Reed J. Cytochrome C: can't live with it – can't live without it. Cell. 1997;91:559–62.
8. Sinha-Hikim A, Swerdloff R. Hormonal and genetic control of germ cell apoptosis in the testis. Rev Reprod. 1999;4:38–47.
9. Sinha-Hikim A, Lue Y, Diaz-Romero M, Yen P, Wang C, Swerdloff R. Deciphering the pathways of germ cell apoptosis in the testis. J Steroid Biochem Mol Biol. 2003;85:175–82.
10. Milligan C, Schwartz L. Programmed cell death during animal development. Br Med Bull. 1997;52(3):570–90.
11. Sharpe R. Regulation of spermatogenesis. In: Knobil E, Neill J, editors. The physiology of reproduction. New York: Raven; 1994. p. 1363–434.
12. Berensztein E, Sciara M, Rivarola M, Belgorosky A. Apoptosis and proliferation of human testicular somatic and germ cells during prepuberty: high rate of testicular growth in newborns mediated by decreased apoptosis. J Clin Endocrinol Metab. 2002;87:5113–8.
13. Sinha-Hikim A, Wang C, Lue Y, Johnson L, Wang X, Swerdloff R. Spontaneous germ cell apoptosis in humans: evidence for ethnic differences in the susceptibility of germ cells to programmed cell death. J Clin Endocrinol Metab. 1998;83:152–6.
14. Tres L, Kierszenbaum A. Cell death patterns of the rat spermatogonial cell progeny induced by Sertoli cell geometric changes and Fas (CD95) agonist. Dev Dyn. 1999;214:361–71.
15. Henriksen K, Hakovirta H, Parvinen M. In-situ quantification of stage-specific apoptosis in the rat seminiferous epithelium: effects of short-term experimental cryptorchidism. Int J Androl. 1995;18:256–62.
16. de Rooij D, Janssen J. Regulation of the density of spermatogonia in the seminiferous epithelium of the Chinese hamster. Anat Rec. 1987;217:124–30.
17. Gandini L, Lombardo F, Paoli D, Caponecchia L, Familiari G, Verlengia C, et al. Study of apoptotic DNA fragmentation in human spermatozoa. Hum Reprod. 2000;15:830–9.
18. Orth J, Gunsalus G, Lamperti A. Evidence from Sertoli cell-depleted rats indicates that spermatid number in adults depends on numbers of Sertoli cells produced during perinatal development. Endocrinology. 1988;122:787–94.
19. Knudson C, Tung K, Tourtellotte W, Brown G, Korsmeyer S. Bax-deficient mice with lymphoid hyperplasia and male germ cell death. Science. 1995;270:96–9.
20. Rodriguez I, Ody C, Araki K, Garcia I, Vasalli P. An early and massive wave of germ cell apoptosis is required for the development of functional spermatogenesis. EMBO J. 1997;16:2262–70.
21. Blanco-Rodriguez J, Martinez-Garcia C. Apoptosis is physiologically restricted to a specialized cytoplasmic compartment in rat spermatids. Biol Reprod. 1999;61:1541–7.
22. Kim E, Barqawi A, Seo J, Meacham R. Apoptosis: its importance in spermatogenic dysfunction. Urol Clin North Am. 2002;29(4):755–65.
23. Furuchi T, Masuko K, Nishimune Y, Obinata M, Matsui Y. Inhibition of testicular germ cell apoptosis and differentiation in mice misexpressing Bcl-2 in spermatogonia. Development. 1996;122:1703–9.

24. Sugihara A, Saiki S, Tsuji M, Tsujimura T, Nakata Y, Kubota A, et al. Expression of Fas and Fas ligand in the testes and testicular germ cell tumors: an immunohistochemical study. Anticancer Res. 1997;17:3861–5.

25. Lee J, Richburg J, Shipp E, Meistrich M, Boekelheide K. The Fas system, a regulator of testicular germ cell apoptosis, is differentially upregulated in Sertoli cell versus germ cell injury of the testis. Endocrinology. 1999;140:852–8.

26. Adachi M, Suematsu S, Kondo T, Ogasawara J, Tanaka T, Yoshida N, et al. Targeted mutation in the Fas gene causes hyperplasia in peripheral lymphoid organs and liver. Nat Genet. 1995;11:294–300.

27. Kane D, Sarafian T, Anton R, Hahn H, Gralla E, Valentine J, et al. Bcl-2 inhibition of neural death: decreased generation of reactive oxygen species. Science. 1993;262:1274–7.

28. Polyak K, Xia Y, Zweier JL, Kinzler K, Vogelstein B. A model for p53-induced apoptosis. Nature. 1997;389:300–5.

29. Salvesen G, Dixit V. Caspases: intracellular signaling by proteolysis. Cell. 1997;91:443–6.

30. Pentikainen V, Erkkila K, Dunkel L. Fas regulates germ cell apoptosis in the human testis in vitro. Am J Physiol. 1999;276:310–6.

31. Tesarik J, Martinez F, Rienzi L, Iacobelli M, Ubaldi F, Mendoza C, et al. In-vitro effects of FSH and testosterone withdrawal on caspase activation and DNA fragmentation in different cell types of human seminiferous epithelium. Hum Reprod. 2002;17:1811–9.

32. Kodaira K, Takahashi R, Hirabayashi M, Suzuki T, Obinata M, Ueda M. Overexpression of c-myc induces apoptosis at the prophase of meiosis of rat primary spermatocytes. Mol Reprod Dev. 1996;45:403–10.

33. Nantel F, Monaco L, Foulkes N, Masquilier D, LeMeur M, Henriksen K, et al. Spermiogenesis deficiency and germ cell apoptosis in CREM-mutant mice. Nature. 1996;380:159–62.

34. Weinbauer G, Nieschlag E. The role of testosterone in spermatogenesis. In: Nieschlag E, Behre H, editors. Testosterone: action, deficiency, substitution. 2nd ed. New York: Springer; 1998. p. 143–68.

35. Sandlow J, Feng H, Zheng L, Sandra A. Migration and ultrastructural localization of the c-kit receptor protein in spermatogenic cells and spermatozoa of the mouse. J Urol. 1999;161:1676–80.

36. Feng H, Sandlow J, Sparks A, Sandra A, Zheng L. Decreased expression of the c-kit receptor is associated with increased apoptosis in subfertile human testes. Fertil Steril. 1999;71:85–9.

37. Blanco-Rodriguez J. A matter of death and life: the significance of germ cell death during spermatogenesis. Int J Androl. 1998;21:236–48.

38. Tramontano F, Malanga M, Farina B, Jones R, Quesada P. Heat stress reduces poly(ADPR) polymerase expression in rat testis. Mol Hum Reprod. 2000;6:575–81.

39. Henriksen K, Hakovirta H, Parvinen M. Testosterone inhibits and induces apoptosis in rat seminiferous tubules in a stage-specific manner: in situ quantification in squash preparations after administration of ethane dimethane sulfonate. Endocrinology. 1995;136:3285–91.

40. Yazawa H, Sasagawa I, Nakada T. Apoptosis of testicular germ cells induced by exogenous glucocorticoid in rats. Hum Reprod. 2000;15:1917–20.

41. Sinha-Hikim A, Wang C, Leung A, Swerdloff R. Involvement of apoptosis in the induction of germ cell degeneration in adult rats after gonadotropin-releasing hormone antagonist treatment. Endocrinology. 1995;136:2770–5.

42. Billig H, Furuta I, Rivier C, Tapanainen J, Parvinen M, Hsueh A. Apoptosis in testis germ cells: developmental changes in gonadotropin dependence and localization to selective tubule stages. Endocrinology. 1995;136:5–12.

43. Johnson L. Spermatogenesis and aging in the human. J Androl. 1986;7:331–54.

44. Wang C, Sinha-Hikim A, Lue Y, Baravarian S, Swerdloff R. Reproductive ageing in the Brown Norway rat is characterized by accelerated germ cell apoptosis and is not altered by luteinizing hormone replacement. J Androl. 1999;20:509–18.

45. Kimura M, Itoh N, Takagi S, Sasao T, Takahashi A, Masumori N, et al. Balance of apoptosis and proliferation of germ cells related to spermatogenesis in aged men. J Androl. 2003;24:185–91.

46. Ku J, Shim H, Kim S, et al. The role of apoptosis in the pathogenesis of varicocele. BJU Int. 2005;96:1092–9.
47. Baccetti B, Collodel G, Piomboni P. Apoptosis in human ejaculated sperm cells (notulae seminologicae 9). J Submicrosc Cytol Pathol. 1996;28:587–96.
48. Saleh R, Agarwal A, Sharma R, Said T, Sikka S, Thomas A. Evaluation of nuclear DNA damage in spermatozoa from infertile men with varicocele. Fertil Steril. 2003;80:1431–6.
49. Bertolla R, Cedenho A, Hassun Filho P, Lima S, Ortiz V, Srougi M. Sperm nuclear DNA fragmentation in adolescents with varicocele. Fertil Steril. 2006;85:625–8.
50. Fujisawa M, Ishikawa T. Soluble forms of Fas and Fas ligand concentrations in the seminal plasma of infertile men with varicocele. J Urol. 2003;170:2363–5.
51. Chen C, Lee S, Chen D, Chien H, Chen I, Chu Y, et al. Apoptosis and kinematics of ejaculated spermatozoa in patients with varicocele. J Androl. 2004;25:348–53.
52. Hendin B, Kolettis P, Sharma R, Thomas A, Agarwal A. Varicocele is associated with elevated spermatozoal reactive oxygen species production and diminished seminal plasma antioxidant capacity. J Urol. 1999;161:1831–4.
53. Simsek F, Turkeri L, Cevik I, Bircan K, Akdas A. Role of apoptosis in testicular tissue damage caused by varicocele. Arch Esp Urol. 1998;51:947–50.
54. Hurley I, Cooper G, Napolitano B, Gilbert B, Marmar J, Benoff S. High testicular cadmium ($Cd^{2+}$) levels in varicocele-associated infertility (VAI). Andrologia. 2000;32:190–6.
55. Benoff S, Millan C, Hurley I, Napolitano B, Marmar J. Bilateral increased apoptosis and bilateral accumulation of cadmium in infertile men with left varicocele. Hum Reprod. 2004;19: 616–27.
56. Fujisawa M, Hiramine C, Tanaka H, Okada H, Arakawa S, Kamidono S. Decrease in apoptosis of germ cells in the testes of infertile men with varicocele. World J Urol. 1999;17:296–300.
57. Tanaka H, Fujisawa M, Tanaka H, Okada H, Kamidono S. Apoptosis-related proteins in the testes of infertile men with varicocele. BJU Int. 2002;89:905–9.
58. O'Donnell L, McLachlan R, Wreford N, de Kretser D, Robertson D. Testosterone withdrawal promotes stage-specific detachment of round spermatids from the rat seminiferous epithelium. Biol Reprod. 1996;55:895–901.
59. Eskild W, Hansson V. Vitamin A functions in the reproductive organs. In: Blomhoff R, editor. Vitamin A in health and disease. New York: Marcel Dekker; 1994. p. 531–59.
60. Akmal K, Dufour J, Kim K. Retinoic acid receptor gene expression in the rat testis: potential role during the prophase of meiosis and in the transition from round to elongating spermatids. Biol Reprod. 1997;56:549–56.
61. Kastner P, Mark M, Leid M, Gansmuller A, Chin W, Grondona J, et al. Abnormal spermatogenesis in RXR mutant mice. Genes Dev. 1996;10:80–92.
62. Roest H, van Klaveren J, de Wit J, van Grup C, Kohen M, Vermey M, et al. Inactivation of the HR6B ubiquitin-conjugating DNA repair enzyme in mice causes male sterility associated with chromatin modification. Cell. 1996;86:799–810.
63. Sassone-Corsi P. Transcriptional checkpoints determining the fate of male germ cells. Cell. 1997;88(2):163–6.
64. Lin W, Lamb D, Wheeler T, Abrams J, Lipshultz L, Kim E. Apoptotic frequency is increased in spermatogenic maturation arrest and the hypospermatogenic states. J Urol. 1997;158(5): 1791–3.
65. Amer M, Soliman E, El-Sadek M, Mendoza C, Tesarik J. Is complete spermiogenesis failure a good indication for spermatid conception? Lancet. 1997;350:116–22.
66. van Engeland M, Kuijpers H, Ramaekers F, Reutelingsperger C, Schutte B. Plasma membrane alterations and cytoskeletal changes in apoptosis. Exp Cell Res. 1997;235:421–30.
67. Tesarik J, Greco E, Cohen-Bacrie P, Mendoza C. Germ cell apoptosis in men with complete and incomplete spermiogenesis failure. Mol Hum Reprod. 1998;4(8):757–62.
68. Tesarik J, Ubaldi F, Rienzi L, Martinez F, Jacobelli M, Mendoza C, et al. Caspase-dependent and independent DNA fragmentation in Sertoli and germ cells from men with primary testicular failure: relationship with histological diagnosis. Hum Reprod. 2004;19(2):254–61.

69. Inaba Y, Fujisawa M, Okada H, Arakawa S, Kamidod S. The apoptotic changes of testicular germ cells in the obstructive azoospermia models of prepubertal and adult rats. Invest Urol. 1998;160(2):540–4.
70. Flickinger C, Herr J, Baran M, Howards S. Testicular development and the formation of spermatic granulomas of the epididymis after obstruction of the vas deferens in immature rats. J Urol. 1995;154:1539–44.
71. Hirsch I, Choi H. Quantitative testicular biopsy in congenital and acquired genital obstruction. J Urol. 1990;143:311–9.

# Chapter 5
# Spermiogenesis in Sperm Genetic Integrity

**Marie-Chantal Grégoire, Frédéric Leduc, and Guylain Boissonneault**

Spermiogenesis is the haploid phase of male germ cell differentiation, spanning from postmeiotic spermatids to their release as spermatozoa into the lumen of the seminiferous tubules. This differentiation is one of the most radical programs found in the eukaryotic world associated with nuclear events never observed in somatic cells. First, the acrosome forms throughout the spermiogenesis by a process depending on the Golgi apparatus. It undergoes several changes from proacrosomal granules to fully developed acrosome, which contains several proteolytic enzymes essential for fertilization. At mid-spermiogenesis, the flagellum starts to develop arising from the centriole pair, which migrate to the nucleus membrane to implant the flagellum on the opposite side of the acrosome, providing the typical polarity of the nucleus [1]. To achieve the highly compacted elongated nucleus, the chromatin is remodeled by a set of abundant transition proteins (TPs) subsequently replaced by the protamines (PRMs). The PRMs bind DNA, neutralizing the phosphodiester backbone of the double helix [2] and allowing a tight compaction of the DNA as torroids [3]. Round spermatids massively synthesize mRNAs under the rigorous control of several cell-specific transcription factors. These mRNAs are stored to be translated at later steps when chromatin remodeling no longer supports transcription.

M.-C. Grégoire, MSc (✉) • F. Leduc, MSc • G. Boissonneault, PhD
Department of Biochemistry, University
of Sherbrooke, Sherbrooke, QC, Canada
e-mail: marie-chantal.gregoire@usherbrooke.ca

A. Zini, A. Agarwal (eds.), *Sperm Chromatin for the Clinician*,
© Springer Science+Business Media New York 2013

## Chromatin Remodeling in Spermatids

### Specific Histones and Histone Variants Present During Spermiogenesis

To achieve the tightly compacted structure of the nucleus, several differentiation steps are needed from the somatic-like histone-bound chromatin structure to the large-scale genome compaction provided by PRMs late during spermiogenesis. In different species, several histone variants are exclusively expressed in male germ cells [4]. Interestingly, incorporation of one of the many testis-specific histone variant is thought to form nucleosomes with lower stability than those containing canonical histones [5–7]. These testis-specific histones include H1 variants [8–10] (H1T, H1T2, HILS1), H2A variants [11, 12] (mouse: H2AL1, H2AL2, H2AL3; human: H2A.Bbd), H2B variants [11, 13–15] (mouse: H2BL1, H2BL2, TH2B ; human: hTSH2B, H2BFWT), and H3 variants [16, 17] (H3T). Apart from these testis-specific structural histones, other noncanonical variants shared by other tissues also exist. For instance, H2AFX plays a role in the DNA damage response [18, 19], while H3F3A and H3F3B are involved in histone replacement and chromatin regulation [20, 21]. Also, CENPA and H2AZ are also present during spermatogenesis, being involved in centromeric structure and gene activation, respectively [22]. The majority of these variants may participate in the progressive inhibition of transcription and in the correct DNA compaction, as well as morphological changes of the spermatid nuclei.

### Posttranslational Modifications and Their Contribution to the Remodeling Program

In addition to the incorporation of histone variants, posttranslational modifications (PTM) of histones, either alone or in combination, are important for the successful completion of spermiogenesis. PTM such as acetylation, ubiquitination, phosphorylation, methylation, and sumoylation may add to the remarkable plasticity of the spermatidal chromatin. It has been shown that massive H3 (unpublished data, Leduc and Boissonneault) and H4 hyperacetylation is observed at chromatin remodeling steps in spermatids, which would provide a better context for histone withdrawal by lowering their affinity for DNA and establish a more open chromatin structure [23–28]. For somatic cells, it has been shown that histone ubiquitination is also associated with destabilization of nucleosomes, in relation to active gene transcription [29]. In elongating spermatids, ubiquitinated forms of H2A and H3 were shown [30, 31] while the absence of the ubiquitin ligase RNF8 has been shown to impair the removal of histones leading to infertility [32]. While the phosphorylation of H2AFX on serine 139 (γH2AFX, previously known as γH2AX) has been observed throughout spermatogenesis [33], elongating spermatids seems to be particularly enriched in this histone variant, at steps associated with detection of DNA strand breaks [18, 19]. Moreover, Krishnamoorthy and colleagues [34] reported that phosphorylation of histone H4 at serine 1 is essential for chromatin compaction in yeast. Interestingly, they also reported that this modification is present during mouse spermiogenesis and disappears in elongating spermatids when TP2 is translated. Finally, lysine methylation, known to be involved in transcriptional regulation and the propagation of chromosome stability [35], was reported in elongating spermatids [35]. More specifically, the onset of spermatid elongation is characterized by mono-, di-, and tri-methylation of lysine 4 on histone H3 (H3K4) accompanied by an increase in the lysine-specific histone demethylase AOF2, also coincident with the chromatin remodeling process [36]. In addition, trimethylation of lysine 9 on histone H3 (H4K9me3) and lysine 20 on histone H4 (H4K20me3) were reported to occur at chromocenters following the onset of nuclear elongation in spermatids [37]. These observations suggest that the timely methylation of histone lysines plays a key role in the chromatin remodeling process. Furthermore, sumoylation pathway is also regulated and expressed in the elongating spermatids, but its contribution remains unclear [38, 39]. Hence, PTM of histones seem to be essential to orchestrate the nucleosome-to-PRM transition leading to efficient compaction of the male haploid genome.

## Nuclear Proteins Transition

While the histone variants incorporation in nucleosomes and the posttranslational histone modification are known to destabilize the nucleosome–DNA interactions, the mechanism controlling the transition from a nucleosome-based chromatin to such a densely packed nucleus is yet unknown. In most mammals, nucleosomes are first replaced by TPs and then PRMs [40]. In vitro studies showed that when the DNA–nucleosome interactions are being disrupted by either histone PTM or histone variants, both the TPs or PRMs are able to replace DNA-bound nucleosome, since they have a higher affinity for DNA [41, 42]. By contrast, in vivo studies have recently shown that histone exchange occur normally in mice lacking both TPs, suggesting that the latter proteins may be accessory to the process [43]. To efficiently pack the genome, haploid cells are expressing positively charged PRMs, which efficiently neutralize the DNA phosphate backbone, allowing to bring adjacent DNA molecules in close juxtaposition. Protamination is, however, necessary, as alteration in the PRM level such as those resulting from haploinsufficiency induced in mice may lead to infertility [44]. Normal protamination of the spermatid nucleus provides both chemical and mechanical stability to the haploid genome [45] throughout their transit to fertilization [46, 47].

# Endogenous DNA Breaks as Part of the Normal Differentiation Program of Spermatids

A topological transition occurs between a nucleosome-based supercoiled chromatin to a PRM-based tightly compacted linear structure, as the cell must remove most of the negative DNA supercoiling in the process [48, 49]. Since DNA is bound to the nuclear matrix and wrapped around nucleosomes, DNA breaks could provide the necessary swivel to relieve torsional stress [50].

## Detection and Characterization of DNA Breaks in Elongating Spermatids

As early as 1981, reports suggested that some DNA damage in the form of strand breaks was associated with the massive chromatin remodeling in elongating spermatids, since endogenous DNA polymerases activity was detected [51–56]. More recently, our group has established that DNA breaks are present in the whole population of fertile mouse and human spermatids and are, therefore, part of the normal differentiation program of these cells [26]. Both nick translation and terminal deoxy-nucleotidyl transferase-mediated dUTP nick-end labeling (TUNEL) were used to demonstrate the presence of free 3'OH groups. As both techniques can potentially label single- and double-strand breaks, earlier reports could not distinguish between these types of DNA damage. However, single-cell gel electrophoresis, also known as the comet assay, performed in either neutral or alkaline conditions suggested that transient double-stranded breaks are created in elongating spermatids [57].

## Possible Origins of DNA Breaks

As stated above, DNA breaks either single- or double-stranded would be expected to relieve the torsional stress induced by the withdrawal of histones leaving free super-coils [58]. One possibility is that the mechanical stress itself could induce the breaks as the chromatin remodeling is extensive and takes place within a few differentiation steps. Enzymatic induction of DNA strand breaks is most likely as they can be end-labeled with enzymes using 3'OH as substrate. Topoisomerases have long been con-sidered as likely candidates to support chromatin remodeling because of their ubiquitous role in chromosome dynamics during the somatic cell cycle.

## Type II Topoisomerases as Likely Candidates

Change in DNA topology can be achieved by single-stranded breaks changing the linking number in steps of one. Single-stranded breaks induced by type I topoisom-erases, would be considered a much smaller threat on the genome's integrity than a DSB generated by type II topoisomerases. However, Roca and Mezquita demonstrated more than 30 years ago that type I topoisomerase activity was largely associated with transcription, whereas type II topoisomerase activity was observed throughout spermatogenesis and particularly present at stages of spermatidal DNA compaction in chicken [59–62]. Similar conclusions were drawn from the study of rat spermatogenesis [52, 53, 63]. The presence of topoisomerases II in rat elongating spermatids was confirmed by immunoblots and its expected nuclear localization by immunofluorescence. Interestingly, it was also demonstrated that elongating spermatids had topoisomerase II of lower molecular weight (142 and 148 kDa), whereas bands of 170 and 177 kDa were observed in round spermatids, which correspond to the $\alpha$ and $\beta$ isoforms, respectively. Although this observation has not yet been confirmed in other species, it raises the possibility of an atypical topoisomerase activity in elongating spermatids (see below).

Using purified elongating spermatids nuclei, we also demonstrated that type II topoisomerase inhibitors, such as suramin and etoposide, abolished TUNEL positivity, suggesting that most DNA strand breaks originate from type II topoisomerase activity [57]. Topoisomerase II$\beta$ foci were observed in elongating spermatids, whereas topoisomerase II$\alpha$ remained undetected [18]. In mammal somatic cells, the topoisomerase $\alpha$ and $\beta$ are differentially expressed; topoisomerase II$\alpha$ is mostly found in replicating cells, whereas topoisomerase II$\beta$ predominates in quiescent cells [64, 65]. Hence, detection of topoisomerase II$\beta$ in elongating spermatids is not surprising, as spermatids are nonreplicative cells. Topoisomerase II$\beta$ was also found in spermatozoa and is considered to be part of the nuclear matrix, supporting a role in the chromatin remodeling of spermatids [66].

Alternatively, one interesting possibility is that DSB could be induced by retrotransposon nucleases that are expressed throughout spermatogenesis and also detected in the nucleus of spermatids [59–61]. The open chromatin induced by the PTM of histones may present an ideal opportunity for such nucleases and retrotransposition in general.

## DNA Breaks and DNA Packaging: The Chicken or the Egg?

Observations in infertile men and transgenic mice models demonstrated that low PRM content in sperm or altered PRM1–PRM2 ratio is associated with infertility [44, 67–71]. In addition, altered sperm chromatin correlates with high level of DNA strand breaks. Since sperm chromatin is preferentially established in elongating spermatids steps, this suggests a link between this important transition and the final genetic integrity of the mature gamete. A less compacted sperm nucleus would be more vulnerable to any chemical or physical insults, such as those resulting from reactive oxygen species [72]. Using a double knockout mouse model, Zhao and colleagues demonstrated that the absence of both TP1 and TP2 seriously compromises chromatin condensation, leading to infertility [43]. Interestingly, DNA breaks were found to persist beyond the normal chromatin remodeling steps. DNA strand breaks were observed primarily in less condensed nuclei of an atypical heterogeneous population of spermatids therefore supporting the link between condensation and DNA integrity. It is noteworthy that mice lacking only one of the TPs were fertile as one TP partially compensates for the absence of the other.

Transition proteins are known to enhance DNA ligation activity in vitro [73]. They may act as a linker and provide the proper scaffold for DNA repair processes in a histone-depleted chromatin environment. So, condensing proteins such as TPs and PRMs may serve a dual purpose by condensing the nucleus and improving DNA repair. Moreover, in vitro interaction assay has recently been used to demonstrate that PARP2, a poly(ADP-ribosyl) polymerase involved in DNA repair and apoptosis, interacts with TP2, whereas PARP1 was found to poly(ADP-ribosyl)ate HSPA2, a newly identified transition protein chaperone of the Hsp70 family. Similarly, PARP family members may also play a dual role in DNA repair and chromatin remodeling. PARPs may facilitate transition proteins incorporation in the spermatidal chromatin by poly(ADP-ribosyl)ation of histones, inducing both chromatin relaxation and modulation of TP chaperones. Although normally present at later steps, it is likely that PRMs play a similar role as the TPs in preserving genetic integrity, as they share the same overall DNA-binding properties.

# DNA Damage Response and DNA Repair Processes in Spermatids

## DNA Damage Response

In higher eukaryotes, γH2AFX is a universal biomarker of double-strand breaks and is considered one of the most reliable signatures of an active DNA damage response [74, 75]. This PTM appears less than 3 min after the occurrence of a DSB and may serve as a recognition pattern to help recruit DNA repair proteins at the break site [75, 76]. γH2AFX foci were initially reported to be detected during the chromatin remodeling steps of rat spermiogenesis [19], and we later confirmed the presence of similar foci during spermiogenesis of both mice [18] and humans (unpublished observations, Leduc and Boissonneault). Based on our recent immunofluorescence data in mouse, γH2AFX immunolabeling is found distributed throughout the nuclei of steps 10 and 11 spermatids [18]. In somatic and germinal cells, this modification spreads up to a megabase surrounding the DSB site [33, 77]. The global distribution of γH2AFX appears not surprising, since to sustain a global change in DNA topology, one would assume that DNA breaks must be distributed throughout most of the genome and that the phosphorylation of H2AFX will follow accordingly. One hypothesis is that such DSB could localize at the bases of matrix attachment regions (MARs) known to be rich in topoisomerase IIβ [78]. In sperm cells, the loops circumscribed by MARs are thought to range between 40 and 50 kb [79]. If a DNA break occurs every 40–50 kb, it is most probable that a majority of the genome would be covered by γH2AFX in elongating spermatids.

Although members of the phosphatidylinositol 3-kinase family, such as ATM, ATR, and DNA-PKcs, are known to phosphorylate H2AFX, other kinases could also spread this PTM in such a unique chromatin context. For example, SSTK (small serine/threonine protein kinase) can phosphorylate in vitro H2AFX amongst other histones [80]. Furthermore, SSTK null mutant mice display a condensation defect during spermiogenesis supporting its role in the chromatin remodeling of spermatids. More research is needed to identify the apical kinase involved.

## Do Topoisomerases Trigger DNA Damage Response?

Topoisomerase II activity should not normally trigger the activation of H2AFX because the enzyme catalytic cycle involves cleavage and ligation with an intermediate where both 5′ termini are covalently attached to the enzyme [81], therefore never really leaving a recognizable DSB. As type II topoisomerases are considered as potential inducers of DSBs in elongating spermatids, there is an interesting possibility that a faulty enzyme variant, unable to carry out the full catalytic cycle, leaves unrepaired DSBs. Such a variant would be generated by (1) alternative splicing or specific proteolytic cleavage leading to lower molecular topoisomerases, (2) PTM, (3) separation of the homodimer due to extended unwinding, or (4) incomplete catalysis because of the chromatin context. Indeed, the presence of the tyrosyl phosphodiesterase (TDP1) distributed as foci in the nuclei of elongating spermatids suggests an atypical topoisomerase activity, as TDP1 is known to remove topoisomerase adducts by efficient cleavage of the 3′-phosphotyrosyl bonds (type I topoisomerase adducts) as well as 5′-phosphotyrosyl bonds of stalled type II topoisomerases albeit to a lower extent [82–84]. We then proposed that TDP1 could remove stalled topoisomerase IIβ, leaving a DSB that can be signaled by the phosphorylation of H2AFX [18]. Recently, TTRAP (TRAF and TNF receptor-associated protein) has been identified in humans as a 5′ tyrosyl phosphodiesterase [85], which may represent a more likely candidate to remove topoisomerase IIβ adducts. The status of spermatidal topoisomerases is clearly in need of further investigations.

## DNA Repair Mechanisms in Spermatids

As spermatids are haploid cells and cannot rely on HR due to the lack of sister chromatid, DSB repair processes must involve error-prone pathways. These pathways include nonhomologous end joining either DNA-PKcs-dependent (NHEJ-D) or its backup pathway (NHEJ-B), single-strand annealing (SSA), or microhomology-mediated end joining (MMEJ) (Table 5.1). The pathways involved in the repair of endogenous DSB in spermatids are still unknown. If a typical end-joining process is identified, this may reveal a new source of genetic instability in these cells, as such processes can induce deletions and insertions. Alternatively, because of the potential for these cells to generate progeny, it is conceivable that they evolved a more reliable end-joining mechanism that would prevent subtle mutations to be

**Table 5.1** Factors associated with known DNA double-strand break repair pathways

| Double-strand break repair pathways | Proteins involved |
| --- | --- |
| Homologous recombination [86] | RPA, RAD51, RAD52, RAD54, BRCA1, BRCA2 |
| Nonhomologous end joining, DNA-PKcs-dependent pathway [86, 87] | KU70, KU80, DNA-PKcs, XRCC4, LIGIV, XFL |
| Nonhomologous end joining, backup pathway [88] | PARP1, XRCC1, LigIII |
| Single-strand annealing [89] | RPA, RAD52, ERCC1/XPF |
| Microhomology-mediated end joining | Unknown |

transmitted to the next generation. The participation of TPs and PRMs in these pathways may enhance reliability of the DNA repair mechanism to be identified.

## Nonhomologous End joining

The end-joining repair processes are repressed throughout the meiotic stages of spermatogenesis to promote HR. Such a repression is no longer present during spermiogenesis [86–88]. Although much remain to be known about the repair of endogenous DSB, round spermatids apparently rely on the NHEJ-B pathway to repair radiation-induced DSBs but with slower kinetics than in somatic cells [88, 89]. DNA-PKcs is an important kinase of the NHEJ-D pathway. The later pathways also seem to be involved in spermatidal DSB repair, as DNA-PKcs-deficient SCid mice demonstrated lower repair rates of $\gamma$H2AFX foci following irradiation.

Evidence of NHEJ-D was reported during spermiogenesis of several grasshopper species as established by the immunofluorescence detection of KU70 and $\gamma$H2AFX nuclear foci [90]. Further confirmation of this pathway will be needed, as KU proteins also play a role in telomere maintenance [91, 92]. Specialized DNA polymerases, such as polymerases of the X family, polymerase $\mu$ and polymerase $\lambda$, are also involved in the repair of DSBs by NHEJ, as they process incompatible ends, fill gaps, and remove unwanted flaps [86]. The sole detection of DNA repair factors by immunological techniques do not implicate that they are functional. However, using in situ incorporation of biotinylated dUTP, we have confirmed an endogenous DNA polymerase activity in elongating spermatids of mice, leading to the conclusion of an active repair process [18].

Polymerases of the PARP family, PARP1 and PARP2, are often referred to as guardians of genome integrity [93, 94]. PARPs are chromatin-associated proteins activated by DNA strand breaks. Upon activation, they catalyze the covalent attachment of ADP-ribose from NAD+ substrate to a number of proteins, such as histones, TP53, topoisomerases, and even themselves. This automodification releases PARPs from DNA and can be reversed by the poly(ADP-ribose) glycohydrolase (PARG). PARP1 participates in the base excision repair (BER) and also in the NHEJ backup pathways.

Considering that PARP1 and PARP2 have overlapping functions and that a double-knockout of these proteins is embryonic lethal, it is difficult to study their individual role during spermiogenesis. Inactivation of PARP2 in mice leads to hypofertility, as pachytene spermatocytes display defective meiotic sex chromosome inactivation.

Compromised differentiation of spermatids can also be observed [95]. Knockout mice for PARP1, PARG (110 kDa isoform) or both displayed abnormal sperm with varying degrees of residual DNA breaks [96]. Not as striking as one could have expected, the perturbation of the poly(ADP-ribose) metabolism clearly impacts the differentiation program of spermatids.

**DNA Repair by Homology in a Haploid Cell**

The two other end-joining pathways, SSA and MMEJ, use repetitive DNA and microhomology, respectively, as a template to repair DSB. Although very different from one another, these two systems inevitably introduce errors in the DNA sequence mostly by deletions. The SSA pathway shares several proteins with HR, and the two pathways usually compete against each other in somatic cells [97], a situation that should not prevail in spermatids. Repair of a DSB by the SSA pathway proceeds from long homologous sequences (>30 nucleotides) and the one copy of the repeat sequence and the intervening sequence serving as a template are destroyed upon completion of the repair [98]. In MMEJ, the KU-independent end joining is mediated by a 5–25 nucleotides homology resulting in deletions of sequences, and sometimes insertions, close to the break site [99]. Although MMEJ deletions are smaller than those usually created by SSA, this will, nonetheless, lead to an alteration of the genome's integrity.

## Highly Conserved Process Among Higher Eukaryotes

A rapid survey of the recent literature points to the highly conserved nature of the DNA damage response to endogenous breaks in spermatids. Evidence of DNA damage response was presented in mammalian models, such as mice and rats, but it can also be extended to human as we have shown. Rahtke and colleagues observed DNA breaks during spermiogenesis of *Drosophila* [100], whereas others demonstrated that spermatids of several grasshopper species displayed KU70 and γH2AFX foci [90]. Most interestingly, γH2AFX foci was also reported in spermatids of the algae *Chara vulgaris* [101], suggesting that a related process extends to plants. Hence, this process could very well be used throughout the eukaryotic world where gametogenesis requires condensation of the genetic material.

## Possible Consequences and Clinical Relevance

### Impairment of Genetic Integrity in the Male Gamete

The generation of a transient more "open" chromatin structure during spermiogenesis and the presence of DSBs in such a striking chromatin-remodeling context make it possible that more important genomic alterations could be observed.

Interestingly, many studies reported that more than 80% of the structural de novo chromosome aberrations are of paternal origin [102–104]. In healthy men's sperm, the spontaneous frequencies of structural chromosomal abnormalities was shown to be higher than those of numerical abnormalities, and chromosomal breaks are more prevalent than partial duplications and deletions [105].

It is well known that lifestyle factors such as smoking, alcohol, and caffeine consumption have been associated with chromosomal aberration and genomic alterations in somatic cells [106–111]. While several studies showed a deleterious effect of lifestyle factors on the male fertility, only a few studies focused on the effect of tobacco smoking and alcohol consumption on male germ cells' genetic integrity and showed unclear correlations with sperm aneuploidy and DNA fragmentation [112–115]. However, Schmid and colleagues showed that caffeine consumption is associated with increased DSBs in sperm [116]. Interestingly, caffeine might lead to inactivation of H2AFX through the inhibition of kinases related to DNA repair, such as ATM, ATR, and DNA-PKcs [117–119].

Aging was associated with increased genetic alterations and chromosomal aberrations in sperm, suggesting a less efficient DNA packaging process [116, 120–122]. Altogether, these studies suggest that some environmental and lifestyle factors may likely result in chromosomal aberrations, persistent DNA breaks, and genetic impairments in mature spermatozoa, leading to dramatic consequences on the reproductive outcome.

Given the peculiar chromatin of spermatids, one can assume that such a context may favor chromosomal translocation due to the proximity of the breaks if generated by a nuclear matrix associated type II topoisomerases and the DNA repair pathways available. Interestingly, the natural rate of chromosomal aberrations as seen in untreated controls and reported by some studies monitoring the effects of some toxicants is quite high ranging from 0.7 to 5% [123–125].

Retrotransposition is another interesting mechanism of genetic instability potentially occurring in spermiogenesis. Testicular expression of the ORF1 and ORF2 proteins encoded by LINE1 sequence has been demonstrated, particularly in the early steps of spermiogenesis [60]. Knowing that ORF2 protein has an endonuclease activity [126, 127], Gasior and colleagues showed that LINE1 ORFs expression leads to a high level of DSB formation and activation of H2AFX [61]. In addition, it was shown that LINE retrotransposition in transformed human cells can lead to a variety of genomic rearrangements [128]. Together, these findings makes it tempting to speculate that the spermatidal chromatin remodeling would offer a suitable context for retrotransposition, increasing the repertoire of possible mutations distributed throughout the millions of sperm cells.

Finally, as the human genome is composed of nearly 50% of repeated DNA, microhomology-based DNA repair pathways such the SSA and MMEJ described above may prove to play an important role in spermatids and be the cause of several genetic diseases and cancers, as mutagenic deletions often share homology at breakpoint junctions, such as Alu and LINE repeats [129, 130]. For instance, microdeletions in the highly repetitive Y chromosome seem important in the etiology of infertility [131, 132] and may bear also the signature of these alternative mutagenic DNA repair systems.

## Impact of This Transient Window of Genetic Instability on Clinical Practices

In contrast to spermatocytes, spermatids are apparently devoid of cell cycle checkpoints. Their differentiation program can be compared to an assembly line where defective products will be discarded through their lack of fitness for fertilization. Moreover, spermatids have a scheduled differentiation program most probably synchronized by Sertoli cells. Any delay in the process is likely to have consequences for the gamete's integrity. Therefore, procedures that bypass the natural selection of gametes, such as ICSI, ROSI, or IVF to a lower extent, bear the risk of selecting unfit gametes.

Although they possess a haploid genome, round spermatids are less compatible with artificial reproduction techniques (ART) as demonstrated by the low successful birth rate following ROSI in mouse (1.7–28.2%) [133, 134]. Recently, it has been shown that 77.5% of the ROSI-generated embryos exhibited abnormal chromosome segregation at the first mitosis, originating from double-strand breakage of the male-derived genomic DNA. ICSI and ROSI procedures resulted in no embryonic development when chromosome segregation was abnormal at the first mitotic division [135]. Therefore, residual DNA breaks in the male gamete may lead to abnormal chromosome segregation and genetic impairment in the developing zygote. Moreover, taking into account that the remodeling process is accompanied with DNA breaks, one can assume that selecting spermatids undergoing this transition should lead to unsuccessful reproductive outcomes. Unfortunately, when ROSI technique is performed in humans, one cannot avoid selecting spermatids undergoing chromatin remodeling, as they have the same apparent morphology that of those immediately preceding or following these crucial steps.

## Potential Recovery by the Oocyte After Fertilization

Autosomal aneuploidies are more frequently of maternal origin, whereas point mutations and chromosomal rearrangements are of paternal origin [136, 137]. Moreover, it was shown that the DNA repair capacity of spermatids declines drastically after the nuclear remodeling and continues to decline until spermiation [138]. On the contrary, the repair capacities of the oocyte are quite stable throughout oogenesis and persist after fertilization and may repair DNA damages from both parental genomes [139, 140]. Using first-cleavage metaphases, it was shown that both NHEJ and HR are used by the oocyte to rescue the genetic integrity of the paternal genome after fertilization. However, not all DNA breaks were efficiently repaired, as many residual chromosomal aberrations were found in controls. Thus, even if the oocyte can repair some paternal DNA lesions, chromosomal aberrations can persist after the first zygotic cell cycle [123]. Moreover, if the DNA repair systems of the spermatid create point mutations or chromosomic rearrangements, these will likely escape the oocyte's damage response and will be transmitted to the next generation.

# Summary

Altogether, this review suggests that spermiogenesis has probably been overlooked as an important source of genetic instability that can provide a repertoire of mutations distributed through millions of spermatozoa, each having the potential to transfer genetic alterations to the next generation. Further investigation will be needed to establish whether this could be considered as a new component of evolution.

**Acknowledgments** Funded by the Natural Sciences and Engineering Research Council of Canada (grant # 155182) to G.B.

# References

1. Loonie D. Russell APSH, Robert Ettlin. Histological and histopathological evaluation of the testis. Clearwate: Cache River Press; 1990.
2. Balhorn R. A model for the structure of chromatin in mammalian sperm. J Cell Biol. 1982; 93(2):298–305.
3. Ward W. Deoxyribonucleic acid loop domain tertiary structure in mammalian spermatozoa. Biol Reprod. 1993;48(6):1193–201.
4. Talbert PB, Henikoff S. Histone variants–ancient wrap artists of the epigenome. Nat Rev Mol Cell Biol. 2010;11(4):264–75.
5. Li A, Maffey AH, Abbott WD, Conde e Silva N, Prunell A, Siino J, et al. Characterization of nucleosomes consisting of the human testis/sperm-specific histone H2B variant (hTSH2B). Biochemistry. 2005;44(7):2529–35.
6. Syed SH, Boulard M, Shukla MS, Gautier T, Travers A, Bednar J, et al. The incorporation of the novel histone variant H2AL2 confers unusual structural and functional properties of the nucleosome. Nucleic Acids Res. 2009;37(14):4684–95.
7. González-Romero R, Méndez J, Ausió J, Eirín-López JM. Quickly evolving histones, nucleosome stability and chromatin folding: all about histone H2A.Bbd. Gene. 2008;413(1–2):1–7.
8. Seyedin SM, Kistler WS. Isolation and characterization of rat testis H1t. An H1 histone variant associated with spermatogenesis. J Biol Chem. 1980;255(12):5949–54.
9. Tanaka H, Iguchi N, Isotani A, Kitamura K, Toyama Y, Matsuoka Y, et al. HANP1/H1T2, a novel histone H1-like protein involved in nuclear formation and sperm fertility. Mol Cell Biol. 2005;25(16):7107–19.
10. Yan W, Ma L, Burns KH, Matzuk MM. HILS1 is a spermatid-specific linker histone H1-like protein implicated in chromatin remodeling during mammalian spermiogenesis. Proc Natl Acad Sci USA. 2003;100(18):10546–51.
11. Govin J, Escoffier E, Rousseaux S, Kuhn L, Ferro M, Thévenon J, et al. Pericentric heterochromatin reprogramming by new histone variants during mouse spermiogenesis. J Cell Biol. 2007;176(3):283–94.
12. Chadwick BP, Willard HF. A novel chromatin protein, distantly related to histone H2A, is largely excluded from the inactive X chromosome. J Cell Biol. 2001;152(2):375–84.
13. Shires A, Carpenter MP, Chalkley R. A cysteine-containing H2B-like histone found in mature mammalian testis. J Biol Chem. 1976;251(13):4155–8.
14. Zalensky AO, Siino JS, Gineitis AA, Zalenskaya IA, Tomilin NV, Yau P, et al. Human testis/sperm-specific histone H2B (hTSH2B). Molecular cloning and characterization. J Biol Chem. 2002;277(45):43474–80.

15. Churikov D, Siino J, Svetlova M, Zhang K, Gineitis A, Morton Bradbury E, et al. Novel human testis-specific histone H2B encoded by the interrupted gene on the X chromosome. Genomics. 2004;84(4):745–56.
16. Franklin SG, Zweidler A. Non-allelic variants of histones 2a, 2b and 3 in mammals. Nature. 1977;266(5599):273–5.
17. Witt O, Albig W, Doenecke D. Testis-specific expression of a novel human H3 histone gene. Exp Cell Res. 1996;229(2):301–6.
18. Leduc F, Maquennehan V, Nkoma GB, Boissonneault G. DNA damage response during chromatin remodeling in elongating spermatids of mice. Biol Reprod. 2008;78(2):324–32.
19. Meyer-Ficca M, Scherthan H, Burkle A, Meyer R. Poly(ADP-ribosyl)ation during chromatin remodeling steps in rat spermiogenesis. Chromosoma. 2005;114(1):67–74.
20. Bramlage B, Kosciessa U, Doenecke D. Differential expression of the murine histone genes H3.3A and H3.3B. Differentiation. 1997;62(1):13–20.
21. Elsaesser SJ, Goldberg AD, Allis CD. New functions for an old variant: no substitute for histone H3.3. Curr Opin Genet Dev. 2010;20(2):110–7.
22. Zalensky AO, Breneman JW, Zalenskaya IA, Brinkley BR, Bradbury EM. Organization of centromeres in the decondensed nuclei of mature human sperm. Chromosoma. 1993;102(8): 509–18.
23. Oliva R, Mezquita C. Histone H4 hyperacetylation and rapid turnover of its acetyl groups in transcriptionally inactive rooster testis spermatids. Nucleic Acids Res. 1982;10(24): 8049–59.
24. Christensen M, Rattner J, Dixon G. Hyperacetylation of histone H4 promotes chromatin decondensation prior to histone replacement by protamines during spermatogenesis in rainbow trout. Nucleic Acids Res. 1984;12(11):4575–92.
25. Grimes S, Henderson N. Hyperacetylation of histone H4 in rat testis spermatids. Exp Cell Res. 1984;152(1):91–7.
26. Marcon L, Boissonneault G. Transient DNA strand breaks during mouse and human spermiogenesis new insights in stage specificity and link to chromatin remodeling. Biol Reprod. 2004;70(4):910–8.
27. Meistrich M, Trostle-Weige P, Lin R, Bhatnagar Y, Allis C. Highly acetylated H4 is associated with histone displacement in rat spermatids. Mol Reprod Dev. 1992;31(3):170–81.
28. Hazzouri M, Pivot-Pajot C, Faure A, Usson Y, Pelletier R, Sele B, et al. Regulated hyperacetylation of core histones during mouse spermatogenesis: involvement of histone deacetylases. Eur J Cell Biol. 2000;79(12):950–60.
29. Li W, Nagaraja S, Delcuve GP, Hendzel MJ, Davie JR. Effects of histone acetylation, ubiquitination and variants on nucleosome stability. Biochem J. 1993;296 (Pt 3):737–44.
30. Baarends W, Hoogerbrugge J, Roest H, Ooms M, Vreeburg J, Hoeijmakers J, et al. Histone ubiquitination and chromatin remodeling in mouse spermatogenesis. Dev Biol. 1999;207(2):322–33.
31. Chen HY, Sun JM, Zhang Y, Davie JR, Meistrich ML. Ubiquitination of histone H3 in elongating spermatids of rat testes. J Biol Chem. 1998;273(21):13165–9.
32. Lu L-Y, Wu J, Ye L, Gavrilina GB, Saunders TL, Yu X. RNF8-dependent histone modifications regulate nucleosome removal during spermatogenesis. Dev cell. 2010;18(3):371–84.
33. Blanco-Rodríguez J. GammaH2AX marks the main events of the spermatogenic process. Microsc Res Tech. 2009;72(11):823–32.
34. Krishnamoorthy T, Chen X, Govin J, Cheung W, Dorsey J, Schindler K, et al. Phosphorylation of histone H4 Ser1 regulates sporulation in yeast and is conserved in fly and mouse spermatogenesis. Genes Dev. 2006;20(18):2580.
35. Sims RJ, Nishioka K, Reinberg D. Histone lysine methylation: a signature for chromatin function. Trends Genet. 2003 Nov 1;19(11):629–39.
36. Godmann, Auger, Ferraroni-Aguiar, Sauro D, Sette, Behr, et al. Dynamic regulation of histone H3 methylation at lysine 4 in mammalian spermatogenesis. Biol Reprod. 2007;77(5):754–764.
37. van der Heijden G, Derijck A, Ramos L, Giele M, van der Vlag J, de Boer P. Transmission of modified nucleosomes from the mouse male germline to the zygote and subsequent remodeling of paternal chromatin. Dev Biol. 2006;298(2):458–69.

38. Vigodner M, Morris P. Testicular expression of small ubiquitin-related modifier-1 (SUMO-1) supports multiple roles in spermatogenesis: silencing of sex chromosomes in spermatocytes, spermatid microtubule nucleation, and nuclear reshaping. Dev Biol. 2005;282(2):480–92.
39. La Salle S, Sun F, Zhang X-D, Matunis MJ, Handel MA. Developmental control of sumoylation pathway proteins in mouse male germ cells. Dev Biol. 2008;321(1):227–37.
40. Balhorn R, Weston S, Thomas C, Wyrobek A. DNA packaging in mouse spermatids. Synthesis of protamine variants and four transition proteins. Exp Cell Res. 1984;150(2):298–308.
41. Marushige K, Marushige Y, Wong TK. Complete displacement of somatic histones during transformation of spermatid chromatin: a model experiment. Biochemistry. 1976;15(10): 2047–53.
42. Oliva R, Mezquita C. Marked differences in the ability of distinct protamines to disassemble nucleosomal core particles in vitro. Biochemistry. 1986;25(21):6508–11.
43. Zhao M, Shirley C, Hayashi S, Marcon L, Mohapatra B, Suganuma R, et al. Transition nuclear proteins are required for normal chromatin condensation and functional sperm development. Genesis. 2004;38(4):200–13.
44. Cho C, Willis WD, Goulding EH, Jung-Ha H, Choi YC, Hecht NB, et al. Haploinsufficiency of protamine-1 or –2 causes infertility in mice. Nat Genet. 2001;28(1):82–6.
45. Sotolongo B, Lino E, Ward W. Ability of hamster spermatozoa to digest their own DNA. Biol Reprod. 2003;69(6):2029–35.
46. Kuretake S, Kimura Y, Hoshi K, Yanagimachi R. Fertilization and development of mouse oocytes injected with isolated sperm heads. Biol Reprod. 1996;55(4):789–95.
47. Tateno H, Kimura Y, Yanagimachi R. Sonication per se is not as deleterious to sperm chromosomes as previously inferred. Biol Reprod. 2000;63(1):341–6.
48. Risley MS, Einheber S, Bumcrot DA. Changes in DNA topology during spermatogenesis. Chrom-osoma. 1986;94(3):217–27.
49. Ward WS. The structure of the sleeping genome: implications of sperm DNA organization for somatic cells. J Cell Biochem. 1994;55(1):77–82.
50. Laberge RM, Boissonneault G. Chromatin remodeling in spermatids: a sensitive step for the genetic integrity of the male gamete. Arch Androl. 2005;51(2):125–33.
51. Hecht N, Parvinen M. DNA synthesis catalysed by endogenous templates and DNA-dependent DNA polymerases in spermatogenic cells from rat. Exp Cell Res. 1981;135(1):103–14.
52. McPherson S, Longo F. Localization of DNase I-hypersensitive regions during rat spermatogenesis: stage-dependent patterns and unique sensitivity of elongating spermatids. Mol Reprod Dev. 1992;31(4):268–79.
53. McPherson S, Longo F. Nicking of rat spermatid and spermatozoa DNA: possible involvement of DNA topoisomerase II. Dev Biol. 1993;158(1):122–30.
54. McPherson S, Longo F. Chromatin structure-function alterations during mammalian spermatogenesis: DNA nicking and repair in elongating spermatids. European journal of histochemistry : EJH. 1993;37(2):109–28.
55. Sakkas D, Manicardi G, Bianchi P, Bizzaro D, Bianchi U. Relationship between the presence of endogenous nicks and sperm chromatin packaging in maturing and fertilizing mouse spermatozoa. Biol Reprod. 1995;52(5):1149–55.
56. Iseki S. DNA strand breaks in rat tissues as detected by in situ nick translation. Exp Cell Res. 1986;167(2):311–26.
57. Laberge R, Boissonneault G. On the nature and origin of DNA strand breaks in elongating spermatids. Biol Reprod. 2005;73(2):289–96.
58. Boissonneault G. Chromatin remodeling during spermiogenesis: a possible role for the transition proteins in DNA strand break repair. FEBS Lett. 2002;514(2–3):111–4.
59. Branciforte D, Martin SL. Developmental and cell type specificity of LINE-1 expression in mouse testis: implications for transposition. Mol Cell Biol. 1994;14(4):2584–92.
60. Ergün S, Buschmann C, Heukeshoven J, Dammann K, Schnieders F, Lauke H, et al. Cell type-specific expression of LINE-1 open reading frames 1 and 2 in fetal and adult human tissues. J Biol Chem. 2004;279(26):27753–63.

61. Gasior SL, Wakeman TP, Xu B, Deininger PL. The human LINE-1 retrotransposon creates DNA double-strand breaks. J Mol Biol. 2006;357(5):1383–93.
62. Roca J, Mezquita C. DNA topoisomerase II activity in nonreplicating, transcriptionally inactive, chicken late spermatids. EMBO J. 1989;8(6):1855–60.
63. Chen J, Longo F. Expression and localization of DNA topoisomerase II during rat spermatogenesis. Mol Reprod Dev. 1996;45(1):61–71.
64. Morse-Gaudio M, Risley MS. Topoisomerase II expression and VM-26 induction of DNA breaks during spermatogenesis in Xenopus laevis. J Cell Sci. 1994;107 ( Pt 10):2887–98.
65. Turley H, Comley M, Houlbrook S, Nozaki N, Kikuchi A, Hickson I, et al. The distribution and expression of the two isoforms of DNA topoisomerase II in normal and neoplastic human tissues. Br J Cancer. 1997;75(9):1340–6.
66. Shaman J, Prisztoka R, Ward W. Topoisomerase IIB and an extracellular nuclease interact to digest sperm DNA in an apoptotic-like manner. Biol Reprod. 2006;75(5):741–8.
67. Balhorn R, Reed S, Tanphaichitr N. Aberrant protamine 1/protamine 2 ratios in sperm of infertile human males. Experientia. 1988;44(1):52–5.
68. Belokopytova IA, Kostyleva EI, Tomilin AN, Vorob'ev VI. Human male infertility may be due to a decrease of the protamine P2 content in sperm chromatin. Mol Reprod Dev. 1993;34(1):53–7.
69. Aoki V, Emery B, Liu L, Carrell D. Protamine levels vary between individual sperm cells of infertile human males and correlate with viability and DNA integrity. J Androl. 2006;27(6):890–8.
70. Ravel C, Chantot-Bastaraud S, El Houate B, Berthaut I, Verstraete L, De Larouziere V, et al. Mutations in the protamine 1 gene associated with male infertility. Mol Hum Reprod. 2007;13(7):461–4.
71. Carrell D, Emery B, Hammoud S. Altered protamine expression and diminished spermatogenesis: what is the link? Hum Reprod Update. 2007;13(3):313–27.
72. Aitken R, De Iuliis G. On the possible origins of DNA damage in human spermatozoa. Mol Hum Reprod. 2010;16(1):3–13.
73. Caron N, Veilleux S, Boissonneault G. Stimulation of DNA repair by the spermatidal TP1 protein. Mol Reprod Dev. 2001;58(4):437–43.
74. Lowndes NF, Toh GW-L. DNA repair: the importance of phosphorylating histone H2AX. Curr Biol. 2005;15(3):R99–R102.
75. Rogakou EP, Pilch DR, Orr AH, Ivanova VS, Bonner WM. DNA double-stranded breaks induce histone H2AX phosphorylation on serine 139. J Biol Chem. 1998;273(10):5858–68.
76. Pilch DR, Sedelnikova OA, Redon C, Celeste A, Nussenzweig A, Bonner WM. Characteristics of gamma-H2AX foci at DNA double-strand breaks sites. Biochem Cell Biol. 2003;81(3):123–9.
77. Srivastava N, Raman M. Homologous recombination-mediated double-strand break repair in mouse testicular extracts and comparison with different germ cell stages. Cell Biochem Funct. 2007;25(1):75–86.
78. Martins RP, Krawetz SA. Decondensing the protamine domain for transcription. Proc Natl Acad Sci USA. 2007;104(20):8340–5.
79. Ward WS. Function of sperm chromatin structural elements in fertilization and development. Mol Hum Reprod. 2010;16(1):30–6.
80. Spiridonov NA, Wong L, Zerfas PM, Starost MF, Pack SD, Paweletz CP, et al. identification and characterization of SSTK, a serine/threonine protein kinase essential for male fertility. Mol Cell Biol. 2005;25(10):4250–61.
81. Deweese J, Osheroff N. The DNA cleavage reaction of topoisomerase II: wolf in sheep's clothing. Nucleic Acids Research. 2009;37(3):738–48.
82. Barthelmes H, Habermeyer M, Christensen M, Mielke C, Interthal H, Pouliot J, et al. TDP1 overexpression in human cells counteracts DNA damage mediated by topoisomerases I and II. J Biol Chem. 2004;279(53):55618–25.
83. Nitiss K, Malik M, He X, White S, Nitiss J. Tyrosyl-DNA phosphodiesterase (Tdp1) participates in the repair of Top2-mediated DNA damage. Proc Natl Acad Sci USA. 2006;103(24):8953–8.

84. Interthal H, Chen H, Champoux J. Human Tdp1 cleaves a broad spectrum of substrates, including phosphoamide linkages. J Biol Chem. 2005;280(43):36518–28.
85. Cortes Ledesma F, El Khamisy SF, Zuma MC, Osborn K, Caldecott KW. A human 5'-tyrosyl DNA phosphodiesterase that repairs topoisomerase-mediated DNA damage. Nature. 2009;461(7264):674–8.
86. Weterings E, Chen DJ. The endless tale of non-homologous end-joining. Cell Res. 2008;18(1): 114–24.
87. Pastwa E, Somiari R, Malinowski M, Somiari S, Winters T. In vitro non-homologous DNA end joining assays-The 20th anniversary. Int J Biochem Cell Biol. 2009;41(6):1254–60.
88. Ahmed EA, de Boer P, Philippens MEP, Kal HB, de Rooij DG. Parp1–XRCC1 and the repair of DNA double strand breaks in mouse round spermatids. Mutat Res. 2010;683(1–2):84–90.
89. Valerie K, Povirk LF. Regulation and mechanisms of mammalian double-strand break repair. Oncogene. 2003;22(37):5792–812.
90. Cabrero J, Palomino-Morales RJ, Camacho JPM. The DNA-repair Ku70 protein is located in the nucleus and tail of elongating spermatids in grasshoppers. Chromosome Res. 2007;15(8): 1093–100.
91. Celli GB, Denchi EL, de Lange T. Ku70 stimulates fusion of dysfunctional telomeres yet protects chromosome ends from homologous recombination. Nat Cell Biol. 2006;8(8): 885–90.
92. Boulton SJ, Jackson SP. Components of the Ku-dependent non-homologous end-joining pathway are involved in telomeric length maintenance and telomeric silencing. EMBO J. 1998;17(6):1819–28.
93. Maymon B, Cohenarmon M, Yavetz H, Yogev L, Lifschitzmercer B, Kleiman S, et al. Role of poly(ADP-ribosyl)ation during human spermatogenesis. Fertil Steril. 2006;86(5):1402–7.
94. Di Meglio S, Denegri M, Vallefuoco S, Tramontano F, Scovassi AI, Quesada P. Poly(ADPR) polymerase-1 and poly(ADPR) glycohydrolase level and distribution in differentiating rat germinal cells. Mol Cell Biochem. 2003;248(1–2):85–91.
95. Dantzer F, Mark M, Quenet D, Scherthan H, Huber A, Liebe B, et al. Poly(ADP-ribose) polymerase-2 contributes to the fidelity of male meiosis I and spermiogenesis. Proc Natl Acad Sci USA. 2006;103(40):14854–9.
96. Meyer-Ficca ML, Lonchar J, Credidio C, Ihara M, Li Y, Wang Z-Q, et al. Disruption of poly(ADP-ribose) homeostasis affects spermiogenesis and sperm chromatin integrity in mice. Biol Reprod. 2009;81(1):46–55.
97. Stark JM, Pierce AJ, Oh J, Pastink A, Jasin M. Genetic steps of mammalian homologous repair with distinct mutagenic consequences. Mol Cell Biol. 2004;24(21):9305–16.
98. Weinstock D, Richardson C, Elliott B, Jasin M. Modeling oncogenic translocations: distinct roles for double-strand break repair pathways in translocation formation in mammalian cells. DNA Repair (Amst). 2006;5(9–10):1065–74.
99. McVey M, Lee SE. MMEJ repair of double-strand breaks (director's cut): deleted sequences and alternative endings. Trends Genet. 2008;24(11):529–38.
100. Rathke C, Baarends WM, Jayaramaiah-Raja S, Bartkuhn M, Renkawitz R, Renkawitz-Pohl R. Transition from a nucleosome-based to a protamine-based chromatin configuration during spermiogenesis in Drosophila. J Cell Sci. 2007;120(Pt 9):1689–700.
101. Wojtczak A, Popłoska K, Kwiatkowska M. Phosp-horylation of H2AX histone as indirect evidence for double-stranded DNA breaks related to the exchange of nuclear proteins and chromatin remodeling in Chara vulgaris spermiogenesis. Protoplasma. 2008;233(3–4):263–7.
102. Thomas NS, Durkie M, Van Zyl B, Sanford R, Potts G, Youings S, et al. Parental and chromosomal origin of unbalanced de novo structural chromosome abnormalities in man. Hum Genet. 2006;119(4):444–50.
103. Chandley AC. On the parental origin of de novo mutation in man. J Med Genet. 1991;28(4):217–23.
104. Olson SB, Magenis, R.E. Preferential paternal origin of de novo structural chromosome rearrangements. In: Daniel A, editor. The cytogenetics of mammalian autosomal rearrangements. New York: Liss; 1988. p. 583–99.

105. Sloter ED, Lowe X, Moore II DH, Nath J, Wyrobek AJ. Multicolor FISH analysis of chromosomal breaks, duplications, deletions, and numerical abnormalities in the sperm of healthy men. Am J Hum Genet. 2000;67(4):862–72.
106. Maffei F, Forti GC, Castelli E, Stefanini GF, Mattioli S, Hrelia P. Biomarkers to assess the genetic damage induced by alcohol abuse in human lymphocytes. Mutat Res. 2002; 514(1–2):49–58.
107. Obe G, Herha J. Chromosomal aberrations in heavy smokers. Hum Genet. 1978;41(3):259–63.
108. Hopkins JM, Evans HJ. Cigarette smoke-induced DNA damage and lung cancer risks. Nature. 1980;283(5745):388–90.
109. Glei M, Habermann N, Osswald K, Seidel C, Persin C, Jahreis G, et al. Assessment of DNA damage and its modulation by dietary and genetic factors in smokers using the Comet assay: a biomarker model. Biomarkers. 2005;10(2–3):203–17.
110. Fedeli D, Fedeli A, Luciani F, Massi M, Falcioni G, Polidori C. Lymphocyte DNA alteration by sub-chronic ethanol intake in alcohol-preferring rats. Clin Chim Acta. 2003;337(1–2):43–8.
111. Katsuki Y, Nakada S, Yokoyama T, Imoto I, Inazawa J, Nagasawa M, et al. Caffeine yields aneuploidy through asymmetrical cell division caused by misalignment of chromosomes. Cancer Sci. 2008;99(8):1539–45.
112. Rubes J, Lowe X, Moore D, Perreault S, Slott V, Evenson D, et al. Smoking cigarettes is associated with increased sperm disomy in teenage men. Fertil Steril. 1998;70(4):715–23.
113. Belcheva A, Ivanova-Kicheva M, Tzvetkova P, Marinov M. Effects of cigarette smoking on sperm plasma membrane integrity and DNA fragmentation. Int J Androl. 2004;27(5):296–300.
114. Martin QS, Evelyn Ko, Leona Barclay, Tina Hoang, Alfred Rademaker, RenÉe. Cigarette smoking and aneuploidy in human sperm. Mol Reprod Dev. 2001;59(4):417–21.
115. Sepaniak S, Forges T, Gerard H, Foliguet B, Bene M-C, Monnier-Barbarino P. The influence of cigarette smoking on human sperm quality and DNA fragmentation. Toxicology. 2006; 223(1–2):54–60.
116. Schmid T, Eskenazi B, Baumgartner A, Marchetti F, Young S, Weldon R, et al. The effects of male age on sperm DNA damage in healthy non-smokers. Hum Reprod. 2007;22(1):180.
117. Rybaczek, Bodys, Maszewski. H2AX foci in late S/G2- and M-phase cells after hydroxyurea- and aphidicolin-induced DNA replication stress in Vicia. Histochem Cell Biol. 2007;128(3):227–41.
118. Block W, Yu Y, Merkle D, Gifford J, Ding Q, Meek K, et al. Autophosphorylation-dependent remodeling of the DNA-dependent protein kinase catalytic subunit regulates ligation of DNA ends. Nucleic Acids Res. 2004;32(14):4351.
119. Sarkaria JN, Busby EC, Tibbetts RS, Roos P, Taya Y, Karnitz LM, et al. Inhibition of ATM and ATR kinase activities by the radiosensitizing agent, caffeine. Cancer Res. 1999;59(17):4375–82.
120. Bosch M, Rajmil O, Egozcue J, Templado C. Linear increase of structural and numerical chromosome 9 abnormalities in human sperm regarding age. Eur J Hum Genet. 2003;11(10):754–9.
121. Sloter E, Nath J, Eskenazi B, Wyrobek AJ. Effects of male age on the frequencies of germinal and heritable chromosomal abnormalities in humans and rodents. Fertil Steril. 2004;81(4):925–43.
122. Tiemann-Boege I, Navidi W, Grewal R, Cohn D, Eskenazi B, Wyrobek AJ, et al. The observed human sperm mutation frequency cannot explain the achondroplasia paternal age effect. Proc Natl Acad Sci USA. 2002;99(23):14952–7.
123. Marchetti F, Essers J, Kanaar R, Wyrobek AJ. Disruption of maternal DNA repair increases sperm-derived chromosomal aberrations. Proc Natl Acad Sci USA. 2007;104(45):17725–9.
124. Marchetti F, Wyrobek AJ. DNA repair decline during mouse spermiogenesis results in the accumulation of heritable DNA damage. DNA Repair (Amst). 2008;7(4):572–81.
125. Kusakabe H, Kamiguchi Y. Chromosome analysis of mouse zygotes after injecting oocytes with spermatozoa treated in vitro with green tea catechin, (–)-epigallocatechin gallate (EGCG). Mutat Res. 2004;564(2):195–200.
126. Feng Q, Moran JV, Kazazian HH, Boeke JD. Human L1 retrotransposon encodes a conserved endonuclease required for retrotransposition. Cell. 1996;87(5):905–16.
127. Goodier JL, Ostertag EM, Engleka KA, Seleme MC, Kazazian HH. A potential role for the nucleolus in L1 retrotransposition. Hum Mol Genet. 2004;13(10):1041–8.

128. Gilbert N, Lutz S, Morrish TA, Moran JV. Multiple fates of L1 retrotransposition intermediates in cultured human cells. Mol Cell Biol. 2005;25(17):7780–95.
129. Deininger PL, Batzer MA. Alu repeats and human disease. Mol Genet Metab. 1999;67(3): 183–93.
130. Wei Y, Sun M, Nilsson G, Dwight T, Xie Y, Wang J, et al. Characteristic sequence motifs located at the genomic breakpoints of the translocation t(X;18) in synovial sarcomas. Oncogene. 2003;22(14):2215–22.
131. Minor A, Wong E, Harmer K, Ma S. Molecular and cytogenetic investigation of Y chromosome deletions over three generations facilitated by intracytoplasmic sperm injection. Prenat Diagn. 2007 May 29.
132. Aitken R, Krausz C. Oxidative stress, DNA damage and the Y chromosome. Reproduction. 2001;122(4):497–506.
133. Ogura A, Matsuda J, Yanagimachi R. Birth of normal young after electrofusion of mouse oocytes with round spermatids. Proc Natl Acad Sci USA. 1994;91(16):7460–2.
134. Kimura Y, Yanagimachi R. Mouse oocytes injected with testicular spermatozoa or round spermatids can develop into normal offspring. Development. 1995;121(8):2397–405.
135. Yamagata K, Suetsugu R, Wakayama T. Assessment of chromosomal integrity using a novel live-cell imaging technique in mouse embryos produced by intracytoplasmic sperm injection. Hum Reprod. 2009;24(10):2490–9.
136. Hassold T, Hunt P. To err (meiotically) is human: the genesis of human aneuploidy. Nat Rev Genet. 2001;2(4):280–91.
137. Crow JF. The origins, patterns and implications of human spontaneous mutation. Nat Rev Genet. 2000;1(1):40–7.
138. Olsen A, Lindeman B, Wiger R, Duale N, Brunborg G. How do male germ cells handle DNA damage? Toxicol Appl Pharmacol. 2005;207(2 suppl.):521–31.
139. Brandriff B, Pedersen RA. Repair of the ultraviolet-irradiated male genome in fertilized mouse eggs. Science. 1981;211(4489):1431–3.
140. Ashwood-Smith MJ, Edwards RG. DNA repair by oocytes. Mol Hum Reprod. 1996;2(1): 46–51.

# Part II
# Clinical Aspects of Sperm Chromatin Damage

# Chapter 6
# Male Subfertility and Sperm Chromatin Damage

Mona Bungum, Aleksander Giwercman, and Marcello Spanò

Infertility is defined as a state in which a couple desiring a child is unable to conceive following 12 months of unprotected intercourse. Infertility represents one of the most common diseases and affects between 17 and 25% of couples [1, 2]. For long, female factors have been regarded as the primary causes of failure to conceive. However, male causes are involved in about half of the cases [3]. Male infertility is a multifactorial disease that can be due to a variety of genetic and acquired factors. However, in about half of the men the aetiology of impaired semen quality remains unexplained [3]. In a high proportion of the cases, no cause-related treatment is possible [4].

The traditional semen analysis where the World Health Organization (WHO) has set criteria in regard to sperm concentration, motility and morphology is the cornerstone procedure used to diagnose male infertility [5]. However, the WHO parameters only address few aspects of sperm quality and function, and thus, the discriminative power in relation to fertility is quite low [6, 7]. Finding better markers of male fertility may have important clinical and biological implications [8–10]. It may improve understanding of mechanisms underlying subfertility and facilitate development of new specific therapies. Moreover, better markers could help in

M. Bungum, MSc, Med Dr, PhD (✉)
Reproductive Medicine Centre, Skåne University Hospital Malmö, Lund University,
Sodra Forstadsgatan, Malmö 20502, Sweden
e-mail: mona.bungumed.lu.se

A. Giwercman, MD, PhD
Reproductive Medicine Centre,
Skåne University Hospital Malmö, Lund University,
Malmö, Sweden

M. Spanò, PhD
Laboratory of Toxicology,
Unit of Radiation Biology and Human Health,
Italian National Agency for New Technologies, Engery,
and Sustainable Economic Development,
Casaccia Research Centre, Casaccia, Rome, Italy

A. Zini, A. Agarwal (eds.), *Sperm Chromatin for the Clinician*,
© Springer Science+Business Media New York 2013

deciding for which couple assisted reproductive technology (ART) is needed and to identify the most effective type of ART treatment for a given couple [11].

Fertility requires fusion of the genomes of an oocyte and a sperm, and the completion of this process and subsequent embryo development depends, in addition to the repair capacity of the oocyte, on the inherent integrity of sperm DNA [12–14]. Animal studies have shown that a male gamete with damaged DNA can transmit genetic defects and in worse cases can lead to pregnancy loss, infant mortality, birth defects and genetic diseases in offspring [15, 16]. Extensive laboratory animal literature unequivocally reports that the genetic integrity of the male gamete is pivotal to ensure normal embryo development [17]. In support to animal studies are the findings relating paternal smoking and sperm DNA damage passed from the father to the offspring following ART [18] and the evidence of an association between paternal smoking and an increased risk of childhood cancer in the offspring [19].

Today, subfertile couples can be helped through ART. However, concerns have been raised about the increasing use of ART and in particular ICSI that bypasses natural biological barriers preventing against fertilization by defective sperm and, as a consequence, chromatin/DNA alterations can be transmitted to the embryo and the offspring. Therefore, during the last decades, a growing attention has gained the assessment of sperm chromatin integrity in the pathophysiology of infertility [20, 21]. In this chapter, we review how sperm chromatin/DNA integrity can impact male fertility.

## Male Infertility/Subfertility

In 20% of involuntary childlessness couple, the predominant cause is solely male related, and in another 27%, anomalies in both partners contribute to the childlessness [3]. Reduced male fertility can be the result of congenital and acquired urogenital abnormalities, infections of the genital tract, varicocele, endocrine disturbances and genetic or immunological factors [3]. Environmental, occupational, lifestyle and therapeutic exposures have also been invoked as possible cofactors hampering male fertility [22–25].

However, the underlying cause of infertility remains unexplained in at least 50% of the infertile men. Genetic abnormalities [26–28] are thought to account for 15–30% of male factor infertility. Approximately 5% of infertile men have chromosomal abnormalities, a prevalence that increases up to 15% in the population of azoospermic males [29, 156].

Recent studies have shown that epigenetic modifications in sperm may also cause infertility [26, 30–34]. One of the main epigenetic mechanisms in sperm appears to be DNA methylation [156]. Several studies indicate that DNA methylation is altered, in at least some imprinted genes, in oligozoospermic men and men with improper histone to protamine replacement [35–37]. Furthermore, methylation defects as well as other epigenetic defects may play an important role in the development and growth of ART offspring [38–41].

Another important cause of male infertility is considered, and this is the main topic of this chapter, the occurrence of chromatin and nuclear abnormalities manifesting themselves as breaks in sperm nuclear DNA [16, 20, 42–45].

## Diagnosis of Male Infertility/Subfertility

Mostly, the diagnosis of male infertility/subfertility is based solely on the presence of an abnormal semen analysis of sperm concentration, motility and morphology [5]. The standard sperm parameters vary significantly between individuals, seasons, countries and regions and even between consecutive samples within the same man [5, 46–50]. As the analysis is mainly performed by standard light microscopy of 100–200 spermatozoa, the analysis implies a high level of subjectivity resulting in a high grade of intra- and interlaboratory variation [51, 52], and thus, a low predictive power of the analysis is seen. Another problem when assessing predictivity of semen parameters is that female factors only rarely are taken into account. Whilst mostly the term infertility are used, most patients are actually subfertile, rather than sterile (infertile), but the degree of subfertility is difficult to predict [53]. A fertile partner may compensate for a less fertile spouse, and thus, in most cases the term subfertility better covers the condition.

During the last decades, several other laboratory tests of sperm function have been developed, such as antisperm antibody test, vital staining, biochemical analysis of semen, hypoosmotic swelling test, sperm penetration assay, hemizona assay, creatine kinase test, reactive oxygen species (ROS) tests and computer-assisted sperm analysis (CASA), to mention the most commonly used [8]. However, the clinical value of these tests has been questioned, and few are implemented in clinical routine [54].

Although the origin and the mechanisms responsible for sperm DNA damage are not yet fully clarified, a bulk of data have accumulated, demonstrating an association between genetic damage and fertility or progeny outcome [16, 20, 43, 45, 55–59, 156]. It has been proposed that sperm DNA integrity could be a possible fertility predictor to be used as a supplement to the traditional sperm parameters [11, 42].

## Assessment of Sperm Chromatin Damage

During the past decades, a variety of new techniques to assess sperm nuclear integrity have been developed [42, 60–62]. This issue is reviewed in depth in other chapters of this book. Briefly, such techniques, using microscopy-based and flow-cytometry-based analyses, can evaluate sperm DNA and chromatin integrity in situ on cell-by-cell basis. Each test uses a different strategy to detect DNA/chromatin damages. Unspecific DNA strand breaks can be detected by the single-cell gel electrophoresis assay (comet assay) in its alkaline, neutral and two-tailed versions [63–65], the terminal deoxynucleotidyl transferase dUTP nick-end labelling (TUNEL) assay [66, 67], in situ nick translation (ISNT) [68] or DNA breakage detection fluorescence in situ hybridization (DBD-FISH) [69]. In addition, DNA breaks can be evaluated indirectly through the DNA denaturability by the sperm chromatin structure assay (SCSA) [42, 70], the sperm chromatin dispersion (SCD) test [71, 72] and the toluidine blue assay [73]. Chromatin integrity can also be assessed with respect to the degree of protamination by the CMA3 assay [68, 74], which relies on the detection of lysine residues as a measure of an excess of histones remaining bound to the sperm DNA, and by measuring the level of compaction due to the formation of inter- and intraprotamine disulphide bridges [75]. More recently, techniques have been developed to assess the epigenetic components of sperm such as the global DNA methylation level [76, 77]. These tests can measure a parameter generally known as sperm DNA fragmentation. For sake of brevity, we use the abbreviation DFI (DNA Fragmentation Index) to identify the fraction of DNA defective sperm independently from the various DNA fragmentation assays used. From studies carried out both in normal and infertile men, it turned out that, with few exceptions, sperm DNA integrity tests generally correlate well with each other, even though the level of correlation between the same techniques can vary across different studies. In Table 6.1, the studies correlating different DNA fragmentation assays, together with their correlation levels, and involving more than 50 individuals are reported.

## Genesis of Sperm DNA Damage

The most common types of sperm DNA damage include single- or double-strand breaks, base modifications and adducts, DNA intra-/interstrand and DNA–protein cross links [16]. Even though the mechanisms leading to the formation of DNA damage in sperm are only partially elucidated, it has generally been proposed that DNA damage in sperm can be produced by unrepaired DNA breaks during the spermiogenetical chromatin packaging [78], by partial or complete protamine deficiency [26, 79, 80], abortive apoptosis during spermatogenesis [81] and the action of (sperm- or leucocyte-derived) oxidative damage [44]. Furthermore, a variety of external factors such as genotoxic agents due to therapeutical, occupational and environmental exposures [44, 45, 82] may cause sperm DNA breaks by some of the mechanisms mentioned above. At least, some of these exposures directly target DNA, whereas others induce oxidative stress. ROS can damage sperm DNA [44, 83], and a reliable biomarker of the oxidative attack on the DNA molecule is the formation of 8-hydroxy-2'-deoxyguanosine (8-OHdG). Higher levels of this adduct have been found in the sperm DNA of infertile men [84, 85]. 8-OHdG adducts representing a modified DNA structure potentially leading to a DNA break and strong

**Table 6.1** Studies (with>50 individuals) correlating different DNA fragmentation assays

| Technique | N Normal men | Infertile men | Results | References |
|---|---|---|---|---|
| SCSA vs. AOT | | 185 | N.S. | Apedaile et al. [110] |
| SCSA vs. AOT | 7 | 60 | N.S. | Chohan et al. [157] |
| SCSA vs. comet (neutral pH 8) | 80 | | N.S. | Schmid et al. [156] |
| SCSA vs. comet (alkaline pH 13) | 80 | | N.S. | Schmid et al. [156] |
| SCSA vs. comet (alkaline pH 12.1) | | 55 | $r = 0.3$ | O'Flaherty et al. [158] |
| SCSA vs. FIM-TUNEL | 7 | 60 | $r = 0.9$ | Chohan et al. [157] |
| SCSA vs. FIM-TUNEL | 25 | 55 | $r = 0.50$ | Smith et al. [131] |
| SCSA vs. FCM-TUNEL | 24 | 96 | $r = 0.41$ | Ståhl et al. [159] |
| SCSA vs. FCM-TUNEL | 666 | | $r = 0.56$ | Toft (personal communication, 2006) |
| SCSA vs. FCM-TUNEL | | 58 | $r = 0.27$ | O'Flaherty et al. [158] |
| SCSA vs. SCD | 7 | 60 | $r = 0.9$ | Chohan et al. [157] |
| SCSA vs. Toluidine Blue | 63 | 79 | $r = 0.47$ | Tsarev et al. [145] |
| M-TUNEL vs. SCD | 30 | 60 | $r = 0.6–0.9$ | Zhang et al. [160] |
| FIM-TUNEL vs. FCM-TUNEL | | 66 | $r = 0.72$ | Domínguez-Fandos et al. [161] |
| FIM-TUNEL vs. SCD | 7 | 60 | $r = 0.9$ | Chohan et al. [157] |
| FIM-TUNEL vs. CMA3 | | 61 | $r = 0.76$ | Plastira et al. [162] |
| FIM-TUNEL vs. CMA3 | | 132 | $r = 0.53$ | Tarozzi et al. [57] |
| FCM-TUNEL vs. FIM-TUNEL | | 68 | $r = 0.94$ | Cohen-Bacrie et al. [112] |
| FCM TUNEL vs. comet (alkaline pH 10) | 42 | 21 | $r = 0.56$ | Bian et al. [163] |
| FCM TUNEL vs. CMA3 (FCM) | 39 | 28 | $r = 0.83–0.96$ | De Iuliis et al. [164] |
| FCM TUNEL vs. 8-OHdG (FCM) | | 94 | $r = 0.25$ ($r = 0.76$ in the high-density Percoll fraction) | De Iuliis et al. [164] |
| SCD vs. CMA3 | | 78 | $r = 0.29$ | Tavalaee et al. [165] |

*SCSA* sperm chromatin structure assay; *AOT* acridine orange test; *TUNEL* terminal deoxynucleotidyl transferase dUTP nick-end labelling; *M-TUNEL* TUNEL assay, bright field microscopy; *FIM-TUNEL* TUNEL assay, fluorescence microscopy; *FCM-TUNEL* flow cytometry TUNEL; *SCD* sperm chromatin dispersion test; *CMA3* chromomycin A3; *ISNT* in situ nick translation; *8-OHdG* 8-hydroxydeoxyguanosine level evaluated by high-performance liquid chromatography; *N.S.* not statistically significant relationships between the two forms of damage have been reported [44]. These issues are reviewed in detail elsewhere in this book. The proposed mechanisms are obviously not mutually exclusive, and recently, a two-step hypothesis has been put forward where faulty spermatogenesis can lead to defective chromatin remodelling with the DNA more susceptible and vulnerable to a variety of stressors [16, 44].

## Factors Reported to Impact Sperm Chromatin Integrity

The personal burden of sperm DNA fragmentation can increase under the influence of variety of stressors [20, 21, 86]. Exposures to physical agents and chemicals including therapeutic drugs, pesticides, metals, air pollutants and tobacco smoking are known to target male germ cells. At least, some of these exposures directly target DNA, whereas others induce oxidative stress. Smokers have an increased level of oxidative damage in their sperm DNA compared to non-smokers [87], and several studies have reported a negative effect of cigarette smoking on sperm DNA [88].

Moreover, recent studies have indicated an association between high body mass index (BMI) and reduced semen quality [89–91]. A higher fraction of sperm with high DNA damage was reported in obese men than in normal-weight men [92]. However, results are conflicting, and so far, no such prospective or intervention studies have been published.

Fever can have marked effects on both the conventional semen parameters and sperm DNA integrity [21, 93, 94]. Also, several studies have reported that the higher is the abstinence period, the higher is the fraction of DNA defective sperm. It seems likely that this correlation stems from a longer exposure of sperm to ROS attacks. A weak positive correlation has been found both in the general population and in infertility patients [43, 95–100]. However, this relation did not emerge in other studies [101, 102], including a study designed to specifically address this issue [103].

Another important source of deterioration of the DNA integrity of spermatozoa is aging. It is known that a major proportion of abnormal reproductive outcomes are associated with paternally transmitted numerical and structural chromosomal abnormalities and advancing paternal age has been implicated in a broad range of abnormal reproductive and genetic outcomes [104]. Older men are reported to have sperm with more DNA fragmentation than younger men [95, 100, 105, 106, 156], a finding well in accordance with the age-dependent decline in standard semen parameters [107]. Increased life expectancies, changes in family-planning practices and advances in ART in industrialized countries are resulting in an increasing number of births in couples aged 34–54 years. The age-related increase of damage in male germ cells raises substantial health concerns regarding the possible long-term consequences of increasing paternal ages on the viability and genetic health of the offspring.

# Male Infertility and Sperm Chromatin Damage

## *The Association Between the Traditional Sperm Parameters and Sperm DNA Integrity*

Although the level will vary, in all men, sperm cells with DNA breaks are always present in the ejaculate. Whilst unselected men planning for their first pregnancy had a mean DFI of 14% [96], infertile men have a mean DFI of 23% as compared to a DFI of 12% observed for fertile men [108].

In Table 6.2, the studies involving more than 100 men reporting prevalence of DNA-defective sperm in infertile men as compared to normal controls are quoted.

Several studies have demonstrated a weak-to-moderate inverse correlation, if any, between sperm DNA fragmentation measured by the various sperm integrity assays and the traditional semen parameters [95, 98, 109–114]. The correlation levels among different studies comparing the same techniques can vary, probably because minor variations in the protocols and in the semen samples can influence the final figures. However, by and large, sperm DNA fragmentation assessment is quite independent from the WHO standard parameters. Motility has generally been the parameter with the highest degree of association to sperm DNA defects, probably because both sperm chromatin compaction and acquisition of motility are parallel differentiation processes culminating during the passage of the maturing male gamete in the epididymal tract.

**Table 6.2** Studies (with >100 individuals) reporting prevalence of DNA defective sperm in infertile men as compared to normal controls

| Technique | Controls, *n* | Infertile, *n* | References |
| --- | --- | --- | --- |
| M-TUNEL | 20 | 236 | Høst et al. [166] |
| FIM-TUNEL | 23 | 87 | Gandini et al. [167] |
| FIM-TUNEL | 49 | 61 | Plastira et al. [162] |
| FCM-TUNEL | 47 | 66 | Sergerie et al. [144] |
| CMA3 | 49 | 61 | Plastira et al. [162] |
| SCSA | 165 | 115 | Evenson et al. [122] |
| SCSA | 13 | 88 | Zini et al. [125] |
| SCSA | 16 | 92 | Saleh et al. [126] |
| SCSA | 13 | 101 | |
| SCSA | 100 | 200 | Pant et al. [168] |
| SCSA | 137 | 127 | Giwercman et al. [108] |
| Aniline Blue | 75 | 90 | Hammadeh et al. [169] |
| Toluidine Blue | 63 | 79 | Tsarev et al. [145] |
| 8-OHdG | 54 | 60 | Shen et al. [85] |

*SCSA* sperm chromatin structure assay; *TUNEL* terminal deoxynucleotidyl transferase dUTP nick-end labelling; *M-TUNEL* TUNEL assay, bright field microscopy; *FIM-TUNEL* TUNEL assay, fluorescence microscopy; *FCM-TUNEL* flow cytometry TUNEL; *CMA3* Chromomycin A3; *8-OHdG* 8-hydroxydeoxyguanosine level evaluated by high-performance liquid chromatography

The relation between the fractions of DNA defective sperm and blood concentration of sexual hormones and other biomarkers of the sexual accessory glands has also been studied. In a study involving 278 young men with no knowledge of their fertility status [115], the DFI as evaluated by the SCSA was weakly correlated, negatively with estradiol and free testosterone and positively correlated with the seminal concentration of zinc and fructose. In another study involving 362 male partners of infertile couples [116], the fraction of sperm with high DNA damage, evaluated by the neutral comet assay, resulted positively associated with free thyroxine (T4) and total triiodothyronine (T3).

## Intraindividual Variation of Sperm Chromatin Parameters

Traditional semen parameters usually exhibit a high intraindividual variability [51, 52] and coefficient of variations (CVs) as high as 54% has been reported [117]. The issue of possible intraindividual changes of sperm chromatin parameters with time has specifically been addressed by some groups, and DFI is demonstrated to be a sperm parameter characterized by a lower level of variability. In a study of 45 men who delivered eight monthly semen samples, the average within-donor CV of DFI as measured by SCSA was around 23% [101]. These results were confirmed by other SCSA studies. Zini et al. [118] measured the DFI in 21 men who provided two semen samples, 2–6 weeks apart and observed a within-subject CV of 21%. In another study, involving 277 men, semen was measured twice during 6 months and a within-subject CV of 23% for DFI was obtained [95]. Altogether, these data point to a lower level of intraindividual variation for SCSA measurements as compared to the standard sperm parameters.

Time stability of sperm DNA integrity was assessed both by the SCSA and the TUNEL assays in a healthy non-smoking fertile volunteer, characterized by a low DFI, over a 10-year period. Compared with TUNEL data, SCSA measurements showed less variation over the data collection period with a DFI within-subject CV of 47.4 and 22.3%, respectively. DFI remained normal, and no trend was observed over the period of observation [119]. Finally, the stability over time of the flow cytometry TUNEL assay, during a 6-month period, was tested in a longitudinal study using 15 men donors who provided monthly multiple semen samples. A good reproducibility of the TUNEL assay was obtained: individual CVs for sperm DFI ranged from 12.9 to 43.9%, whereas parallel measurements on cell counts showed within-donor CVs ranging from 16.7 up to 63.2% [120].

In a study of 282 patients undergoing ART with repeated (between 2 and 5) SCSA measurements, CV of DFI was a bit higher than previously reported, about 29%, showing that intraindividual variability in DFI could be of significance. Repeated measurements were recommended in men having a DFI >20% [121], since a switch of DFI to a higher level may have implications for the selection of the ART treatment [11].

## Impact of Sperm DNA Damage on Fecundity in General Population

Whether sperm chromatin integrity parameters, independently from the WHO parameters, could predict the chances of spontaneous pregnancy was a question addressed by two almost concomitant SCSA studies, one carried out in USA (the Georgetown study, 165 couples) and the other carried out in Europe (the Danish first pregnancy planners study, 215 couples). Both demonstrated that in couples from the general population, the chance of spontaneous pregnancy, measured by the time-to-pregnancy (TTP), decreases when DFI exceeded 20–30% [96, 122]. If the DFI was more than 30%, TTP tended to become infinite and the chances of spontaneous pregnancies were quite negligible [96, 122]. Stratifying the population into two groups, below and above a DFI threshold at 30%, the probability of pregnancy for the group with DFI <30% was significantly higher than that for the group with DFI >30%. These two in vivo studies showed that the pregnancy rates are significantly higher for the group with DFI below the thresholds of 30% [123]. In the same population of Danish first-pregnancy planners [96], the likelihood of pregnancy occurring in a single menstrual cycle was inversely associated with the level of 8-OHdG [124], corroborating the result of the previous SCSA analysis and reinforcing the notion that oxidative DNA damage can play a major role in the genesis of DNA breaks [44].

## Impact of Sperm DNA Damage on Fecundity in Subfertile Men

There are few studies addressing the issue of prevalence of high levels of sperm DNA damage among infertile men. Such prevalence was reported to be 17% when the 30% SCSA derived DFI threshold was used [125], and 58% using a 24% SCSA-DFI threshold [126]. On the other hand, Verit and coworkers did not find increased DFI levels among infertile men with normal conventional semen parameters, as compared to fertile donors [127].

The prevalence of sperm DNA damage in 350 men from infertile couples with both normal and abnormal semen parameters was studied to investigate whether sperm DNA fragmentation, assessed by the SCSA, could add to the information obtained by routine semen analysis when explaining the causes of infertility [128]. In this study, 28% of men had a DFI >20%, while 12% had a DFI >30%. In the subgroup of 224 men with abnormal semen parameters, 35% had a DFI >20% and 16% had a DFI >30%, whereas these figures were 15 and 5%, respectively, in the subgroup of men with normal semen parameters. Men with low sperm motility and abnormal morphology had significantly higher odds ratios (OR) for having a DFI >20% (4.0 for motility and 1.9 for morphology) and DFI >30% (6.2 for motility and 2.8 for morphology) compared with men with normal sperm motility and morphology.

In a more recent study, 127 men from infertile couples where female factors contributing to the infertility problem were excluded, and 137 men with proven fertility were considered. Also in this work, DFI was assessed using SCSA. The risk of being infertile was increased when DFI >20% (OR 5.1) in men with normal standard semen parameters, whereas if one of the WHO parameters were abnormal, the OR for infertility was increased already at DFI above 10% (OR 16). DFI above 20% was found in 40% of men with otherwise normal standard parameters. Thus, the DFI as measured by SCSA adds to the value of semen analysis in prediction of the chance of natural conception [108]. Furthermore, in almost 50% of so-called "unexplained" cases of infertility, sperm DNA defects seem to be at least a contributing factor to the problem.

Moreover, a SCSA derived DFI threshold at 30% has been observed in two large ART studies where ORs of 8–14 were observed in the probability of delivery after intrauterine insemination [11, 129]. Thus, DFI was found to be an independent predictor of fertility in vivo. The role of sperm DNA fragmentation in ART is reviewed in another chapter of this book.

In addition to the relationship between sperm DNA fragmentation and pregnancy outcome, sperm DNA integrity has also been started to be used in sperm quality assessment in other andrological pathologies, such as varicocele, cancer and infections, providing valuable information on disease severity and therapeutic efficacy. Usually, a higher percentage of defective sperm is found in varicocele patients, probably attributable to oxidative stress [65, 130–132]. In many cases, sperm chromatin quality was improved after surgery [133–135] or by antioxidant therapy [136].

Patients with genitourinary infection by *Chlamydia trachomatis* or *Mycoplasma* showed an increased DFI in comparison with fertile controls and antibiotic therapy resulted important in providing a remedy for infection-induced high DNA fragmentation levels [137]. This is consistent with the results from another study where patients with bacteriospermia had improvement in DFI results after antibiotic treatment [136].

Among pathologies unrelated with andrology disturbances where the fraction of sperm with fragmented DNA was higher in patients than in suitable controls, thalassemia major [138], spinal cord injury [139] and type I diabetes mellitus [140] should be mentioned. In the latter, DFI measured by the alkaline comet assay and levels of oxidative DNA modification were evaluated in spermatozoa of diabetic and non-diabetic men. A positive correlation was observed between DFI and concentrations of 8-OHdG, again supporting the hypothesis that oxidative stress may play a major role in the genesis of DNA breaks.

Studies on patients with testicular cancer have shown that sperm DNA might be damaged already before irradiation or chemotherapy [141]. However, cancer therapy was shown to further contribute to increased DNA damage [142].

# Future Perspectives

There is an urgent call for better methods of assessing male fertility potential. A more precise diagnosing would enable clinicians to better counsel the infertile couple and may also result in improvement and further development of cause-related therapy, which is very little used in today's clinical practice.

Unfortunately, few of the assays used to assess sperm DNA integrity have been standardized sufficiently, and there remain wide variations in results obtained from different laboratories [58, 62]. Statistically validated threshold values could be of help in the future clinical applications of sperm DNA integrity tests. So far, SCSA has been the only method providing thresholds of clinical relevance for in vivo and in vitro pregnancy [11, 42, 96, 122, 123, 129, 143]. Other tests in which clinical thresholds for infertility have been suggested are the comet [58], the TUNEL [144] assays, the SCD [72] and the toluidine blue tests [145]. However, differently from the SCSA, none of these other assays has provided stable thresholds based on large study populations. Each of the techniques seems to have its own specificity and limitations and it is still not clear what is unequivocally measured by each test. Thus, we can choose from a variety of assays, often proposing some variations of the application protocol, but so far, we cannot comfortably decide which is the best and the most robust and why. It should be noted that all these tests can detect only a subgroup of the possible alterations of the DNA molecule [16]. Likely, only a "tip of the iceberg" of the overall DNA damage is measured [93]. An array of methods measuring "potential" DNA damage, in terms of precursors to actual strand breaks, combined with DNA fragmentation assays, may give a more complete picture of the extent of total DNA damage [146]. The predictive value of sperm DNA fragmentation assays could also depend on a variety of other unknown factors such as the extent of DNA damage per sperm, the location of DNA damage in coding or noncoding regions, the association of DNA breaks to other type of DNA lesions and how much sperm DNA damage an oocyte can deal with [16, 45, 62, 64, 146]. Further fundamental research is mandatory to solve these key questions.

Cause-related therapy is almost non-existent in male subfertility. As oxidative damage is considered one of the main, if not the most important, factors underlying the induction of sperm DNA damage, the effects of antioxidant therapy (generally based on antioxidants such as vitamin C, vitamin E, carotene, selenium, zinc, etc.) on sperm DNA quality has been attempted to verify the theoretical possibility of an amelioration of the DNA damage caused by oxidative stress [64, 83, 136, 147–151]. However, the studies have been small and conflicting. Further trials are needed to investigate whether such therapy and other types of causal treatment are effective.

## Conclusions and Clinical Recommendations

It can be concluded that infertile men generally have more sperm DNA damage than fertile men. Studies of both fertile and infertile men have shown that DFI as measured by SCSA is an independent predictor of male subfertility. Despite this, there is no worldwide consensus if sperm chromatin integrity testing should be implemented as a routine in infertility work-up and in ART [59, 62, 64]. Although there seem to be insufficient data to recommend an indiscriminate application of sperm DNA testing, there are specific conditions where men would certainly benefit from this analysis. These could be male partners of couples planning to undergo

ART to evaluate the impact of sperm DNA damage on reproductive outcomes (fertilization, embryo development, pregnancy, miscarriage, post-natal development) and to select which type of ART should be preferable. Also, male partners of couples with unexplained infertility or recurrent pregnancy loss could benefit from SCSA analysis [59].

So far, SCSA is the only method which has demonstrated clear and clinically useful cut-off levels for inferring male infertility potential [96, 108, 122], and its prognostic value in ART has also been shown [11, 129]. The SCSA can be used as a tool to discriminate among the different treatment options, IUI, IVF and ICSI. In men having WHO sperm parameters that indicate ICSI, there are no therapeutic advantages of performing SCSA [11, 129, 151–153]. However, in the group of men with unexplained infertility causes, 40% may have a DFI level that exceeds 20%, and thus the chances of in vivo fertility are reduced [11, 108]. In these men, the SCSA analysis, in adjunct to the standard semen quality parameters, can be valuable to disclose the causes of their infertility. In cases where a traditional semen quality analysis shows one or no abnormality, a SCSA check should be performed as the chance of spontaneous pregnancy is significantly reduced for DFI above 10% [108]. In these "unexplained" infertile couples, provided that female age is <35 years and the duration of infertility is short, IUI should be the treatment of first choice. In long-standing unexplained infertility (>5 years) and a female partner above 35 years, where DFI is above 20%, a direct referral to IVF may be the best alternative [154]. It is worth to stress again the combined impact of both female and male reproductive capability determining the cumulative fertility of a couple. A highly fertile partner can often compensate for a less fertile one. Female factors, not at least age [155] and duration of infertility [154], should always be taken into consideration when evaluating sperm DNA integrity in counselling a couple seeking ART.

Despite the fact that DFI, as other sperm parameters, but to a lesser extent, is subject of intraindividual variation, SCSA analysis was found to be a strong predictor of infertility in vivo [108]. However, in men seeking ART having a DFI above 20%, there is a 27% risk of having a DFI above 30% in the next semen sample, and this could influence the result of the ART-treatment negatively [11]. Thus, these men having a DFI above 20% should have their SCSA analysis repeated close to their ART treatment [121].

Lastly, human studies relating sperm DNA defects to health of the offspring is not yet published. However, successful mammalian reproduction depends partly on the inherent integrity of the sperm DNA, as sperm DNA damage may adversely impact reproductive outcomes. From a clinical long-term perspective, we cannot overlook the message from extensive animal experiments providing unequivocal links between DNA damage in spermatozoa and defects in embryonic development or in the health of the offspring. Therefore, a sort of "precautionary principle" should be adopted deploying all possible strategies aiming at reducing the involvement of defective sperm in the fertilization process. Sperm DNA integrity testing has also demonstrated to be potentially useful beyond the framework of fertility assessment and should be used as an adjunct tool for the sperm quality assessment in andrological pathologies, such as varicocele, cancer and infections, providing precious information on disease severity and therapeutic efficacy.

**Acknowledgements** We wish to thank all the authors whose papers have been quoted and apologize to those whose contributions could not be cited because of lack of space.

# References

1. de Kretser DM. Male infertility. Lancet. 1997;349:787–90.
2. Dunson DB, Baird DD, Colombo B. Increased infertility with age in men and women. Obstet Gynecol. 2004;103:51–6.
3. WHO. WHO manual for the standardised investigation, diagnosis and management of the infertile male. Cambridge: Cambridge University Press; 2000.
4. Skakkebæk NE, Giwercman A, de Kretser D. Pathogenesis and management of male infertility. Lancet. 1994;343:1473–9.
5. World Health Organisation. WHO laboratory manual for examination of human semen and semen-cervical mucus interaction. Cambridge: Cambridge University Press; 1999. p. 1–20.
6. Bonde JP, Ernst E, Jensen TK, Hjøllund NHI, Kolstad H, Henriksen TB, et al. Relation between semen quality and fertility: a population-based study of 430 first-pregnancy planners. Lancet. 1998;352:1172–7.
7. Guzick DS, Overstreet JW, Factor-Litvak P, Brazil CK, Nakajima ST, Coutifaris C, et al. Sperm morphology, motility, and concentration in fertile and infertile men. New Engl J Med. 2001;345:1388–93.
8. Aitken RJ. Sperm function tests and fertility. Int J Androl. 2006;29:69–75.
9. Lewis SE. Is sperm evaluation useful in predicting human fertility? Reproduction. 2007;134:31–40.
10. Agarwal A, Bragais FM, Sabanegh E. Assessing sperm function. Urol Clin North Am. 2008;35:157–71.
11. Bungum M, Humaidan P, Axmon A, Spano M, Bungum L, Erenpreiss J, et al. Sperm DNA integrity assessment in prediction of assisted reproduction technology outcome. Hum Reprod. 2007;22:174–9.
12. Twigg JP, Irvine DS, Aitken RJ. Oxidative damage to DNA in human spermatozoa does not preclude pronucleus formation at intracytoplasmic sperm injection. Hum Reprod. 1998;13:1864–71.
13. Ahmadi A, Ng SC. Fertilizing ability of DNA-damaged spermatozoa. J Exp Zool. 1999;284:696–704.
14. Marchetti F, Essers J, Kanaar R, Wyrobek AJ. Disruption of maternal DNA repair increases sperm-derived chromosomal aberrations. Proc Natl Acad Sci USA. 2007;104:17725–9.
15. Fernández-Gonzalez R, Moreira PN, Pérez-Crespo M, Sánchez-Martín M, Ramirez MA, Pericuesta E, et al. Long-term effects of mouse intracytoplasmic sperm injection with DNA-fragmented sperm on health and behavior of adult offspring. Biol Reprod. 2008;78:761–72.
16. Aitken RJ, De Iuliis GN, McLachlan RI. Biological and clinical significance of DNA damage in the male germ line. Int J Androl. 2009;32:46–56.
17. Marchetti F, Wyrobek AJ. Mechanisms and consequences of paternally-transmitted chromosomal abnormalities. Birth Defects Res C Embryo Today. 2005;75:112–29.
18. Zenzes MT. Smoking and reproduction: gene damage to human gametes and embryos. Hum Reprod Update. 2000;6:122–31.
19. Chang JS. Parental smoking and childhood leukemia. Methods Mol Biol. 2009;472:103–37.
20. Erenpreiss J, Spano M, Erenpreisa J, Bungum M, Giwercman A. Sperm chromatin structure and male fertility: biological and clinical aspects. Asian J Androl. 2006;8:11–29.

21. Evenson DP, Jost LK, Corzett M, Balhorn R. Characteristics of human sperm chromatin structure following an episode of influenza and high fever: a case study. J Androl. 2000;21:739–46.
22. Perry MJ. Effects of environmental and occupational pesticide exposure on human sperm: a systematic review. Hum Reprod Update. 2008;14:233–42.
23. Varghese AC, du Plessis SS, Agarwal A. Male gamete survival at stake: causes and solutions. Reprod Biomed Online. 2008;17:866–80.
24. Wigle DT, Arbuckle TE, Turner MC, Bérubé A, Yang Q, Liu S, et al. Epidemiologic evidence of relationships between reproductive and child health outcomes and environmental chemical contaminants. J Toxicol Environ Health B Crit Rev. 2008;11:373–517.
25. Bonde JP. Male reproductive organs are at risk from environmental hazards. Asian J Androl. 2010;12:152–6.
26. Carrell DT, Emery BR, Hammoud S. The aetiology of sperm protamine abnormalities and their potential impact on the sperm epigenome. Int J Androl. 2008;31:537–45.
27. Matzuk MM, Lamb DJ. The biology of infertility: research advances and clinical challenges. Nat Med. 2008;14:1197–213.
28. O'Flynn O'Brien KL, Varghese AC, Agarwal A. The genetic cause of male factor infertility: a review. Fertil Steril 2010;93:1–12.
29. Ferlin A, Raicu F, Gatta V, Zuccarello D, Palka G, Foresta C. Male infertility: role of genetic background. Reprod Biomed Online. 2007;14:734–45.
30. Jirtle RL, Skinner MK. Environmental epigenomics and disease susceptibility. Nat Rev Genet. 2007;8:253–62.
31. Sasaki H, Matsui Y. Epigenetic events in mammalian germ-cell development: reprogramming and beyond. Nat Rev Genet. 2008;9:129–40.
32. Nanassy L, Carrell DT. Paternal effects on early embryogenesis. J Exp Clin Assist Reprod. 2008;5:2.
33. Carrell DT, Hammoud SS. The human sperm epigenome and its potential role in embryonic development. Mol Hum Reprod. 2010;16:37–47.
34. Miller D, Brinkworth M, Iles D. Paternal DNA packaging in spermatozoa: more than the sum of its parts? Reproduction. 2010;139:287–301.
35. Houshdaran S, Cortessis VK, Siegmund K, Yang A, Laird PW, Sokol RZ. Widespread epigenetic abnormalities suggest a broad DNA methylation erasure defect in abnormal human sperm. PLoS One. 2007;2:e1289.
36. Kobayashi H, Sato A, Otsu E, Hiura H, Tomatsu C, Utsunomiya T, et al. Aberrant DNA methylation of imprinted loci in sperm from oligospermic patients. Hum Mol Genet. 2007;16:2542–51.
37. Filipponi D, Feil R. Perturbation of genomic imprinting in oligozoospermia. Epigenetics. 2009;4:27–30.
38. Bowdin S, Allen C, Kirby G, Brueton L, Afnan M, Barratt C, et al. A survey of assisted reproductive technology births and imprinting disorders. Hum Reprod. 2007;22:3237–40.
39. Doornbos ME, Maas SM, McDonnell J, Vermeiden JP, Hennekam RC. Infertility, assisted reproduction technologies and imprinting disturbances: a Dutch study. Hum Reprod. 2007;22:2476–80.
40. Kobayashi H, Hiura H, John RM, Sato A, Otsu E, Kobayashi N, et al. DNA methylation errors at imprinted loci after assisted conception originate in the parental sperm. Eur J Hum Genet. 2009;17:1582–91.
41. Manipalviratn S, DeCherney A, Segars J. Imprinting disorders and assisted reproductive technology. Fertil Steril. 2009;91:305–15.
42. Evenson DP, Larson KL, Jost LK. Sperm chromatin structure assay: its clinical use for detecting sperm DNA fragmentation in male infertility and comparisons with other techniques. J Androl. 2002;23:25–43.
43. Spanò M, Seli E, Bizzaro D, Manicardi GC, Sakkas D. The significance of sperm nuclear DNA strand breaks on reproductive outcome. Curr Opin Obstet Gynecol. 2005; 17:255–60.

44. Aitken RJ, De Iuliis GN. On the possible origins of DNA damage in human spermatozoa. Mol Hum Reprod. 2010;16:3–13.
45. Sakkas D, Alvarez JG. Sperm DNA fragmentation: mechanisms of origin, impact on reproductive outcome, and analysis. Fertil Steril. 2010;93:1027–36.
46. Chia SE, Tay SK, Lim ST. What constitutes a normal seminal analysis? Semen parameters of 243 fertile men. Hum Reprod. 1998;13:3394–8.
47. Auger J, Eustache F, Andersen AG, Irvine DS, Jorgensen N, Skakkebaek NE, et al. Sperm morphological defects related to environment, lifestyle and medical history of 1001 male partners of pregnant women from four European cities. Hum Reprod. 2001;16:2710–7.
48. Jorgensen N, Andersen AG, Eustache F, Irvine DS, Suominen J, Petersen JH, et al. Regional differences in semen quality in Europe. Hum Reprod. 2001;16:1012–9.
49. Chen Z, Toth T, Godfrey-Bailey L, Mercedat N, Schiff I, Hauser R. Seasonal variation and age-related changes in human semen parameters. J Androl. 2003;24:226–31.
50. Jorgensen N, Asklund C, Carlsen E, Skakkebaek NE. Coordinated European investigations of semen quality: results from studies of Scandinavian young men is a matter of concern. Int J Androl. 2006;29:54–61; discussion 105–8.
51. Neuwinger J, Behre HM, Nieschlag E. External quality control in the andrology laboratory: an experimental multicenter trial. Fertil Steril. 1990;54:308–14.
52. Cooper TG, Neuwinger J, Bahrs S, Nieschlag E. Internal quality control of semen analysis. Fertil Steril. 1992;58:172–8.
53. Baker HWG. Male infertility. Philadelphia: Saunders; 2001.
54. Muller CH. Rationale, interpretation, validation, and uses of sperm function tests. J Androl. 2000;21:10–30.
55. Evenson DP, Wixon R. Clinical aspects of sperm DNA fragmentation detection and male infertility. Theriogenology. 2006;65:979–91.
56. Zini A, Libman J. Sperm DNA damage: importance in the era of assisted reproduction. Curr Opin Urol. 2006;16:428–34.
57. Tarozzi N, Bizzaro D, Flamigni C, Borini A. Clinical relevance of sperm DNA damage in assisted reproduction. Reprod Biomed Online. 2007;14:746–57.
58. Lewis SE, Agbaje IM. Using the alkaline comet assay in prognostic tests for male infertility and assisted reproductive technology outcomes. Mutagenesis. 2008;23:163–70.
59. Zini A, Sigman M. Are tests of sperm DNA damage clinically useful? Pros and cons. J Androl. 2009;30:219–29.
60. Perreault SD, Aitken RJ, Baker HW, Evenson DP, Huszar G, Irvine DS, et al. Integrating new tests of sperm genetic integrity into semen analysis: breakout group discussion. Adv Exp Med Biol. 2003;518:253–68.
61. Aitken RJ, De Iuliis GN. Value of DNA integrity assays for fertility evaluation. Soc Reprod Fertil Suppl. 2007;65:81–92.
62. Barratt CL, Aitken RJ, Björndahl L, Carrell DT, de Boer P, Kvist U, et al. Sperm DNA: organization, protection and vulnerability: from basic science to clinical applications–a position report. Hum Reprod. 2010;25:824–38.
63. Singh NP, Danner DB, Tice RR, McCoy MT, Collins GD, Schneider EL. Abundant alkali-sensitive sites in DNA of human and mouse sperm. Exp Cell Res. 1989;184:461–70.
64. Lewis SE, Agbaje I, Alvarez J. Sperm DNA tests as useful adjuncts to semen analysis. Syst Biol Reprod Med. 2008;54:111–25.
65. Enciso M, Muriel L, Fernández JL, Goyanes V, Segrelles E, Marcos M, et al. Infertile men with varicocele show a high relative proportion of sperm cells with intense nuclear damage level, evidenced by the sperm chromatin dispersion test. J Androl. 2006;27:106–11.
66. Gorczyca W, Traganos F, Jesionowska H, Darzynkiewicz Z. Presence of DNA strand breaks and increased sensitivity of DNA in situ to denaturation in abnormal human sperm cells: analogy to apoptosis of somatic cells. Exp Cell Res. 1993;207:202–5.
67. Mitchell LA, De Iuliis GN, Aitken RJ. The TUNEL assay consistently underestimates DNA damage in human spermatozoa and is influenced by DNA compaction and cell vitality: development of an improved methodology. Int J Androl. 2011;3:2–13.

68. Bianchi PG, Manicardi GC, Bizzaro D, Bianchi U, Sakkas D. Effect of deoxyribonucleic acid protamination on fluorochrome staining and in situ nick-translation of murine and human mature spermatozoa. Biol Reprod. 1993;49:1083–8.

69. Fernández JL, Vázquez-Gundín F, Delgado A, Goyanes VJ, Ramiro-Díaz J, de la Torre J, et al. DNA breakage detection-FISH (DBD-FISH) in human spermatozoa: technical variants evidence different structural features. Mutat Res. 2000;453:77–82.

70. Evenson DP, Darzynkiewicz Z, Melamed MR. Relation of mammalian sperm chromatin heterogeneity to fertility. Science. 1980;210:1131–3.

71. Fernandez JL, Muriel L, Rivero MT, Goyanes V, Vazquez R, Alvarez JG. The sperm chromatin dispersion test: a simple method for the determination of sperm DNA fragmentation. J Androl. 2003;24:59–66.

72. Fernández JL, Muriel L, Goyanes V, Segrelles E, Gosálvez J, Enciso M, et al. Simple determination of human sperm DNA fragmentation with an improved sperm chromatin dispersion test. Fertil Steril. 2005;84:833–42.

73. Erenpreiss J, Bars J, Lipatnikova V, Erenpreisa J, Zalkalns J. Comparative study of cytochemical tests for sperm chromatin integrity. J Androl. 2001;22:45–53.

74. Manicardi GC, Bianchi PG, Pantano S, Azzoni P, Bizzaro D, Bianchi U, et al. Presence of endogenous nicks in DNA of ejaculated human spermatozoa and its relationship to chromomycin A3 accessibility. Biol Reprod. 1995;52:864–7.

75. Zubkova EV, Wade M, Robaire B. Changes in spermatozoal chromatin packaging and susceptibility to oxidative challenge during aging. Fertil Steril. 2005;84:1191–8.

76. Benchaib M, Ajina M, Lornage J, Niveleau A, Durand P, Guerin JF. Quantitation by image analysis of global DNA methylation in human spermatozoa and its prognostic value in in vitro fertilization: a preliminary study. Fertil Steril. 2003;80:947–53.

77. Benchaib M, Braun V, Ressnikof D, Lornage J, Durand P, Niveleau A, et al. Influence of global sperm DNA methylation on IVF results. Hum Reprod. 2005;20:768–73.

78. Leduc F, Nkoma GB, Boissonneault G. Spermiogenesis and DNA repair: a possible etiology of human infertility and genetic disorders. Syst Biol Reprod Med. 2008;54:3–10.

79. Oliva R. Protamines and male infertility. Hum Reprod Update. 2006;12:417–35.

80. Carrell DT, Emery BR, Hammoud S. Altered protamine expression and diminished spermatogenesis: what is the link? Hum Reprod Update. 2007;13:313–27.

81. Sakkas D, Seli E, Bizzaro D, Tarozzi N, Manicardi GC. Abnormal spermatozoa in the ejaculate: abortive apoptosis and faulty nuclear remodelling during spermatogenesis. Reprod Biomed Online. 2003;7:428–32.

82. Delbès G, Hales BF, Robaire B. Toxicants and human sperm chromatin integrity. Mol Hum Reprod. 2010;16:14–22.

83. Kefer JC, Agarwal A, Sabanegh E. Role of antioxidants in the treatment of male infertility. Int J Urol. 2009;16:449–57.

84. Kodama H, Yamaguchi R, Fukuda J, Kasai H, Tanaka T. Increased oxidative deoxyribonucleic acid damage in the spermatozoa of infertile male patients. Fertil Steril. 1997;68:519–24.

85. Shen HM, Chia SE, Ong CN. Evaluation of oxidative DNA damage in human sperm and its association with male infertility. J Androl. 1999;20:718–23.

86. Aitken RJ, De Iuliis GN. Origins and consequences of DNA damage in male germ cells. Reprod Biomed Online. 2007;14:727–33.

87. Fraga CG, Motchnik PA, Wyrobek AJ, Rempel DM, Ames BN. Smoking and low antioxidant levels increase oxidative damage to DNA. Mutat Res. 1996;351:199–203.

88. Sepaniak S, Forges T, Gerard H, Foliguet B, Bene MC, Monnier-Barbarino P. The influence of cigarette smoking on human sperm quality and DNA fragmentation. Toxicology. 2006;223:54–60.

89. Pauli EM, Legro RS, Demers LM, Kunselman AR, Dodson WC, Lee PA. Diminished paternity and gonadal function with increasing obesity in men. Fertil Steril. 2008;90:346–51.

90. Aggerholm AS, Thulstttrup AM, Toft G, Ramlau-Hansen CH, Bonde JP. Is overweight a risk factor for reduced semen quality and altered serum sex hormone profile? Fertil Steril. 2008;90:619–26.

91. Hammoud AO, Wilde N, Gibson M, Parks A, Carrell DT, Meikle W. Male obesity and alterations in sperm parameters. Fertil Steril. 2008;90:2222–5.
92. Chavarro JE, Toth TL, Wright DL, Meeker JD, Hauser R. Body mass index in relation to semen quality, sperm DNA integrity, and serum reproductive hormone levels among men attending an infertility clinic. Fertil Steril. 2009;93:2222–31.
93. Evenson D, Jost L. Sperm chromatin structure assay is useful for fertility assessment. Methods Cell Sci. 2000;22:169–89.
94. Sergerie M, Mieusset R, Croute F, Daudin M, Bujan L. High risk of temporary alteration of semen parameters after recent acute febrile illness. Fertil Steril. 2007;88:970.e1–7.
95. Spanò M, Kolstad AH, Larsen SB, Cordelli E, Leter G, Giwercman A, et al. The applicability of the flow cytometric sperm chromatin structure assay in epidemiological studies. Asclepios. Hum Reprod. 1998;13:2495–505.
96. Spanò M, Bonde JP, Hjøllund HI, Kolstad HA, Cordelli E, Leter G. Sperm chromatin damage impairs human fertility. The Danish First Pregnancy Planner Study Team. Fertil Steril. 2000;73:43–50.
97. Bonde JP, Joffe M, Apostoli P, Dale A, Kiss P, Spano M, et al. Sperm count and chromatin structure in men exposed to inorganic lead: lowest adverse effect levels. Occup Environ Med. 2002;59:234–42.
98. Giwercman A, Richthoff J, Hjøllund H, Bonde JP, Jepson K, Frohm B, et al. Correlation between sperm motility and sperm chromatin structure assay parameters. Fertil Steril. 2003;80:1404–12.
99. Rignell-Hydbom A, Rylander L, Giwercman A, Jönsson BA, Lindh C, Eleuteri P, et al. Exposure to PCBs and p, p'-DDE and human sperm chromatin integrity. Environ Health Perspect. 2005;113:175–9.
100. Wyrobek AJ, Eskenazi B, Young S, Arnheim N, Tiemann-Boege I, Jabs EW, et al. Advancing age has differential effects on DNA damage, chromatin integrity, gene mutations, and aneuploidies in sperm. Proc Natl Acad Sci USA. 2006;103:9601–6.
101. Evenson DP, Jost LK, Baer RK, Turner TW, Schrader SM. Individuality of DNA denaturation patterns in human sperm as measured by the sperm chromatin structure assay. Reprod Toxicol. 1991;5:115–25.
102. Sun JG, Jurisicova A, Casper RF. Detection of deoxyribonucleic acid fragmentation in human sperm: correlation with fertilization in vitro. Biol Reprod. 1997;56:602–7.
103. De Jonge C, LaFromboise M, Bosmans E, Ombelet W, Cox A, Nijs M. Influence of the abstinence period on human sperm quality. Fertil Steril. 2004;82:57–65.
104. Kühnert B, Nieschlag E. Reproductive functions of the ageing male. Hum Reprod Update. 2004;10:327–39.
105. Moskovtsev SI, Willis J, Mullen JB. Age-related decline in sperm deoxyribonucleic acid integrity in patients evaluated for male infertility. Fertil Steril. 2006;85:496–9.
106. Belloc S, Benkhalifa M, Junca AM, Dumont M, Bacrie PC, Ménézo Y. Paternal age and sperm DNA decay: discrepancy between chromomycin and aniline blue staining. Reprod Biomed Online. 2009;19:264–9.
107. Sartorius GA, Nieschlag E. Paternal age and reproduction. Hum Reprod Update. 2010;16:65–79.
108. Giwercman A, Lindstedt L, Larsson M, Bungum M, Spano M, Levine RJ, et al. Sperm chromatin structure assay as an independent predictor of fertility in vivo: a case-control study. Int J Androl. 2010;33:e221–7.
109. Zini A, Bielecki R, Phang D, Zenzes MT. Correlations between two markers of sperm DNA integrity, DNA denaturation and DNA fragmentation, in fertile and infertile men. Fertil Steril. 2001;75:674–7.
110. Apedaile AE, Garrett C, Liu DY, Clarke GN, Johnston SA, Baker HW. Flow cytometry and microscopic acridine orange test: relationship with standard semen analysis. Reprod Biomed Online. 2004;8:398–407.
111. Trisini AT, Singh NP, Duty SM, Hauser R. Relationship between human semen parameters and deoxyribonucleic acid damage assessed by the neutral comet assay. Fertil Steril. 2004;82:1623–32.

112. Cohen-Bacrie P, Belloc S, Ménézo YJ, Clement P, Hamidi J, Benkhalifa M. Correlation between DNA damage and sperm parameters: a prospective study of 1,633 patients. Fertil Steril. 2009;91:1801–5.
113. de Jager C, Aneck-Hahn NH, Bornman MS, Farias P, Leter G, Eleuteri P, et al. Sperm chromatin integrity in DDT-exposed young men living in a malaria area in the Limpopo Province, South Africa. Hum Reprod. 2009;24:2429–38.
114. Moskovtsev SI, Willis J, White J, Mullen JB. Sperm DNA damage: correlation to severity of semen abnormalities. Urology. 2009;74:789–93.
115. Richthoff J, Spano M, Giwercman YL, Frohm B, Jepson K, Malm J, et al. The impact of testicular and accessory sex gland function on sperm chromatin integrity as assessed by the sperm chromatin structure assay (SCSA). Hum Reprod. 2002;17:3162–9.
116. Meeker JD, Singh NP, Hauser R. Serum concentrations of estradiol and free T4 are inversely correlated with sperm DNA damage in men from an infertility clinic. J Androl. 2008;29:379–88.
117. Keel BA. Within- and between-subject variation in semen parameters in infertile men and normal semen donors. Fertil Steril. 2006;85:128–34.
118. Zini A, Kamal K, Phang D, Willis J, Jarvi K. Biologic variability of sperm DNA denaturation in infertile men. Urology. 2001;58:258–61.
119. Sergerie M, Mieusset R, Daudin M, Thonneau P, Bujan L. Ten-year variation in semen parameters and sperm deoxyribonucleic acid integrity in a healthy fertile man. Fertil Steril. 2006;86:1513.e11–8.
120. Sergerie M, Laforest G, Boulanger K, Bissonnette F, Bleau G. Longitudinal study of sperm DNA fragmentation as measured by terminal uridine nick end-labelling assay. Hum Reprod. 2005;20:1921–7.
121. Erenpreiss J, Bungum M, Spano M, Elzanaty S, Orbidans J, Giwercman A. Intra-individual variation in sperm chromatin structure assay parameters in men from infertile couples: clinical implications. Hum Reprod. 2006;21:2061–4.
122. Evenson DP, Jost LK, Marshall D, Zinaman MJ, Clegg E, Purvis K, et al. Utility of the sperm chromatin structure assay as a diagnostic and prognostic tool in the human fertility clinic. Hum Reprod. 1999;14:1039–49.
123. Evenson DP, Wixon R. Data analysis of two in vivo fertility studies using sperm chromatin structure assay-derived DNA fragmentation index vs. pregnancy outcome. Fertil Steril. 2008;90:1229–31.
124. Loft S, Kold-Jensen T, Hjollund NH, Giwercman A, Gyllemborg J, Ernst E, et al. Oxidative DNA damage in human sperm influences time to pregnancy. Hum Reprod. 2003;18:1265–72.
125. Zini A, Fischer MA, Sharir S, Shayegan B, Phang D, Jarvi K. Prevalence of abnormal sperm DNA denaturation in fertile and infertile men. Urology. 2002;60:1069–72.
126. Saleh RA, Agarwal A, Nelson DR, Nada EA, El-Tonsy MH, Alvarez JG, et al. Increased sperm nuclear DNA damage in normozoospermic infertile men: a prospective study. Fertil Steril. 2002;78:313–8.
127. Verit FF, Verit A, Kocyigit A, Ciftci H, Celik H, Koksal M. No increase in sperm DNA damage and seminal oxidative stress in patients with idiopathic infertility. Arch Gynecol Obstet. 2006;274:339–44.
128. Erenpreiss J, Elzanaty S, Giwercman A. Sperm DNA damage in men from infertile couples. Asian J Androl. 2008;10:786–90.
129. Bungum M, Humaidan P, Spano M, Jepson K, Bungum L, Giwercman A. The predictive value of sperm chromatin structure assay (SCSA) parameters for the outcome of intrauterine insemination, IVF and ICSI. Hum Reprod. 2004;19:1401–8.
130. Saleh RA, Agarwal A, Sharma RK, Said TM, Sikka SC, Thomas Jr AJ. Evaluation of nuclear DNA damage in spermatozoa from infertile men with varicocele. Fertil Steril. 2003;80:1431–6.
131. Smith R, Kaune H, Parodi D, Madariaga M, Rios R, Morales I, et al. Increased sperm DNA damage in patients with varicocele: relationship with seminal oxidative stress. Hum Reprod. 2006;21:986–93.

132. Blumer CG, Fariello RM, Restelli AE, Spaine DM, Bertolla RP, Cedenho AP. Sperm nuclear DNA fragmentation and mitochondrial activity in men with varicocele. Fertil Steril. 2008;90:1716–22.
133. Zini A, Blumenfeld A, Libman J, Willis J. Beneficial effect of microsurgical varicocelectomy on human sperm DNA integrity. Hum Reprod. 2005;20:1018–21.
134. Werthman P, Wixon R, Kasperson K, Evenson DP. Significant decrease in sperm deoxyribonucleic acid fragmentation after varicocelectomy. Fertil Steril. 2008;90:1800–4.
135. Nasr-Esfahani MH, Abasi H, Razavi S, Ashrafi S, Tavalaee M. Varicocelectomy: semen parameters and protamine deficiency. Int J Androl. 2009;32:115–22.
136. Moskovtsev SI, Lecker I, Mullen JB, Jarvi K, Willis J, White J, et al. Cause-specific treatment in patients with high sperm DNA damage resulted in significant DNA improvement. Syst Biol Reprod Med. 2009;55:109–15.
137. Gallegos G, Ramos B, Santiso R, Goyanes V, Gosálvez J, Fernández JL. Sperm DNA fragmentation in infertile men with genitourinary infection by *Chlamydia trachomatis* and *Mycoplasma*. Fertil Steril. 2008;90:328–34.
138. Perera D, Pizzey A, Campbell A, Katz M, Porter J, Petrou M, et al. Sperm DNA damage in potentially fertile homozygous beta-thalassaemia patients with iron overload. Hum Reprod. 2002;17:1820–5.
139. Brackett NL, Ibrahim E, Grotas JA, Aballa TC, Lynne CM. Higher sperm DNA damage in semen from men with spinal cord injuries compared with controls. J Androl. 2008;29: 93–9.
140. Agbaje IM, McVicar CM, Schock BC, McClure N, Atkinson AB, Rogers D, et al. Increased concentrations of the oxidative DNA adduct 7,8-dihydro-8-oxo-2-deoxyguanosine in the germ-line of men with type 1 diabetes. Reprod Biomed Online. 2008;16:401–9.
141. Kobayashi H, Larson K, Sharma RK, Nelson DR, Evenson DP, Toma H, et al. DNA damage in patients with untreated cancer as measured by the sperm chromatin structure assay. Fertil Steril. 2001;75:469–75.
142. Ståhl O, Eberhard J, Cavallin-Ståhl E, Jepson K, Friberg B, Tingsmark C, et al. Sperm DNA integrity in cancer patients: the effect of disease and treatment. Int J Androl. 2009;32: 695–703.
143. Evenson D, Wixon R. Meta-analysis of sperm DNA fragmentation using the sperm chromatin structure assay. Reprod Biomed Online. 2006;12:466–72.
144. Sergerie M, Laforest G, Bujan L, Bissonnette F, Bleau G. Sperm DNA fragmentation: threshold value in male fertility. Hum Reprod. 2005;20:3446–51.
145. Tsarev I, Bungum M, Giwercman A, Erenpreisa J, Ebessen T, Ernst E, et al. Evaluation of male fertility potential by Toluidine Blue test for sperm chromatin structure assessment. Hum Reprod. 2009;24:1569–74.
146. Alvarez JG. The predictive value of sperm chromatin structure assay. Hum Reprod. 2005;20:2365–7.
147. Greco E, Iacobelli M, Rienzi L, Ubaldi F, Ferrero S, Tesarik J. Reduction of the incidence of sperm DNA fragmentation by oral antioxidant treatment. J Androl. 2005;26:349–53.
148. Greco E, Romano S, Iacobelli M, Ferrero S, Baroni E, Minasi MG, et al. ICSI in cases of sperm DNA damage: beneficial effect of oral antioxidant treatment. Hum Reprod. 2005;20:2590–4.
149. Silver EW, Eskenazi B, Evenson DP, Block G, Young S, Wyrobek AJ. Effect of antioxidant intake on sperm chromatin stability in healthy nonsmoking men. J Androl. 2005;26:550–6.
150. Song GJ, Norkus EP, Lewis V. Relationship between seminal ascorbic acid and sperm DNA integrity in infertile men. Int J Androl. 2006;29:569–75.
151. Gandini L, Lombardo F, Paoli D, Caruso F, Eleuteri P, Leter G, et al. Full-term pregnancies achieved with ICSI despite high levels of sperm chromatin damage. Hum Reprod. 2004;19:1409–17.
152. Virro MR, Larson-Cook KL, Evenson DP. Sperm chromatin structure assay (SCSA) parameters are related to fertilization, blastocyst development, and ongoing pregnancy in in vitro fertilization and intracytoplasmic sperm injection cycles. Fertil Steril. 2004;81:1289–95.

153. Ménézo YJ, Hazout A, Panteix G, Robert F, Rollet J, Cohen-Bacrie P, et al. Antioxidants to reduce sperm DNA fragmentation: an unexpected adverse effect. Reprod Biomed Online. 2007;14:418–21.
154. Hull MG, Glazener CMA, Kelly NJ, Conway DI, Foster PA, Hinton RA, et al. Population study of causes, treatment, and outcome of infertility. BMJ. 1985;291:1693–7.
155. Hull MG, Fleming CF, Hughes AO, McDermott A. The age-related decline in female fecundity: a quantitative controlled study of implanting capacity and survival of individual embryos after in vitro fertilization. Fertil Steril. 1996;65:783–90.
156. Schmid TE, Eskenazi B, Baumgartner A, Marchetti F, Young S, Weldon R, et al. The effects of male age on sperm DNA damage in healthy non-smokers. Hum Reprod. 2007;22:180–7.
157. Chohan KR, Griffin JT, Lafromboise M, De Jonge CJ, Carrell DT. Comparison of chromatin assays for DNA fragmentation evaluation in human sperm. J Androl. 2006;27:53–9.
158. O'Flaherty C, Vaisheva F, Hales BF, Chan P, Robaire B. Characterization of sperm chromatin quality in testicular cancer and Hodgkin's lymphoma patients prior to chemotherapy. Hum Reprod. 2008;23:1044–52.
159. Ståhl O, Eberhard J, Jepson K, Spano M, Cwikiel M, Cavallin-Ståhl E, et al. Sperm DNA integrity in testicular cancer patients. Hum Reprod. 2006;21:3199–205.
160. Zhang LH, Qiu Y, Wang KH, Wang Q, Tao G, Wang LG. Measurement of sperm DNA fragmentation using bright-field microscopy: comparison between sperm chromatin dispersion test and terminal uridine nick-end labeling assay. Fertil Steril. 2010;94:1027–32.
161. Domínguez-Fandos D, Camejo MI, Ballescà JL, Oliva R. Human sperm DNA fragmentation: correlation of TUNEL results as assessed by flow cytometry and optical microscopy. Cytom A. 2007;71:1011–8.
162. Plastira K, Msaouel P, Angelopoulou R, Zanioti K, Plastiras A, Pothos A, et al. The effects of age on DNA fragmentation, chromatin packaging and conventional semen parameters in spermatozoa of oligoasthenoteratozoospermic patients. J Assist Reprod Genet. 2007;24:437–43.
163. Bian Q, Xu LC, Wang SL, Xia YK, Tan LF, Chen JF, et al. Study on the relation between occupational fenvalerate exposure and spermatozoa DNA damage of pesticide factory workers. Occup Environ Med. 2004;61:999–1005.
164. De Iuliis GN, Thomson LK, Mitchell LA, Finnie JM, Koppers AJ, Hedges A, et al. DNA damage in human spermatozoa is highly correlated with the efficiency of chromatin remodeling and the formation of 8-hydroxy-2'-deoxyguanosine, a marker of oxidative stress. Biol Reprod. 2009;81:517–24.
165. Tavalaee M, Razavi S, Nasr-Esfahani MH. Influence of sperm chromatin anomalies on assisted reproductive technology outcome. Fertil Steril. 2009;91:1119–26.
166. Høst E, Lindenberg S, Smidt-Jensen S. DNA strand breaks in human spermatozoa: correlation with fertilization in vitro in oligozoospermic men and in men with unexplained infertility. Acta Obstet Gynecol Scand. 2000;79:189–93.
167. Gandini L, Lombardo F, Paoli D, Caponecchia L, Familiari G, Verlengia C, et al. Study of apoptotic DNA fragmentation in human spermatozoa. Hum Reprod. 2000;15:830–9.
168. Pant N, Shukla M, Kumar Patel D, Shukla Y, Mathur N, Kumar Gupta Y, et al. Correlation of phthalate exposures with semen quality. Toxicol Appl Pharmacol. 2008; 231:112–6.
169. Hammadeh ME, Zeginiadov T, Rosenbaum P, Georg T, Schmidt W, Strehler E. Predictive value of sperm chromatin condensation (aniline blue staining) in the assessment of male fertility. Arch Androl 2001;46:99–104.

# Chapter 7
# Aging and Sperm DNA Damage

**Fábio F. Pasqualotto and Eleonora B. Pasqualotto**

It has become more socially acceptable to delay fatherhood, but the heritable consequences of this trend remain poorly understood. Approximately 15% of couples of
reproductive age experience infertility, and approximately 1/3 to half of infertility
cases may be attributed to male factors [1]. It is well known that maternal age is a
significant contributor to human infertility [2], primarily due to the precipitous loss
of functional oocytes in women by their late 30s [3]. Human spermatogenesis, on
the contrary, continues well into advanced ages, allowing men to reproduce during
senescence. Although very little is known about the topic, paternal age may also
contribute to human infertility.

It is well known that practically no children are born to mothers aged >50 years
and it is common to all older fathers that they have younger partners. The discrepancy in the reproductive arena between males and females is astonishing, and
reduced fertility and higher reproductive risks associated with advancing maternal
age raise the question whether advanced paternal age is also associated with compromised fertility and increasing risks. In addition, it is well documented that
because of a progressive decrease of fertility due to both quantitative and qualitative
loss of oocytes, eventually ending in menopause, women experience an age-
dependent increase of miscarriages, obstetric morbidities, and chromosomal anomalies of the fetus [4]. This question should be discussed with younger age groups,
since increasing numbers of couples postpone parenthood into their fourth or fifth
decade of life.

F.F. Pasqualotto, MD, PhD (✉)
Department of Urology, University of Caxias do Sul,
Rua Pinheiro Machado, 2569, sl 23/24,
Bairro São Pelegrino, Caxias do Sul, RS, Brazil
e-mail: fabio@conception-rs.com.br

E.B. Pasqualotto, MD, PhD
Department of Gynecology, University of Caxias do Sul,
Caxias do Sul, RS, Brazil

A. Zini, A. Agarwal (eds.), *Sperm Chromatin for the Clinician*,
© Springer Science+Business Media New York 2013

In contrast to the female, male reproductive functions do not cease abruptly, but androgen production and spermatogenesis continue lifelong. However, evaluating a possible decline in the semen quality is a little bit difficult. Some men are reluctant to provide semen samples unless actively concerned about their fertility. For instance, population-based studies typically recruit at least 20% of young men willing to provide semen samples [5], constituting an inevitable participation bias in such studies [6, 7]. In addition, most of the published studies on sperm output in older men are largely restricted to patients attending infertility clinics, where few are older than 50 years [8]. An uncertain, but probably high, proportion of such men have unrecognized defects in sperm production and/or function. Furthermore, access to such specialized medical services may be strongly influenced by nonbiological factors, and the results from infertility clinics may not be reliably extrapolated to the general male population.

Anyway, the effects of paternal age on a couple's fertility are real and may be greater than have previously been thought. Ford et al. [9] stated that, after adjustments for other factors, the probability that a fertile couple will take >12 months to conceive nearly doubles from 8% when the man is <25 years to 15% when he is >35 years; thus, paternal age is a further factor to be taken into account when deciding the prognosis of infertile couples. It has been demonstrated that in men between 26 and 59 years of age and who undergo IVF or ICSI treatment, the rising age is detrimental to sperm DNA integrity and ejaculate volume [10]. Furthermore, Dutch men showed a significantly poorer sperm quality based on a higher DFI compared to migrants. In fact, the age-related decrease in sperm quality below 59 years of age – based on increased sperm DNA damage and decreased ejaculate volume – suggests that delaying childbearing, not only in women but also in men, contributes to a reduced reproductive capacity. The significantly higher DFI in Dutch men compared to migrants could not be explained by differences in age and the most prominent unhealthy lifestyles.

To explain the age-dependent changes observed in semen quality, two issues should be considered [8–12]. First, cellular or physiological changes due to aging have been described in testicles, seminal vesicles, prostate, and epididymis. Age-related narrowing and sclerosis of the testicular tubular lumen, decreases in spermatogenic activity, increased degeneration of germ cells, and decreased numbers and function of Leydig cells have been found in autopsies of men who died from accidental causes [13]. Smooth muscle atrophy and a decrease in protein and water content, which occur in the prostate with aging, may contribute to decreased semen volume and sperm motility. Also, the epididymis, a hormonally sensitive tissue, may undergo age-related changes. The hormonal or epididymal senescence may lead to decreased motility in older men. Second, increasing age implies more frequent exposure to exogenous damage or disease [8]. In addition to age per se, factors such as urogenital infections, vascular diseases, or an accumulation of toxic substances (cigarettes) may be responsible for worsening semen parameters. Indeed, a retrospective cross-sectional study in 3,698 infertile men showed an infection rate of the accessory glands in 6.1% in patients aged <25 years but in 13.6% of patients

>40 years, and total sperm counts were significantly lower in patients with an infection of the accessory glands [14]. In addition, an age-dependent increase of polychlorinated biphenyls (PBC) in men has been described, and in men with normal semen parameters, the PBC concentration is inversely correlated with sperm count and progressive motility [15]. The concentration of cadmium also increases with age in the human testis, epididymis, and prostate, although lead and selenium remain constant over the whole age range in the reproductive organs [16, 17].

Handelsman and Staraj [18] demonstrated that after exclusion of men with different diseases associated with diminishing testicular size, the specific effects of age on testicular volume appears only in the eighth decade of life. In healthy men of this age group, the testis volume is 31% lower than in 18–40-year-old men [19]. However, recently a study has shown a decline in testicular volume over time, specifically, after the age of 45 [20].

Morphological characteristics of aging testes varies from Sertoli cells accumulating cytoplasmic lipid droplets to the cells with reduced number of the droplets [21], as are the Leydig cells [22], which may also be multinucleated [23]. Tubule involution is associated with an enlargement of the tunica propria, leading to progressive sclerosis parallel to a reduction of the seminiferous epithelium with complete tubular sclerosis as an end point [24]. Testicular sclerosis is associated with defective vascularization of the testicular parenchyma and with systemic arteriosclerosis of affected men [25]. Arteriographic patterns of the epididymis and the testes support these findings and are correlated with the degree of systemic arteriosclerosis [25]. In addition, age-dependent alterations of the prostate are well known [26] and are detectable histologically in 50% of 50 year-old men, but in 90% of men aged >90 years [27].

## Semen Analysis

Considering the age-dependent changes in reproductive organs of men, variations in semen parameters over time are not surprising; however, only few studies are controlled for abstinence time and other possible factors that may influence semen quality such as hypertension or smoking habits. Most studies are retrospective and rarely include males with more than 60 or 70 years old. Pasqualotto et al. [20] have recently described a decrease in semen volume across the groups evaluated in the study. In fact, reports in the literature have shown a decrease in semen volume with aging [8, 28, 29]. The higher number of days' abstinence in men over 50 years old could explain these results. In the studies where the analyses were adjusted for abstinence days, a decrease in semen volume of 3–22% was observed [9].

Regarding sperm motility, many studies adjusted for time of abstinence found a significant decrease in sperm motility associated with age and a yearly decrease ranging between 0.17 [30] and 0.7% [31]. However, these studies were performed in sperm donors [30–33] as well as infertile patients [34, 35]. Pasqualotto et al. are on the same page as others showing that sperm motility tends to decrease over time. Those studies that have been adjusted for duration of abstinence have reported statistically significant effects, such as negative linear relationships and decreases in motility ranging from 0.17 to 0.6% for each year of age [8, 30, 36, 37].

Computer-assisted semen analysis (CASA) has been developed as a specific tool to make the assessment of semen quality more objective and detailed [38]. Several specific motility parameters describing the movements of spermatozoa in a more detailed manner can be obtained with CASA. In addition, the classification into motile and immotile spermatozoa can be based on well-defined velocity thresholds. However, no correlations are detected between specific motion parameters as evaluated with CASA and the aging effect in the study by Pasqualotto et al. [20].

When focusing on sperm concentration, abstinence-adjusted studies do not provide a uniform picture. Even though some studies have reported a decrease in sperm concentration with increased age, several other studies have reported an increase in sperm concentration with age or found little or no association between age and sperm concentration [9, 12, 36, 39]. In fact, there are two different populations that we have to be considered before evaluating the results: fertile vs. infertile men. A significant age-dependent decrease [31, 33] as well as constant values over the age range [32] or even a nonsignificant age-dependent increase with age [30] has been detected in healthy men. Regarding the infertile population, sperm concentration increases [34, 35] or remains unaltered [14], as indicated in abstinence-adjusted studies.

One of the good indicators of the germinal epithelium status is the sperm morphology. Degenerative changes in the germinal epithelium because of aging may affect spermatogenesis and, thus, sperm morphology. Pasqualotto et al. [20], based on a linear regression analysis, stated that normal sperm morphology tends to decrease by 0.039% each year. Auger et al. [33], in a linear regression model, have shown that the normal sperm morphology decreases 0.9% yearly. Thus, as compared to an average 30-year-old man, an average 50-year-old man had a 18% decrease in normally shaped sperm [34]. Ng et al. [29] showed that older men had more abnormal sperm morphology with decreasing numbers of normal forms and reduced vitality, as well as increased numbers of cytoplasmic droplets and sperm tail abnormalities (30% vs. 17%) compared to younger men. The aberrant sperm morphology in older men was most evident in defects of tail morphology, possibly reflecting the complex cellular structural assembly process of the axoneme. Such increasing proportion of defects may reflect degenerative changes with aging in the germinal epithelium and/or in the intrinsic program directing spermiogenesis. In fact, the decrease per year varies from 0.2 [37] to 0.9% [33].

All reported changes of histological and seminal parameters develop gradually without a sudden age threshold. The alterations in semen parameters fall within normal ranges. Nevertheless, the age-dependent alterations of testicular histology and semen parameters are accompanied by a significant increase in FSH [20, 40] and a slight but significant decrease in inhibin B [19, 41], which are also found in men with apparently normal semen parameters.

# Fertility of Aging Men

Without any type of doubt, male fertility is basically maintained until very late in life, and it has been documented scientifically up to more than 90 years of age [42]. Besides female age, further confounders, such as reduced coital frequency, an increasing incidence of erectile dysfunction, and smoking habits have to be considered in studies analyzing male fertility. All studies focused on a nonclinical population found a significant negative relationship between male age and couples' fertility.

A retrospective study of a large sample of European couples analyzed the risk of difficulties (due to adverse pregnancy outcome, such as ectopic pregnancy, miscarriage, or stillbirth, or due to delayed conception) and the risk of delay in pregnancy onset [43]. Age-related changes were also found in a prospective study that estimated day-specific probabilities for pregnancy relative to ovulation [44]. Frequency of sexual intercourse was monitored by sexual diaries, and ovulation was based on basal body temperature measurements. According to this study, fertility for men aged >35 years is significantly reduced and the age effect of men aged 35–40 years is about the same as when intercourse frequency drops from twice per week to once per week [45]. In studies dealing with subfertile couples, a significant decrease in pregnancy rates [34] or an increase in TTP [46] was observed with female, but not with male, age, possibly indicating that male age-dependent alterations are masked by the infertility as such.

With methods of assisted reproduction, prerequisites for natural conception such as motility or fertilizing capacity are circumvented. In fact, the more invasive the treatment, the less important male age appears. Therefore, the success rates of ISCI [47] or IVF [48–50] are not associated with male age. On the contrary, the success rate of intrauterine insemination (IUI), a method requiring much higher quality and capability of sperm, is without question related to male age [51, 52].

## *Genetic Risks of the Aging Male*

A maternal age effect has been found for all trisomy conditions but varies among chromosomes, with an exponential increase in chromosome 21 and a linear increase, for instance, in chromosome 16 [53]. Early observations also associate paternal age with certain syndromes [54]. Meanwhile, it has become evident that some mutations, consisting of single-base substitutions in three different genes, namely, RET, FGFR2 (fibroblast growth factor receptor 2), and FGFR3 (fibroblast growth factor receptor 3), are exclusively of paternal origin and may increase with male age [55].

A possible explanation for this male-specific age effect is the much higher number of germ cell divisions in males than in females: in the fetal ovary, germ cells undergo 22 mitotic divisions before they enter the meiotic prophase [56]. They remain in meiotic arrest and continue meiosis in adulthood when ovulation has taken place. Thus, while it was formerly believed that in women germ cell divisions are completed before birth, a recent publication has suggested that adult mouse ovaries still possess mitotically active germ cells [57].

On the contrary, male germ cells divide continuously. It has been estimated that 30 spermatogonial stem cell divisions take place before puberty, when they begin to undergo meiotic divisions. From then on, 23 mitotic divisions per year occur, result- ing in 150 replications by the age of 20 years and 840 replications by the age of 50 years [55]. Therefore, due to these numerous divisions of stem cells, older men may have an increased risk of errors in DNA transcription. Consequently, the association between elevated paternal age and serious birth defects is the reason why the age of semen donors is limited to 40 years in certain countries [58, 59]. On the contrary, male age is not an indicator for prenatal diagnosis.

## Numerical Chromosome Disorders

Aneuploidy, the presence of an extra or missing chromosome, is the leading genetic cause of pregnancy loss. Aneuploidies are detected in 35% of spontaneous abortions, in 4% of stillbirths, and in 0.3% of live births [60]. Among spontaneous abortions, Turner's syndrome (45,X) and trisomy 16, 21, and 22 are the most prev- alent aneuploidies. In general, aneuploidies arise by the process of nondisjunction, for instance, the failure of paired chromosomes to separate in the first meiotic divi- sion of maternal meiosis [61, 62]. Sperm reveal an aneuploidy incidence of 2% with a high variability of disomy frequency of individual sperm from different fluorescence in situ hybridization (FISH) studies [61]. The disomy frequency was calculated to be 0.26% for the sex chromosomes and 0.15% for the autosomes with an exception for chromosomes 14, 21, and 22, which display higher disomy frequencies [63].

Studies analyzing the age-dependent alteration of aneuploidy frequency in chro- mosomes are highly limited due to low case numbers. Interestingly, the age- dependent increase of XY disomy was also detected in sperm from fathers of boys with Klinefelter's syndrome [64], irrespective of paternal or maternal inheritance of the extra X chromosome [31]. Fifty percent of Klinefelter's syndrome cases are of paternal origin, and other gonosomal aneuploidies are even more often paternally inherited in live births, as are 80% of Turner's syndrome cases (45,X) and 100% of XYY karyotypes [65, 66]. However, none of these syndromes are related to paternal age [67]. Similarly, the incidence of autosomal aneuploidies, such as trisomy 13, 16, and 18, is independent of paternal age [66, 68]. Therefore, the paternal age effect for trisomy 21 remains to be elucidated.

Early studies with small sample sizes reflect different results in the same study population depending on the method of statistical analysis [68, 69]. In spontaneous abortions, a nonsignificant paternal age effect was detected [66], and in live births, no age effect [70, 71] or a significant paternal age effect [72, 73] was evident. It should be kept in mind that only 10% of Down's syndrome patients receive the excess chromosome from their father [74], so an age effect could be confined to this small category of cases and subtle age effects might go undetected unless those derived paternally are considered separately. However, with respect to paternally inherited Down's syndrome cases, no paternal age effect became evident [75]. Paternal age effect was seen in association with a maternal age lower than 35 years, so a paternal age effect in aged couples can no longer be neglected concerning trisomy 21, whereas other autosomal or sex chromosomal aneuploidies are not associated with increased paternal age [72].

## Structural Chromosomal Anomalies

Structural chromosomal anomalies result from chromosomal breakage and the following abnormal rearrangement within the same or within different chromosomes. In 84% of cases, de novo structural aberrations are of paternal origin [76], and they are found in 2% of spontaneous abortions and in 0.6% of live births [77]. Cytogenetic studies on structural chromosomal anomalies in sperm are rare but consistently describe an increase of mutations with age [78].

FISH was used for the structural analysis of individual chromosomes: duplications and deletions for the centromeric and subtelomeric regions of chromosome 9 increase significantly with age [79]. In spite of these age-dependent structural alterations in sperm, no increase of de novo structural chromosomal anomalies has been detected in newborns of older fathers [74].

## Autosomal Dominant Diseases

There is a direct relationship between paternal aging and offspring development. Considerable evidence shows a connection between aging and offspring learning and cognition.

Achondroplasia, the most common form of dwarfism, is the first genetic disorder that was hypothesized to have a paternal age component [55]. Apert's syndrome and achondroplasia have been amenable to direct sperm DNA mutation analysis [80, 81], and both are characterized by an age-dependent increase of mutations in sperm, but there are some peculiarities. For sporadic cases of Crouzon's or Pfeiffer's syndrome, 11 different mutations of the FGFR2 gene are responsible, indicating that, unlike Apert's syndrome or achondroplasia, these are genetically heterogeneous conditions [82]. These mutations also arise in the male germ line, and advanced paternal age was noted for fathers of those patients.

The relationship between mutation frequency and paternal age is heterogeneous among autosomal dominantly inherited diseases [83]. In contrast to the above-mentioned diseases, osteogenesis imperfecta, neurofibromatosis, or bilateral retinoblastoma shows a weak paternal age effect [84]. This may be due to the fact that a significant fraction of new mutations is not base substitutions [55]. Many of the mutations of the neurofibromatosis gene are intragenic deletions. These deletions are not age-dependent because they occur by mechanisms other than the base substitutions and are maternally derived in 16 of 21 cases [85].

Owing to this heterogeneity of the paternal age effect in autosomal dominant diseases, the risk estimates proposed by Friedman for paternal age and autosomal dominant mutations may be overestimated [86]. Friedman calculated a risk for autosomal dominant diseases of 0.3–0.5% among offspring of fathers aged >40 years. This risk is comparable with the risk of Down's syndrome for 35–40 year old women. However, the calculation was based on the assumption that the paternal age effect found in achondroplasia is typical of all autosomal dominant diseases.

There are conflicting are the data for Alzheimer's disease. Few studies conclude that paternal age is a risk factor [87]. However, the inconsistent results may be due to small sample sizes of the studies or due to the genetic heterogeneity of the disease.

Regarding schizophrenia, there are more conclusive data. In fact, the studies identified an increased risk of schizophrenia with paternal age [88]. Patients without a family history of schizophrenia had significantly older fathers than familial patients, so de novo mutations were considered responsible [89]. Preeclampsia, which is considered to be a risk factor for schizophrenia, is also associated with paternal age [90].

A recent study, by using 1997–2004 data from the National Birth Defects Prevention Study, has performed a logistic regression models with paternal and maternal age as continuous variables while adjusting for demographic and other factors. They demonstrated elevated odds ratios (ORs) for each year increase in paternal age in the following congenital malformation: cleft palate (OR, 1.02, 95% confidence interval [95% CI], 1.00–1.04), diaphragmatic hernia (OR, 1.04; 95% CI, 1.02–1.06), right ventricular outflow tract obstruction (OR, 1.03; 95% CI, 1.01–1.04), and pulmonary valve stenosis (OR, 1.02, 95% CI, 1.01–1.04). At younger paternal ages, each year increase in paternal age correlated with increased OR of having offspring with encephalocele, cataract, esophageal atresia, anomalous pulmonary venous return, and coarctation of the aorta, but these increased ORs were not observed at older paternal ages. The effect of paternal age was modified by maternal age for gastroschisis, omphalocele, spina bifida, all orofacial clefts, and septal heart defects. This study suggested that paternal age may be a risk factor for some multifactorial birth defects [91].

One very important point we should never forget is that advanced paternal age increases the risk of other cancers in offspring. According to the Swedish Family-Cancer Database, there is an effect of paternal age on the incidence of sporadic breast and sporadic nervous system cancer in offspring [92]. Interestingly, an association between paternal age and the son's risk of prostate cancer was found [93]. The association of paternal age with early-onset prostate cancer (<65 years) was greater than that with late-onset prostate cancer. In fact, older men are having children, but the reality of a male biological clock makes this trend worrisome [94].

# Sperm DNA Damage

Sperm chromatin and DNA integrity is essential to ensure that the fertilizing sperm can support normal embryonic development of the zygote. To better inform treatment pathways and, more importantly, to ensure a generation of healthy children from assisted reproductive technologies (ART), we urgently require tests of sperm function, including the normalcy of sperm DNA, that provide high quality and robust diagnostic and prognostic information.

Understanding the effects of male age on sperm DNA damage is especially relevant for men attending reproductive clinics because of the increasing reliance on modern technologies, especially among marginally fertile older men. ICSI and IVF enhance the probability of achieving fatherhood, yet they also circumvent the natural barriers against fertilization by damaged sperm.

Schmid et al. [95] demonstrated an association between male age and sperm DNA strand damage in a nonclinical sample of active healthy nonsmoking workers and retirees. Sperm of older men had significantly higher frequencies of sperm with DNA damage measured under alkaline conditions, which is thought to represent alkali labile DNA sites and single-strand DNA breaks. However, age was not associated with sperm DNA damage under neutral conditions, which is thought to represent double-strand DNA breaks. The observations of differential effects of age on genomic damage is consistent with the recent finding of Wyrobek et al. [96] who reported age-related effects on DNA fragmentation and achondroplasia mutations, but not on aneuploidy, Apert syndrome mutations, or sex ratio.

The finding of age-related increases in DNA strand damage under alkaline conditions is consistent with the findings of Morris [97] who studied 60 men participating in an IVF program. They reported that sperm DNA damage was positively correlated with donor age and with impairment of postfertilization embryo cleavage following ICSI, indicating an overall decline in the integrity of sperm DNA in older men. The findings by Schmid et al. of no association between age and sperm DNA damage under neutral conditions are in contrast with the study of Singh et al. [98] who studied 66 men, aged 20–57 years, from an infertility clinic and a nonclinical group. However, Singh et al. [98] did not investigate sperm DNA damage under alkaline conditions in sperm, and Morris [97] did not investigate sperm damage under neutral conditions. Using a different assay for measuring DNA strand damage in sperm, the SCSA, Spano et al. [99] found a strong association of DFI with age among men 18–55 year olds, a finding confirmed by Wyrobek et al. [96] using a larger group of men that spanned 20–80 years of age.

Older men may produce more sperm with DNA damage as a consequence of age-associated increased oxidative stress in their reproductive tracts [100, 101]. Oxidative stress can damage sperm DNA as well as mitochondrial and nuclear membranes [102, 103]. Kodama et al. [103] reported an association between oxidative DNA damage in sperm and male infertility. Alternatively, apoptotic functions of spermatogenesis may be less effective in older males resulting in the release of more sperm with DNA damage [104, 105]. While apoptosis has been identified in the testes of elderly men [104], there have been no comparisons on rates of apoptosis among men of different ages. Increased sperm DNA damage has been associated with chromosomal abnormalities, developmental loss, and birth defects in mouse model systems [106, 107] and with increases in the percentage of human embryos that failed to develop after ICSI [97].

Increasing oxidative stress levels associated with aging might be responsible for this increase in DNA damage with age. Oxidative stress-mediated DNA damage may be an etiology for repeated ART failures in older men. Increasing male age may have an influence on DNA fragmentation in the form of single-strand breaks. This may not have any effect on fertilization because the oocyte can repair single-strand breaks. However, if the oocyte repair mechanisms are dysfunctional, this may result in poor, if not failed, blastocyst formation. Thus, oxidative stress-induced DNA damage can lead to various genomic defects [108].

## Oxidative Stress and Aging

Mitochondria play an important role in cellular energy generation, apoptosis regulation, and calcium homeostasis [109]. Coupled to the tricarboxylic acid cycle, the electron transport chain (ETC) and adenosine triphosphate (ATP) synthase in the mitochondria generate ATP, a source of most cellular energy. Since reactive oxygen species (ROS) are continually produced in the mitochondria of spermatozoa, they play an important role in age-related male reproductive pathophysiology.

Mitochondria are more susceptible to oxidative damage because of the active production of ROS, as mtDNA is not protected by histones. Consequently, mitochondrial ROS production damages the mitochondria themselves. Mutations or deletions in mtDNA lead to defects in oxidative phosphorylations, defective cellular calcium dyshomeostasis, and other related mtDNA diseases. A dysfunctional mitochondrial respiratory chain would lead to more ROS production. Oxidative damage is more prevalent in mtDNA and protein in vivo than in other cell components.

The increased ROS level in semen observed with aging is associated with a possible decrease in antioxidant enzyme activity. This imbalance between prooxidants and antioxidants induces oxidative damage, resulting in abnormalities in telomeres and telomerase in sperm cells [110–112]. This sequence of events may explain the decrease in sperm concentration seen with aging. ROS-induced telomere shortening may be due to direct injury to guanine repeat telomere DNA by ROS. The addition of an antioxidant suppresses the rate of telomere shortening in somatic cells. The telomere shortening rate slowed after enrichment by ascorbic acid, a strong antioxidant. The rate of telomere shortening in sheep and humans is directly related to the cellular oxidative stress levels [109].

Oxidative stress in aging male reproductive system may inhibit sperm axonemal phosphorylation and increase lipid peroxidation, which can decrease sperm motility. This oxidative stress can also lead to lipofuscin and amyloid accumulation in the male reproductive tract, potentially the cause of decreased Leydig cell function and a subsequent decrease in blood testosterone levels. A higher rate of lipofuscin accumulation in turn may increase the amount of dysfunctional mitochondria in spermatozoa, thus increasing ROS formation. Along with its negative effect on the fertilizing potential of spermatozoa, ROS also leads to offspring malformation (if fertilization is successful). Oxidative stress-induced mtDNA damage and nuclear DNA damage in aging men may put them at a higher risk for transmitting multiple genetic and chromosomal defects [109].

Therefore, ROS might play a central role in decreased male fertility with aging. This hypothesis provides guidance for future study and experiments, focusing on specific biomarkers of aging in men (telomere function, lipofuscin, amyloid) and their comparison with semen parameters and male fertility.

## Conclusion

Couples are waiting longer to have children, and advances in reproductive technology are allowing older men and women to consider having children. The lack of appreciation among both medical professionals and the lay public for the reality of a male biological clock makes these trends worrisome. The age-related changes associated with the male biological clock affect sperm quality, fertility, hormone levels, and a lot of nonreproductive physiological issues. Although based on a small number of cases, the data presented for testicular morphology, semen parameters, and fertility in aging males are conclusive and reflect a gradual deterioration with age within a broad individual spectrum. Most studies suggest that reduced fertility begins to become evident in the late 30s in men. Increased male age is associated with an increased risk of miscarriages, and both the risk of infertility and the risk of miscarriage strongly depend on female age. Advancing paternal age is associated with an increased risk for trisomy 21 and with diseases of complex etiology such as schizophrenia.

Advanced paternal age increases the risk for spontaneous abortion as well as genetic abnormalities in offspring due to multiple factors, including DNA damage from abnormal apoptosis and ROS. Older men considering parenthood should have a thorough history and physical examination focused on their sexual and reproductive capacity. Such examination should entail disclosure of any sexual dysfunction and the use of medications, drugs, or lifestyle factors that might impair fertility or sexual response.

Couples should be aware of these age-dependent alterations in fertility and predisposition to genetic risks. Although at the moment increased paternal age is not an indication for prenatal diagnosis, there may be further developments in the future.

# References

1. Templeton A. Infertility – epidemiology, aetiology and effective management. Health Bull (Edinb). 1995;53(5):294–8.
2. Joffe M, Li Z. Male and female factors in fertility. Am J Epidemiol. 1995;141(11):1107–8.
3. Lansac J. Delayed parenting. Is delayed childbearing a good thing? Hum Reprod. 1995;10(5): 1033–5.
4. Lubna P, Santoro N. Age-related decline in fertility. Endocrinol Metab Clin N Am. 2003; 32:669–88.
5. Jensen TK, Jorgensen N, Punab M, Haugen TB, Suominen J, Zilaitiene B, et al. Association of in utero exposure to maternal smoking with reduced semen quality and testis size in adulthood: a cross-sectional study of 1770 young men from the general population in five European countries. Am J Epidemiol. 2004;159:49–58.
6. Handelsman DJ. Sperm output of healthy men in Australia: magnitude of bias due to self-selected volunteers. Hum Reprod. 1997;12:2701–5.
7. Cohn BA, Overstreet JW, Fogel RJ, Brazil CK, Baird DD, Cirillo PM. Epidemiologic studies of human semen quality: considerations for study design. Am J Epidemiol. 2002;155: 664–71.
8. Kidd SA, Eskenazi B, Wyrobek AJ. Effects of male age on semen quality and fertility: a review of the literature. Fertil Steril. 2001;75:237–48.
9. Ford WCL, North K, Taylor H, Farrow A, Hull MGR, Golding J and the ALSPAC Study Team. Increasing paternal age is associated with delayed conception in a large population of fertile couples: evidence for declining fecundity in older men. Hum Reprod. 2000;15:1703–8.
10. Hammiche F, Laven JSE, Boxmeer JC, Dohle GR, Steegers EAP, Steegers-Theunissen RPM. Sperm quality decline among men below 60 years of age undergoing IVF or ICSI treatment. J Androl. 2011;32(1):70–6.
11. Eskenazi B, Wyrobek AJ, Sloter E, Kidd SA, Moore L, Young S, et al. The association of age and semen quality in healthy men. Hum Reprod. 2003;18:447–54.
12. Hassan MAM, Killick SR. Effect of male age on fertility: evidence for the decline in male fertility with increasing age. Fertil Steril. 2003;79:1520–7.
13. Neaves WB, Johnson L, Porter JC, Parker CR, Petty S. Leydig cell numbers, daily sperm production and serum gonadotropin levels in aging men. J Clin Endocrinol Metab. 1984;59: 756–63.
14. Rolf C, Kenkel S, Nieschlag E. Age-related disease pattern in infertile men: increasing incidence of infections in older patients. Andrologia. 2002;34:209–17.
15. Dallinga JW, Moonen EJ, Dumoulin JC, Evers JL, Geraedts JP, Kleinjans JC. Decreased human semen quality and organochlorine compounds in blood. Hum Reprod. 2002;17: 1973–99.
16. Oldereid NB, Thomassen Y, Attramadal A, Olaisen B, Purvis K. Concentrations of lead, cadmium and zinc in the tissues of reproductive organs of men. J Reprod Fertil. 1993;99:421–55.
17. Oldereid NB, Thomassen Y, Purvis K. Selenium in human male reproductive organs. Hum Reprod. 1998;13:2172–6.
18. Handelsman DJ, Staraj S. Testicular size: the effects of aging, malnutrition, and illness. J Androl. 1985;6:144–51.
19. Mahmoud AM, Goemaere S, El-Garem Y, Van Pottelbergh I, Comhaire FH, Kaufman JM. Testicular volume in relation to hormonal indices of gonadal function in community-dwelling elderly men. J Clin Endocrinol Metab. 2003;88:179–84.
20. Pasqualotto FF, Sobreiro BP, Hallak J, Pasqualotto EB, Lucon AM. Sperm concentration and normal sperm morphology decrease and follicle-stimulating hormone level increases with age. BJU Int. 2005;96:1087–91.
21. Harbitz TB. Morphometric studies of the Sertoli cells in elderly men with special reference to the histology of the prostate. Acta Pathol Microbiol Scand A Pathol. 1973;81:703–17.
22. Johnson L. Spermatogenesis and aging in the human. J Androl. 1986;7:331–54.

23. Paniagua R, Amat P, Nistal M, Martin A. Ultrastructure of Leydig cells in human ageing testes. J Anat. 1986;146:173–83.
24. Paniagua R, Nistal M, Amat P, Rodriguez MC, Martin A. Seminiferous tubule involution in elderly men. Biol Reprod. 1987;36:939–47.
25. Regadera J, Nistal M, Paniagua R. Testis, epididymis, and spermatic cord in elderly men. Correlation of angiographic and histologic studies with systemic arteriosclerosis. Arch Pathol Lab Med. 1985;109:663–7.
26. Hermann M, Untergasser G, Rumpold H, Berger P. Aging of the male reproductive system. Exp Gerontol. 2000;35:1267–79.
27. Coffey DS, Berry SJ, Ewing LL. An overview of current concepts in the study of benign prostate hyperplasia. In: Rodgers CH, Coffey DS, Cunha G, Grayhack JT, Hinman F, Horton R, editors. Benign prostatic hyperplasia, vol II. NIH publication No. 87-2881; 1987. p. 1–13.
28. Kühnert B, Nieschlag E. Reproductive functions of the ageing male. Hum Reprod Update. 2004;10:327–39.
29. Ng KK, Donat R, Chan L, Lalak A, Di Pierro I, Handelsman DJ. Sperm output of older men. Hum Reprod. 2004;8:1811–5.
30. Fisch H, Goluboff ET, Olson JH, Feldshuh J, Broder SJ, Barad DH. Semen analysis in 1,283 men from the United States over a 25-year period: no decline in quality. Fertil Steril. 1996;65:1009–14.
31. Eskenazi B, Wyrobek AJ, Kidd SA, Lowe X, Moore II D, Weisiger K, et al. Sperm aneuploidy in fathers of children with paternally and maternally inherited Klinefelter syndrome. Hum Reprod. 2002;17:576–83.
32. Schwartz D, Mayaux MJ, Spira A, Moscato ML, Jouannet P, Czyglik F, et al. Semen characteristics as a function of age in 833 fertile men. Fertil Steril. 1983;39:530–5.
33. Auger J, Kunstmann JM, Czyglik F, Jouannet P. Decline in semen quality among fertile men in Paris during the past 20 years. N Engl J Med. 1995;332:281–5.
34. Rolf C, Behre HM, Nieschlag E. Reproductive parameters of older couples compared to younger men of infertile couples. Int J Androl. 1996;19:135–42.
35. Andolz P, Bielsa MA, Vila J. Evolution of semen quality in North-eastern Spain: a study in 22 759 infertile men over a 36 year period. Hum Reprod. 1999;14:731–5.
36. Berling S, Wolner-Hanssen P. No evidence of deteriorating semen quality among men in infertile relationships during the last decade: a study of males from southern Sweden. Hum Reprod. 1997;12:1002–5.
37. Carlsen E, Giwercman A, Keiding N, Skakkebaek NE. Evidence for decreasing quality of semen during past 50 years. BMJ. 1992;305:609–13.
38. Agarwal A, Ozturk E, Loughlin KR. Comparison of semen analysis between the two Hamilton-Thorn semen analysers. Andrologia. 1992;24:327–9.
39. Hommonai ZT, Fainman N, David MP, Paz GF. Semen quality and sex hormone pattern of 29 middle aged men. Andrologia. 1982;14:164–70.
40. Nieschlag E, Lammers U, Freischem CW, Langer K, Wickings EJ. Reproductive functions in young fathers and grandfathers. J Clin Endocrinol Metab. 1982;55:676–81.
41. Baccarelli A, Morpurgo PS, Corsi A, Vaghi I, Fanelli M, Cremonesi G, et al. Activin A serum levels and aging of the pituitary–gonadal axis: a cross-sectional study in middle-aged and elderly healthy subjects. Exp Gerontol. 2001;36:1403–12.
42. Seymour FI, Duffy C, Koerner A. A case of authenticated fertility in a man, aged 94. J Am Med Assoc. 1935;105:1423–4.
43. de la Rochebrochard E, Thonneau P. Paternal age and maternal age are risk factors for miscarriage; results of a multicentre European study. Hum Reprod. 2002;17:1649–56.
44. Dunson DB, Colombo B, Baird D. Changes with age in the level and duration of fertility in the menstrual cycle. Hum Reprod. 2002;17:1399–403.
45. Dunson DB, Baird DD, Colombo B. Increased infertility with age in men and women. Obstet Gynecol. 2004;103:51–6.
46. Olson J. Subfecundity according to the age of the mother and the father. Dan Med Bull. 1990;37:281–2.

47. Spandorfer SD, Avrech OM, Colombero LT, Palermo GD, Rosenwaks Z. Effect of parental age on fertilization and pregnancy characteristics in couples treated by intracytoplasmic sperm injection. Hum Reprod. 1998;13:334–8.
48. Piette C, de Mouzon J, Bachelot A, Spira A. In-vitro fertilization: influence of women's age on pregnancy rates. Hum Reprod. 1990;5:56–9.
49. Gallardo E, Simón C, Levy M. Effect of age on sperm fertility potential: oocyte donation as a model. Fertil Steril. 1996;66:260–4.
50. Paulson RJ, Milligan RC, Sokol RZ. The lack of influence of age on male fertility. Am J Obstet Gynecol. 2001;184:818–22.
51. Mathieu C, Ecochard R, Bied V, Lornage J, Czyba JC. Cumulative conception rate following intrauterine artificial insemination with husband's spermatozoa: influence of husband's age. Hum Reprod. 1995;10:1090–7.
52. Brzechffa PR, Buyalos RP. Female and male partner age and menotrophin requirements influence pregnancy rates with human menopausal gonadotrophin therapy in combination with intrauterine insemination. Hum Reprod. 1997;12:29–33.
53. Wyrobek AJ, Aardema M, Eichenlaub-Ritter U, Ferguson L, Marchetti F. Mechanisms and targets involved in maternal and paternal age effects on numerical aneuploidy. Environ Mol Mutagen. 1996;28:254–64.
54. Penrose LS. Parental age and mutation. Lancet. 1955;269:312–3.
55. Crow JF. The origins, patterns and implications of human spontaneous mutation. Nat Rev Genet. 2000;1:40–7.
56. Drost JB, Lee WR. Biological basis of germline mutation: comparisons of spontaneous germ-line mutation rates among drosophila, mouse, and human. Environ Mol Mutagen. 1995;25 Suppl 26:48–64.
57. Johnson J, Canning J, Kaneko T, Pru JK, Tilly JL. Germline stem cells and follicular renewal in the postnatal mammalian ovary. Nature. 2004;428:145–50.
58. American Society for Reproductive Medicine. Guidelines for therapeutic donor insemination: sperm. Fertil Steril. 1998;70 Suppl 3:1S–3.
59. British Andrology Society. British Andrology Society guidelines for the screening of semen donors for donor insemination. Hum Reprod. 1999;14:1823–6.
60. Hassold T, Hunt P. To err (meiotically) is human: the genesis of human aneuploidy. Nat Rev Genet. 2001;2:280–91.
61. Griffin DK. The incidence, origin, and etiology of aneuploidy. Int Rev Cytol. 1996;167: 263–96.
62. Eichenlaub-Ritter U. Parental age-related aneuploidy in human germ cells and offspring: a story of past and present. Environ Mol Mutagen. 1996;28:211–36.
63. Shi Q, Martin RH. Aneuploidy in human sperm: a review of the frequency and distribution of aneuploidy, effects of donor age and lifestyle factors. Cytogenet Cell Genet. 2000;90: 219–26.
64. Lowe X, Eskenazi B, Nelson DO, Kidd S, Alme A, Wyrobek AJ. Frequency of XY sperm increases with age in fathers of boys with Klinefelter syndrome. Am J Hum Genet. 2001;69:1046–54.
65. Lorda-Sanchez I, Binkert F, Maechler M, Robinson WP, Schinzel AA. Reduced recombination and paternal age effect in Klinefelter syndrome. Hum Genet. 1992;89:524–30.
66. Hatch M, Kline J, Levine B, Hutzler M, Wartburton D. Paternal age and trisomy among spon-taneous abortions. Hum Genet. 1990;85:355–61.
67. Bordson BL, Leonardo VS. The appropriate upper age limit for semen donors: a review of the genetic effects of paternal age. Fertil Steril. 1991;56:397–401.
68. Stene E, Stene J, Stengel-Rutkowski S. A reanalysis of the New York State prenatal diagnosis data on Down's syndrome and paternal age effects. Hum Genet. 1987;77:299–302.
69. Hook EB, Cross PK. Paternal age and Down's syndrome genotypes diagnosed prenatally: no association in New York state data. Hum Genet. 1982;62:167–74.
70. de Michelena MI, Burstein E, Lama JR, Vasquez JC. Paternal age as a risk factor for Down syndrome. Am J Med Genet. 1993;45:679–82.

71. Stoll C, Alembik Y, Dott B, Roth MP. Study of Down syndrome in 238 942 consecutive births. Ann Génét. 1998;41:44–51.
72. Fisch H, Hyun G, Golden R, Hensle TW, Olsson CA, Liberson GL. The influence of paternal age on Down syndrome. J Urol. 2003;169:2275–8.
73. McIntosh GC, Olshan AF, Baird PA. Paternal age and the risk of birth defects in offspring. Epidemiology. 1995;6:282–8.
74. Hassold T, Sherman S. Down syndrome: genetic recombination and the origin of the extra chromosome 21. Clin Genet. 2000;57:95–100.
75. Hook EB, Regal RR. A search for a paternal-age effect upon cases of 47, þ 21 in which the extra chromosome is of paternal origin. Am J Hum Genet. 1984;36:413–21.
76. Olsen SD, Magenis RE. Preferential paternal origin of de novo structural chromosome rearrangements. In: Daniel A, editor. The cytogenetics of mammalian autosomal rearrangements. New York: Alan R. Liss; 1988. p. 583–99.
77. Jacobs PA. The chromosome complement of human gametes. Oxf Rev Reprod Biol. 1992;14:47–72.
78. Sartorelli EM, Mazzucatto LF, de Pina-Neto JM. Effect of paternal age on human sperm chromosomes. Fertil Steril. 2001;76:1119–23.
79. Bosch M, Rajmil O, Martinez-Pasarell O, Egozcue J, Templado C. Linear increase of diploidy in human sperm with age: a four-colour FISH study. Eur J Hum Genet. 2001;9:533–8.
80. Glaser RL, Broman KW, Schulman RL, Eskenazi B, Wyrobek AJ, Jabs EW. The paternal-age effect in Apert syndrome is due, in part, to the increased frequency of mutations in sperm. Am J Hum Genet. 2003;73:939–47.
81. Goriely A, McVean GA, Rojmyr M, Ingemarsson B, Wilkie AO. Evidence for selective advantage of pathogenic FGFR2 mutations in the male germ line. Science. 2003;301:643–6.
82. Glaser RL, Jiang W, Boyadjiev SA, Tran AK, Zachary AA, Van Maldergem L, et al. Paternal origin of FGFR2 mutations in sporadic cases of Crouzon syndrome and Pfeiffer syndrome. Am J Hum Genet. 2000;66:768–77.
83. Risch N, Reich EW, Wishnick MM, McCarthy JG. Spontaneous mutation and parental age in humans. Am J Hum Genet. 1987;41:218–48.
84. Sivakumaran TA, Ghose S, Kumar HAS, Kucheria K. Parental age in Indian patients with sporadic hereditary retinoblastoma. Ophthalmic Epidemiol. 2000;7:285–91.
85. Lazaro C, Gaona A, Ainsworth P, Tenconi R, Vidaud D, Kruyer H, et al. Sex differences in the mutation rate and mutational mechanism in the NF gene in neurofibromatosis type 1 patients. Hum Genet. 1996;98:696–9.
86. Friedman JM. Genetic disease in the offspring of older fathers. Obstet Gynecol. 1981; 57:745–9.
87. Bertram L, Busch R, Spiegl M, Lautenschlager NT, Müller U, Kurz A. Paternal age is a risk factor for Alzheimer disease in the absence of a major gene. Neurogenetics. 1998;1:277–80.
88. Dalman C, Allebeck P. Paternal age and schizophrenia: further support for an association. Am J Psychiatry. 2002;159:1591–2.
89. Malaspina D, Corcoran C, Fahim C, Berman A, Harkavy-Friedman J, Yale S, et al. Paternal age and sporadic schizophrenia: evidence for de novo mutations. Am J Med Genet. 2002;114:299–303.
90. Green RF, Devine O, Crider KS, Olney RS, Archer N, Olshan AF, Shapira SK, National Birth Defects prevention study. Association of paternal age and risk for major congenital anomalies from the National Birth Defects Prevention Study, 1997 to 2004. Ann Epidemiol. 2010; 20(3):241–9.
91. Harlap S, Paltiel O, Deutsch L, Knaanie A, Masalha S, Tiram E, et al. Paternal age and pre-eclampsia. Epidemiology. 2002;13:660–7.
92. Hemminki K, Kyyronen P. Parental age and risk of sporadic and familial cancer in offspring: implications for germ cell mutagenesis. Epidemiology. 1999;10:747–51.
93. Zhang Y, Kreger BE, Dorgan JF, Cupples LA, Myers RH, Splansky GL, et al. Parental age at child's birth and son's risk of prostate cancer. The Framingham Study. Am J Epidemiol. 1999;150:1208–12.

94. Fisch H. Older men are having children, but the reality of a male biological clock makes this trend worrisome. Geriatrics. 2009;64(1):14–7.
95. Schmid TE, Eskenazi B, Baumgartner A, Marchetti F, Young S, Weldon R, et al. The effects of male age on sperm DNA damage in healthy non-smokers. Hum Reprod. 2007;22(1): 180–7.
96. Wyrobek AJ, Evenson D, Arnheim N, Jabs EW, Young S, Pearson F, et al. Advancing male age increase the frequencies of sperm with DNA fragmentation and certain gene mutations, but not aneuploidies or diploidies. Proc Natl Acad Sci USA. 2006;103(25):9601–6.
97. Morris ID. Sperm DNA damage and cancer treatment. Int J Androl. 2002;25(5):255–61.
98. Singh NP, Muller CH, Berger RE. Effects of age on DNA doublestrand breaks and apoptosis in human sperm. Fertil Steril. 2003;80(6):1420–30.
99. Spano M, Kolstad AH, Larsen SB, Cordelli E, Leter G, Giwercman A, et al. The applicability of the flow cytometric sperm chromatin structure assay in epidemiological studies. Hum Reprod. 1998;13(9):2495–505.
100. Barnes CJ, Hardman WE, Maze GL, Lee M, Cameron IL. Age-dependent sensitization to oxidative stress by dietary fatty acids. Aging (Milano). 1998;10(6):455–62.
101. Barroso G, Morshedi M, Oehninger S. Analysis of DNA fragmentation, plasma membrane translocation of phosphatidylserine and oxidative stress in human spermatozoa. Hum Reprod. 2000;15(6):1338–44.
102. Aitken RJ, Baker MA, Sawyer D. Oxidative stress in the male germ line and its role in the aetiology of male infertility and genetic disease. Reprod Biomed Online. 2003;7(1):65–70.
103. Kodama H, Yamaguchi R, Fukuda J, Kasai H, Tanaka T. Increased oxidative deoxyribonucleic acid damage in the spermatozoa of infertile male patients. Fertil Steril. 1997;68(3): 519–24.
104. Brinkworth MH, Weinbauer GF, Bergmann M, Nieschlag E. Apoptosis as a mechanism of germ cell loss in elderly men. Int J Androl. 1997;20(4):222–8.
105. Print CG, Loveland KL. Germ cell suicide: new insights into apoptosis during spermatogenesis. Bioessays. 2000;22(5):423–30.
106. Marchetti F, Lowe X, Bishop J, Wyrobek J. Induction of chromosomal aberrations in mouse zygotes by acrylamide treatment of male germ cells and their correlation with dominant lethality and heritable translocations. Environ Mol Mutagen. 1997;30:410–7.
107. Marchetti F, Bishop JB, Cosentino L, Moore II D, Wyrobek AJ. Paternally transmitted chromosomal aberrations in mouse zygotes determine their embryonic fate. Biol Reprod. 2004;70:616–24.
108. Barratt CLR, Aitken J, Bjorndahl L, Carrell DT, de Boer P, Kvist U, et al. Sperm DNA: organization, protection and vulnerability: from basic science to clinical applications – a position report. Hum Reprod. 2010;25(4):824–38.
109. Desai N, Sabanegh Jr E, Kim T, Agarwal A. Free radical theory of aging: implications in male infertility. Urology. 2010;75(1):14–9.
110. Pasqualotto FF, Sharma RK, Nelson DR, Thomas Jr AJ, Agarwal A. Relationship between oxidative stress, semen characteristics and clinical diagnosis in men undergoing infertility investigation. Fertil Steril. 2000;73:459–64.
111. Pasqualotto FF, Sharma RK, Kobayashi H, Nelson DR, Thomas Jr AJ, Agarwal A. Oxidative stress in normospermic men undergoing fertility evaluation. J Androl. 2001;22:316–22.
112. Sharma RK, Pasqualotto FF, Nelson DR, Thomas Jr AJ, Agarwal Jr A. ROS-TAC is a novel marker of oxidative stress. Hum Reprod. 1999;14:2801–7.

# Chapter 8
# Cancer in Males: Implications for Sperm Quality, Fertility, and Progeny Outcome

Peter Chan and Bernard Robaire

Recent epidemiological studies indicate that there is a worldwide rise in the incidence of many cancers that affect boys and young men [1–3]. Simultaneously, with the advances in medical technology for early detection of cancer and the improvement in the efficacy of cancer therapies, the survival rates of many of these cancer patients have improved dramatically in the past decades. Many of young cancer survivors have not started or completed forming a family. Thus, the impact of cancer and cancer therapies on male reproductive health and the options for fertility preservation are important issues in survivorship for young cancer patients.

In this chapter, we first provide an overview of the epidemiology of cancers in boys and young men of reproductive age with an emphasis on the various issues that arise in the management and counseling of these patients. The biological data on the impact of chemotoxic cancer therapies on sperm chromatin structures are reviewed. Finally, we present fertility preservation and restoration strategies that are currently clinically available and under development for patients in the near future.

## Epidemiology of Cancer in Boys and Young Men

Common cancers in men that receive most attention in the public media include lung, colon, prostate, skin, and liver cancers. These cancers, however, tend to affect men who have passed the reproductive age. For boys and young men, the common cancers include testis cancer, lymphomas, leukemia, sarcoma, and brain cancers.

P. Chan, MD (✉)
Department of Surgery, McGill University and the Research Institute of the MUHC, Montréal, QC, Canada
e-mail: mcgillsperminator@yahoo.com

B. Robaire, PhD
Department Pharmacology and Therapeutics, Department of Obstetrics and Gynecology, McGill University, Montréal, QC, Canada

A. Zini, A. Agarwal (eds.), *Sperm Chromatin for the Clinician*,
© Springer Science+Business Media New York 2013

The incidence of childhood cancer worldwide has been steadily increasing over the past 50 years [1–3]. With an estimated cumulative incidence of 1,720 per million, equivalent to a risk of 1 in 581, childhood cancer is indeed one of the leading causes of death among children younger than 15 years of age [4, 5]. According to recent data from the National Cancer Institute of USA [4], 10,400 children were newly diagnosed with cancer in 2007. Interestingly, boys were affected 1.2 times more frequently than girls [6].

Fortunately, thanks to tremendous strides in cancer management, including early detection strategies and advances in various treatment modalities such as surgeries, radiation, and combination chemotherapy regimens, the survival rates of many childhood cancers have increased dramatically over the past 40 years [7, 8]. In particular, testis cancer, which is the most commonly diagnosed solitary cancer in young men between the ages of 18 and 35 years [9], has a 5-year survival rate of over 90%, even in cases with metastasis, making testis cancer one of the most curable malignancies.

Approximately half of childhood cancers are hematologic malignancies (leukemia and lymphoma) with an anticipated long-term survival greater than 75%. Improvements in prognosis and survival rates have also been observed for many other childhood malignancies, including Wilm's tumor, malignant bone tumors, and rhabdomyosarcomas. The latest statistics in Canada indicate that the relative 5-year survival rate for all childhood cancers combined is approximately 82% [3]. It is estimated that today in North America approximately 1 in 900 of the population aged 20–45 years is a childhood cancer survivor [10]. In Canada, this translates to approximately 10,000 people who are survivors of childhood cancer and are expected to have 70 years or more of life after successful treatment [11].

## Fertility After Cancer Therapy

While many of these young cancer survivors can expect a good quality of life, they may also face a series of undesired consequences related to their cancer and cancer therapies. Impairment in reproductive health is a well-known complication of cancer therapy; it occurs in a significant proportion of cancer survivors due to the spermatotoxicity of cancer treatments such as chemotherapy and radiation therapy. Many young cancer survivors have not initiated or completed forming a family. Interestingly, surveys indicated that almost 80% of childless cancer survivors report the desire to have children and believe that their experience of surviving cancer will make them better parents [12–14].

For the majority of cancer survivors who desire to have children but have poor sperm quantity and quality, assisted reproductive technologies (ART), including in vitro fertilization (IVF) and intracytoplasmic sperm injection (ICSI), are sought to help them to father their own children [15]. While ART is becoming more popular and available, and our knowledge and experience in its efficacy and safety have expanded tremendously in recent years, it does carry significant risks, including an increased risk of congenital malformations, genetic anomalies, low birth weight, and multiple pregnancies [16–19]. Health-care professionals counseling cancer patients and survivors must be prepared to provide them with precise and up-to-date options on postcancer fertility.

## Cancer Management Strategies

Generally, cancer management involves three major modalities, namely, surgery, radiation, and chemotherapy. The choice of treatment depends on the nature and stage of the cancer and the comorbidity of the subject. Not uncommonly, a combination of these modalities in various orders may be required to achieve optimal cancer control. Complications of each modality also vary. Mechanisms of how each treatment modality may potentially compromise male reproductive health are discussed in this section.

### Reproductive Health Before Cancer Treatment

It should be pointed out that the reproductive health of many cancer patients may be suboptimal even before receiving specific cancer therapies, as revealed by studies on the sperm density and morphology of prechemotherapy sperm banked samples and on case–control studies of their natural fecundity [20–23]. The reason for the impaired fertility status may, in part, be due to the decline in the physical state (poor nutrition, fever, cachexia, pain, etc.) of the patients due to cancer. The psychosocial stress attributed to the cancer diagnosis may play a role in the well-being of the subject. Prolonged periods of sexual abstinence may also contribute to the poor sperm quality before chemotherapy. In testis cancer, poor sperm profile may be explained by the fact that there is only one remaining contralateral noncancerous testis to produce sperm. Indeed, some studies have shown that the contralateral noncancerous testis may have compromised reproductive function due to a higher risk of coexisting intraepithelial germ cell tumors and abnormal spermatogenesis, both quantitatively and qualitatively [24].

Using a complementary panel of molecular genetic assays, including the AO/SCSA®, TUNEL, and comet assays to determine sperm DNA damage and mBBr-SH labeling and the CMA3 assay to assess chromatin packaging, we have recently reported that, prior to chemotherapy, 37% of men with testis cancer and 81% of men with Hodgkin's lymphoma demonstrated abnormal sperm chromatin structure despite having normal sperm density and motility [23]. Our findings suggest that with subsequent cytotoxic cancer therapy, their sperms are at risk for further genetic damage.

## Impact of Surgical Management for Cancer on Male Reproductive Status

The purpose of surgical resection of tumor is to remove the tumor with adequate surgical margins to aim for cure or to debulk the volume of tumor to facilitate the effect of adjuvant therapy with radiation or chemotherapy and thus control the cancer. A common surgical management for testicular cancer in young males is radical orchiectomy. Removal of one testis may affect the total spermatogenic activity in an individual. Indeed, men with testis cancer are at risk of having decreased spermatogenic activity in the contralateral testis.

Other surgical managements for cancers in young males may result in damage to the autonomic nervous system required for semen emission. Pelvic and lower intestine surgeries, retroperitoneal lymph node dissection for advanced testicular cancer, or any procedures involving the spine and other parts of the central nervous system may result in postoperative anejaculation. Despite the fact that spermatogenic function is generally not affected in these patients, they are at risk of having impaired fertility due to the absence of semen emission.

Although it is well established in several animal models, including the monkey, that compensatory hypertrophy of the remaining testis occurs in the adult when one testis is removed prior to puberty [25–27], in human subjects, clinical studies indicate that this occurs only to a limited extent [28, 29] and is insufficient to compensate for the loss of one testis.

## Radiation Therapy

Germ cells and somatic cells in testes are prone to damage post radiation. The usual clinical dosage of radiation therapy for cancer ranges from 0.2 to 70 Gy, depending on the nature, stage, and anatomical location of the tumor. A cumulative dosage of 2.5–6 Gy directly to the testes may permanently damage germ cells, leading to prolonged or permanent azoospermia [30]. Even for radiation therapy outside the pelvic areas (e.g., paraaortic lymph nodes) with gonadal shielding to reduce the extent of gonadal toxicity, the scattering effects of radiation may still contribute to impaired fertility post irradiation. Such damage to sperm production may be further attributed to damage to cells in the somatic compartment of the testis. Using spermatogonial stem cell (SCC) transplantation in rat, Zhang et al. [31] demonstrated that transplantation of SCCs from irradiated animals into testes of irradiated nude mice (which had normal differentiation of their own spermatogonia) permitted differentiation of the donor spermatogonia to spermatozoa. Conversely, transplantation of SCCs from untreated prepubertal rats into irradiated rat testes showed that the donor spermatogonia were able to colonize along the seminiferous tubules, but could not differentiate. Their findings suggest that the defect caused by radiation in the rat testes that hinder spermatogonial differentiation is due to damage to the somatic compartment [31].

**Chemotherapy**

Chemotherapy is generally indicated in advanced and metastatic cancer, although its use in certain cancers, such as germ cell tumors at an early, localized stage, may help to lower the risks of subsequent metastasis. In addition to malignant cells, any rapidly dividing cells, including germ cells at various phases of spermatogenesis, are targets of chemotherapy. Gonadotoxicity of chemotherapy to an individual depends on at least three factors: (1) the nature of the malignancy, which dictates the type of chemotherapeutic agents to be used, (2) the stage of the disease, which dictates the duration and dosages of chemotherapy, (3) host factors, such as the baseline reproductive health of the individual. The impact of chemotherapy on male reproductive health is discussed in the next section.

## Impact of Chemotherapy on Male Reproductive Health

### Animal Studies

Using rodents (rats and mice) as models, a large body of evidence has emerged demonstrating that treatment with chemotherapeutic agents that act by blocking cell . division usually have dramatic effects on the production of male germ cells [32, 33]. Depending on the mechanism by which such agents act on the different phases of spermatogenesis (spermatogonial mitotic cell division, meiosis, or spermiogenesis), consequences can range from complete elimination of germ cells from the testis, resulting in Sertoli-cell-only syndrome, to no apparent histological effects on spermatogenesis, but functional effects on germ cells (their motility, fertilizing ability, or capacity to produce normal viable offspring).

Over the past 20 years, studies on male mediated adverse effects of chemotherapeutic drugs, such as cyclophosphamide (CPA), bleomycin, cisplatin, or procarbazine, on fertility and progeny outcome have clearly established some of the underlying molecular mechanisms that result in loss of fertility and altered progeny outcome [34–37]. Using CPA or the combination of drugs used for treating testicular cancer (bleomycin, etoposide, and cisplatin, BEP) as model drugs and the rat as the model animal, it has been demonstrated that paternal exposures result in adverse reproductive outcomes that range from increased preimplantation and postimplantation loss or early postnatal death, to growth retardation and congenital malformation; significantly, some of these outcomes are transmitted to subsequent generations [38–40]. It is particularly noteworthy that the action of such drugs on germ cells not only affects the number of germ cells that the testis can produce but also alters markers of chromatin structure (Comet, acridine orange, TUNEL, MBBr, and CMA3 assays, nuclear proteome) in spermatozoa [41, 42]. It is clear from animal studies that spermatozoa that have damaged chromatin as a result of paternal drug treatment are capable of fertilizing oocytes [38, 43–45].

Animal studies have also revealed that the effects of paternal exposure on progeny can be wide ranging. While treatment with BEP caused a decrease in both sperm production and sperm motility, no apparent effects were observed on progeny at the end of gestation, yet postnatal death rates were dramatically increased [43]. By contrast, chronic CPA treatment had minimal effects on sperm number and motility, yet a wide range of effects were observed in progeny, ranging from abnormalities at birth to learning deficits as adults and in subsequent generations as well as abnormal reproductive capacity [35, 38, 46].

## Clinical Studies

The assessment of the consequences on progeny outcome of exposure of men to chemotherapeutic drugs presents remarkable challenges. Chemotherapy often results in transient or permanent azoospermia or oligozoospermia in cancer patients [47]. Large epidemiological studies, discussed above, have revealed that there is clearly an effect on fertility and time to pregnancy [14]. In addition, the standard semen parameters (sperm number, motility, and morphology, as established by the World Health Organization (WHO) [48]) are not sufficiently reliable predictors of male fertility [23, 49–51]. Consequently, the focus has shifted in recent years to assessing the nature and quality of chromatin in spermatozoa. In a recent comprehensive review and position paper, Barratt et al. [52] have outlined our current clinical understanding and uncertainties related to the many assays used to ascertain sperm chromatin quality.

Aneuploidy, an abnormal number of chromosomes, is one of the more striking consequences of anticancer drugs on sperm chromatin quality. Using multicolor fluorescent in situ hybridization to detect sperm aneuploidy for chromosomes 13, 21, X, and Y in testicular cancer and Hodgkin's lymphoma patients before and up to 24 months after the initiation of chemotherapy, Tempest et al. [53] found that at 6 months, all cancer patients showed significantly increased frequencies of XY disomy and nullisomy for chromosomes 13 and 21. Although frequencies of aneuploidy generally declined over time after termination of treatment, increased aneuploidy frequencies persisted in some chromosomes for up to 24 months.

Using a series of assays that provide complementary information on sperm chromatin structure, e.g., extent of single- and double-strand breaks, degree of protamination, cross-linking of sulfhydryl bonds, O'Flaherty et al. [23] have shown that, prior to initiation of chemotherapy, sperm chromatin integrity was poorer in cancer patients than in a control population. After treatment with chemotherapeutics, not only was there the expected decline in sperm production and chromatin quality but also, up to 2 years later, a reduction in spermatozoal chromatin integrity in over 40% of the patients who had a return of spermatogenesis [54, 55].

Based on the limited studies to date, it is clear that the presence of several cancers in young men results, to varying degrees, in sperm chromatin with reduced integrity. Furthermore, treatment of cancer may cause transient partial or complete loss of spermatozoa. Under some conditions, it is clear that the germ cells that eventually return to repopulate the seminiferous epithelium are still damaged, while under others, they appear to be normal. Whether SCCs are able repair all the damage caused by radiation or chemotherapy or not remains to be established.

## Male Fertility Preservation and Restoration Strategies

Fertility preservation has become recognized as part of the important global care of cancer patients at the time of cancer diagnosis. This has come about because of the potential long-term negative impact of cytotoxic cancer therapies on male reproductive health and the express desire of many young cancer survivors to have children. Continuing research efforts are being made to contribute to the development of multidisciplinary counseling strategies to best advise cancer patients and survivors regarding their potential risks for adverse pregnancy and progeny outcomes.

### Sperm Cryopreservation

Sperm cryopreservation or sperm "banking" is currently the only available strategy to preserve male fertility. ideally, sperm samples should be collected before any cytotoxic cancer therapies, through ejaculation by masturbation after 2–4 days of sexual abstinence. Then, sperm samples should be analyzed, frozen, and stored in aliquots in liquid nitrogen for future use. With the advances in and increased access to ART, such as IVF/ICSI, a very low number of living spermatozoa are required to achieve fertilization; therefore, even sperm samples that are far from meeting the semen parameters set by the WHO may still be used to achieve fertilization.

Sperm cryopreservation does have its limitations as a fertility preservation strategy. First, only subjects beyond the state of physical maturity of adolescence, when "spermarche" begins within the testes, can have spermatozoa in the semen for cryopreservation. One study of 62 attempts by adolescents to bank sperm before cancer therapy resulted in totally normal semen in only four subjects [56]. Semen procurement by masturbation may not always be feasible among adolescents, even for those who have spermatogenesis. In fact, for cultural and religious reasons, the act of masturbation may be viewed as inappropriate by parents of young adolescent cancer patients [57]. Alternative methods to obtain mature sperms in adolescents using high-frequency penile vibratory stimulus, electroejaculation, or surgical testicular sperm extraction will require sedation/anesthesia and are deemed too invasive for youngsters. Thus, sperm banking is not universally practiced in pediatric-oncology centers, and few adolescent friendly facilities exist.

For preadolescent boys with cancer, there is currently no feasible option for fertility preservation. Early investigators held the view that being prepubertal during anticancer therapy conferred protection against gonadal damage. However, a study evaluating 12 men who survived childhood malignancy revealed that although puberty had progressed apparently normally in all 12, 8 patients were azoospermic, and only 1 had normal semen analysis 2–16.5 years post chemotherapy [58]. In addition, following treatment of Hodgkin's lymphoma in childhood, severe germ cell damage was observed in the majority of patients, even 17 years after chemotherapy [55, 59]. Evidently, there is no gonadal protection in the prepubertal male against chemotherapy-induced damage [60, 61]. In fact, some investigators believe that prepubertal testes are more vulnerable to the cytotoxic effects of chemotherapy than adult testes [62].

## Pharmacological Strategies

The hypothesis that blocking the hypothalamic-pituitary-gonadal axis prior to the initiation of chemotherapy to preserve the nondividing germ cell population was first proposed by Glode et al. [63]. Hormonal manipulation, including the use of exogenous GnRH (gonadotropin-releasing hormone) analogs and steroids (testosterone) to suppress the gonadotropin release, has been investigated as a potential fertility preservation strategy. Since cytotoxic treatment acts mainly on rapidly dividing cells, germ cells have been postulated to be less susceptible to cytotoxic effects if hormone treatments are used to render the testes quiescent. This technique has been successful in some rodents (rats, but not mice) [64, 65]; in addition, in rats the extent of the damage of chemotherapeutic agents has been shown to extend beyond the germ cells to the somatic cells surrounding them [66]. There is no evidence of a similar spermatogonial block in monkeys [67]. Thus far, clinical trials have not shown any benefit of this method [60, 68]. Furthermore, this approach would be ineffective for prepubertal children as the proliferation of germ cells in prepubertal primates appears to be gonadotropin-independent [69]. Clearly, there is an urgent need for novel strategies that are effective and minimally invasive for fertility preservation in young male cancer patients.

## Fertility Restoration with Germ-Cell Transplantation

Stem cells of the male germ line, termed SSCs, exist in the testis prior to birth. Harvesting either SSCs or tissue blocks from testes for cryopreservation before anti-cancer therapies offers the hope for prepubertal boys with cancer to preserve fertility and form their family in the future [70]. After the patient is cured and is at an appropriate state of maturity, preserved SSCs, or SSCs derived from frozen tissue blocks, could be autotransplanted back to the seminiferous tubules to regenerate complete spermatogenesis. Cryopreservation of testis tissue from prepubertal boys has revealed that germ cells can be preserved [71]. An important feature of this strategy is that instead of just preserving fertility, it aims to "restore" fertility. This fertility restoration scheme, based on germ cell or tissue transplantation, has been established with mice and other species [66, 70–78] and is currently under investigation to extend its application to humans.

## *Looking to the Future*

While the risks of impaired fertility after cancer therapy have long been recognized, the biological mechanisms and the nature and extent of sperm damage at the molecular level have only been revealed recently. The importance of fertility after cancer is gradually being accepted as an essential survivorship issue for young cancer survivors. The establishment of effective fertility preservation protocols and counseling strategies represents the ongoing efforts of researchers and clinicians.

A multidisciplinary approach, including input from oncologists, reproductive biologists, social workers, ethicists, geneticists, and embryologists, is the essence of successful development and implementation of any fertility management plan for young cancer survivors. Many questions remain to be answered: What is the potential of further recovery of sperm quality in long-term post chemotherapy? How long should a patient wait post chemotherapy before he can safely use his fresh sperm for procreation? What is the nature and extent of risk of adverse reproductive outcomes using sperm with impaired sperm chromatin post chemotherapy? What are the transgenerational risks? To what extent would such risks be reduced by using sperm cryopreserved prior to chemotherapy for procreation? What sperm biological markers and what assays provide the best clinical prediction of the risks of adverse reproductive outcomes when using sperm with impaired chromatin quality? Further research to address these and other related questions is clearly needed to help health-care professionals and health policy makers to enhance the quality of counseling and to establish practice guidelines on the subject of fertility after cancer.

## References

1. Burns KC, Boudreau C, Panepinto JA. Attitudes regarding fertility preservation in female adolescent cancer patients. J Pediatr Hematol Oncol. 2006;28:350–4.
2. Richiardi L, Bellocco R, Adami HO, Torrang A, Barlow L, Hakulinen T, et al. Testicular cancer incidence in eight northern European countries: secular and recent trends. Cancer Epidemiol Biomark Prev. 2004;13:2157–66.
3. Canadian Cancer Society, National Cancer Institute of Canada. Canadian cancer statistics 2010. www.cancer.ca (2010). Accessed 23 July 2010.
4. National Cancer Institute. National Cancer Institute research on childhood cancers: fact sheet. http://www.cancer.gov/cancertopics/factsheet/NCI-childhood-cancers-research (2009). Accessed 2 Jan 2009.
5. Stiller CA. Epidemiology and genetics of childhood cancer. Oncogene. 2004;23:6429–44.
6. Stiller CA, Allen MB, Eatock EM. Childhood cancer in Britain: the National Registry of Childhood Tumours and incidence rates 1978–1987. Eur J Cancer. 1995;31A:2028–34.
7. Waring AB, Wallace WH. Subfertility following treatment for childhood cancer. Hosp Med. 2000;61:550–7.
8. National Cancer Institute. Surveillance epidemiology and end results program of the National Cancer Institute research: fact sheet. http://SEER.Cancer.gov (2009). Accessed 2 Jan 2009.
9. Garner MJ, Turner MC, Ghadirian P, Krewski D. Epidemiology of testicular cancer: an overview. Int J Cancer. 2005;116:331–9.

162 P. Chan and B. Robaire

10. Bhatia S. Cancer survivorship–pediatric issues. Hematology Am Soc Hematol Educ Program. 2005:507–15.
11. Meadows AT. Pediatric cancer survivorship: research and clinical care. J Clin Oncol. 2006;24:5160–5.
12. Schover LR, Brey K, Lichtin A, Lipshultz LI, Jeha S. Oncologists' attitudes and practices regarding banking sperm before cancer treatment. J Clin Oncol. 2002;20:1890–7.
13. Schover LR, Rybicki LA, Martin BA, Bringelsen KA. Having children after cancer. A pilot survey of survivors' attitudes and experiences. Cancer. 1999;86:697–709.
14. Green DM, Lange JM, Peabody EM, Grigorieva NN, Peterson SM, Kalapurakal JA, et al. Pregnancy outcome after treatment for Wilms tumor: a report from the national Wilms tumor long-term follow-up study. J Clin Oncol. 2010;28:2824–30.
15. Chan PT, Palermo GD, Veeck LL, Rosenwaks Z, Schlegel PN. Testicular sperm extraction combined with intracytoplasmic sperm injection in the treatment of men with persistent azoospermia postchemotherapy. Cancer. 2001;92:1632–7.
16. Hansen M, Bower C, Milne E, de Klerk N, Kurinczuk JJ. Assisted reproductive technologies and the risk of birth defects–a systematic review. Hum Reprod. 2005;20:328–38.
17. Schieve LA, Cohen B, Nannini A, Ferre C, Reynolds MA, Zhang Z, Jeng G, Macaluso M, Wright VC; Massachusetts Consortium for Assisted Reproductive Technology Epidemiologic Research (MCARTER). A population-based study of maternal and perinatal outcomes associated with assisted reproductive technology in Massachusetts. Matern Child Health J. 2007;11:517–25.
18. Schieve LA, Meikle SF, Ferre C, Peterson HB, Jeng G, Wilcox LS. Low and very low birth weight in infants conceived with use of assisted reproductive technology. N Engl J Med. 2002;346:731–7.
19. Steel AJ, Sutcliffe A. Long-term health implications for children conceived by IVF/ICSI. Hum Fertil (Camb). 2009;12:21–7.
20. Meirow D, Schenker JG. Cancer and male infertility. Hum Reprod. 1995;10:2017–22.
21. Meseguer M, Molina N, García-Velasco JA, Remohí J, Pellicer A, Garrido N. Sperm cryopreservation in oncological patients: a 14-year follow-up study. Fertil Steril. 2006;85:640–5.
22. Baker JA, Buck GM, Vena JE, Moysich KB. Fertility patterns prior to testicular cancer diagnosis. Cancer Causes Control. 2005;16:295–9.
23. O'Flaherty C, Vaisheva F, Hales BF, Chan P, Robaire B. Characterization of sperm chromatin quality in testicular cancer and Hodgkin's lymphoma patients prior to chemotherapy. Hum Reprod. 2008;23:1044–52.
24. Dieckmann KP, Linke J, Pichlmeier U, Kulejewski M, German Testicular Cancer Study Group. Spermatogenesis in the contralateral testis of patients with testicular germ cell cancer: histological evaluation of testicular biopsies and a comparison with healthy males. BJU Int. 2007;99:1079–85.
25. Cunningham GR, Tindall DJ, Huckins C, Means AR. Mechanisms for the testicular hypertrophy which follows hemicastration. Endocrinology. 1978;102:16–23.
26. Medhamurthy R, Aravindan GR, Moudgal NR. Hemiorchidectomy leads to dramatic and immediate alterations in pituitary follicle-stimulating hormone secretion and the functional activity of the remaining testis in the adult male bonnet monkey (Macaca radiata). Biol Reprod. 1993;49:743–9.
27. Tsutsui T, Kurita A, Kirihara N, Hori T, Kawakami E. Testicular compensatory hypertrophy related to hemicastration in prepubertal dogs. J Vet Med Sci. 2004;66:1021–5.
28. Laron Z, Dickerman Z, Ritterman I, Kaufman H. Follow-up of boys with unilateral compensatory testicular hypertrophy. Fertil Steril. 1980;33:297–301.
29. Lin WW, Kim ED, Quesada ET, Lipshultz LI, Coburn M. Unilateral testicular injury from external trauma: evaluation of semen quality and endocrine parameters. J Urol. 1998;159:841–3.
30. Clifton DK, Bremner WJ. The effect of testicular x-irradiation on spermatogenesis in man. A comparison with the mouse. J Androl. 1983;4:387–92.

31. Zhang Z, Shao S, Meistrich ML. The radiation-induced block in spermatogonial differentiation is due to damage to the somatic environment, not the germ cells. J Cell Physiol. 2007;211:149–58.
32. Robaire B, Hales BF, editors. Advances in male-mediated reproductive toxicology. New York: Kluwer Academic/Plenum; 2003.
33. Anderson D, Brinkworth MH, editors. Male mediated developmental toxicity. London: Royal Society of Chemistry; 2006.
34. Hales BF, Barton TS, Robaire B. Impact of paternal exposure to chemotherapy on offspring in the rat. J Natl Cancer Inst Monogr. 2005;34:28–31.
35. Hales BF, Crosman K, Robaire B. Increased postimplantation loss and malformations among the F2 progeny of male rats chronically treated with cyclophosphamide. Teratology. 1992;45:671–8.
36. Anderson D. Male-mediated developmental toxicity. Toxicol Appl Pharmacol. 2005;207(2 Suppl):506–13.
37. Meistrich ML. Male gonadal toxicity. Pediatr Blood Cancer. 2009;53:261–6.
38. Trasler JM, Hales BF, Robaire B. Paternal cyclophosphamide treatment of rats causes fetal loss and malformations without affecting male fertility. Nature. 1985;316:144–6.
39. Qiu J, Hales BF, Robaire B. Effects of chronic low-dose cyclophosphamide exposure on the nuclei of rat spermatozoa. Biol Reprod. 1995;52:33–40.
40. Harrouk W, Codrington A, Vinson R, Robaire B, Hales BF. Paternal exposure to cyclophosphamide induces DNA damage and alters the expression of DNA repair genes in the rat preimplantation embryo. Mutat Res. 2000;461:229–41.
41. Codrington AM, Hales BF, Robaire B. Chronic cyclophosphamide exposure alters the profile of rat sperm nuclear matrix proteins. Biol Reprod. 2007;77:303–11.
42. Delbès G, Hales BF, Robaire B. Toxicants and human sperm chromatin integrity. Mol Hum Reprod. 2010;16:14–22.
43. Bieber AM, Marcon L, Hales BF, Robaire B. Effects of chemotherapeutic agents for testicular cancer on the male rat reproductive system, spermatozoa, and fertility. J Androl. 2006;27:189–200.
44. Ménézo Y, Dale B, Cohen M. DNA damage and repair in human oocytes and embryos: a review. Zygote. 2010;21:1–9.
45. Sakkas D, Alvarez JG. Sperm DNA fragmentation: mechanisms of origin, impact on reproductive outcome, and analysis. Fertil Steril. 2010;93:1027–36.
46. Auroux M, Dulioust E, Selva J, Rince P. Cyclophosphamide in the F0 male rat: physical and behavioral changes in three successive adult generations. Mutat Res. 1990;229:189–200.
47. Gandini L, Sgro P, Lombardo F, Paoli D, Culasso F, Toselli L, et al. Effect of chemo- or radiotherapy on sperm parameters of testicular cancer patients. Hum Reprod. 2006;21:2882–9.
48. World Health Organization. WHO laboratory manual for examination and processing of human semen. 5th ed. Cambridge: University Press Cambridge; 2010.
49. Spano M, Bonde JP, Hjollund HI, Kolstad HA, Cordelli E, Leter G. Sperm chromatin damage impairs human fertility. The Danish First Pregnancy Planner Study Team. Fertil Steril. 2000;73:43–50.
50. Virro MR, Larson-Cook KL, Evenson DP. Sperm chromatin structure assay (SCSA) parameters are related to fertilization, blastocyst development, and ongoing pregnancy in in vitro fertilization and intracytoplasmic sperm injection cycles. Fertil Steril. 2004;81: 1289–95.
51. Payne JF, Raburn DJ, Couchman GM, Price TM, Jamison MG, Walmer DK. Redefining the relationship between sperm deoxyribonucleic acid fragmentation as measured by the sperm chromatin structure assay and outcomes of assisted reproductive techniques. Fertil Steril. 2005;84:356–64.
52. Barratt CL, Aitken RJ, Björndahl L, Carrell DT, de Boer P, Kvist U, et al. Sperm DNA: organization, protection and vulnerability: from basic science to clinical applications–a position report. Hum Reprod. 2010;25:824–38.

53. Tempest HG, Ko E, Chan P, Robaire B, Rademaker A, Martin RH. Sperm aneuploidy frequencies analysed before and after chemotherapy in testicular cancer and Hodgkin's lymphoma patients. Hum Reprod. 2008;23:251–8.
54. O'Flaherty C, Hales BF, Chan P, Robaire B. Impact of chemotherapeutics and advanced testicular cancer or Hodgkin lymphoma on sperm deoxyribonucleic acid integrity. Fertil Steril. 2010;94:1374–9.
55. Heikens J, Behrendt H, Adriaanse R, Berghout A. Irreversible gonadal damage in male survivors of pediatric Hodgkin's disease. Cancer. 1996;78:2020–4.
56. Postovsky S, Lightman A, Aminpour D, Elhasid R, Peretz M, Arush MW. Sperm cryopreservation in adolescents with newly diagnosed cancer. Med Pediatr Oncol. 2003;40:355–9.
57. Rosoff PM, Katsur ML. Preserving fertility in young cancer patients: a medical, ethical and legal challenge. J Philos Sci Law. 2003;3. http://www6.miami.edu/ethics/jpsl/archives/papers/preservingFert.html. Accessed 4 September 2010.
58. Mustieles C, Muñoz A, Alonso M, Ros P, Yturriaga R, Maldonado S, et al. Male gonadal function after chemotherapy in survivors of childhood malignancy. Med Pediatr Oncol. 1995;24:347–51.
59. Shafford EA, Kingston JE, Malpas JS, Plowman PN, Pritchard J, Savage MO, et al. Testicular function following the treatment of Hodgkin's disease in childhood. Br J Cancer. 1993;68:1199–204.
60. Thomson AB, Anderson RA, Irvine DS, Kelnar CJ, Sharpe RM, Wallace WH. Investigation of suppression of the hypothalamic-pituitary-gonadal axis to restore spermatogenesis in azoospermic men treated for childhood cancer. Hum Reprod. 2002;17:1715–23.
61. van Casteren NJ, van der Linden GH, Hakvoort-Cammel FG, Hählen K, Dohle GR, van den Heuvel-Eibrink MM. Effect of childhood cancer treatment on fertility markers in adult male long-term survivors. Pediatr Blood Cancer. 2009;52:108–12.
62. Revel A, Revel-Vilk S. Pediatric fertility preservation: is it time to offer testicular tissue cryopreservation? Mol Cell Endocrinol. 2008;282:143–9.
63. Glode LM, Robinson J, Gould SF. Protection from cyclophosphamide-induced testicular damage with an analogue of gonadotropin-releasing hormone. Lancet. 1981;1(8230):1132–4.
64. Kurdoglu B, Wilson G, Parchuri N, Ye WS, Meistrich ML. Protection from radiation-induced damage to spermatogenesis by hormone treatment. Radiat Res. 1994;139:97–102.
65. Meistrich ML, Shetty G. Hormonal suppression for fertility preservation in males and females. Reproduction. 2008;136:691–701.
66. Zhang X, Ebata KT, Nagano MC. Genetic analysis of the clonal origin of regenerating mouse spermatogenesis following transplantation. Biol Reprod. 2003;69:1872–8.
67. Boekelheide K, Schoenfeld H, Hall SJ, Weng CCY, Shetty G, Leith J, et al. Gonadotropin-releasing hormone antagonist (cetrorelix) therapy fails to protect non human primates (*Macaca arctoides*) from radiation-induced spermatogenic failure. J Androl. 2009;26:222–34.
68. Waxman JH, Ahmed R, Smith D, Wrigley PF, Gregory W, Shalet S, et al. Failure to preserve fertility in patients with Hodgkin's disease. Cancer Chemother Pharmacol. 1987;19:159–62.
69. Kelnar CJ, McKinnell C, Walker M, Morris KD, Wallace WH, Saunders PT, et al. Testicular changes during infantile 'quiescence' in the marmoset and their gonadotrophin dependence: a model for investigating susceptibility of the prepubertal human testis to cancer therapy? Hum Reprod. 2002;17:1367–78.
70. Nagano MC. A surgical strategy using spermatogonial stem cells for restoring male fertility. In: Tulandi T, Gosden RG, editors. Preservation of fertility. London: Taylor & Francis; 2004. p. 125–40.
71. Keros V, Hultenby K, Borgström B, Fridström M, Jahnukainen K, Hovatta O. Methods of cryopreservation of testicular tissue with viable spermatogonia in pre-pubertal boys undergoing gonadotoxic cancer treatment. Hum Reprod. 2007;22:1384–95.
72. Oatley JM, Brinster RL. Regulation of spermatogonial stem cell self-renewal in mammals. Annu Rev Cell Dev Biol. 2008;24:263–86.
73. Nagano MC. Homing efficiency and proliferation kinetics of male germ line stem cells following transplantation in mice. Biol Reprod. 2003;69:701–7.

74. Ebata KT, Yeh JR, Zhang X, Nagano MC. The application of biomarkers of spermatogonial stem cells for restoring male fertility. Dis Markers. 2008;24:267–76.
75. Ebata KT, Zhang X, Nagano MC. Expression patterns of cell-surface molecules on male germ line stem cells during postnatal mouse development. Mol Reprod Dev. 2005;72:171–81.
76. Ebata T, Zhang X, Nagano MC. Male germ line stem cells have an altered potential to proliferate and differentiate during postnatal development in mice. Biol Reprod. 2007;76:841–7.
77. Yeh JR, Zhang X, Nagano MC. Establishment of a short-term in vitro assay for mouse spermatogonial stem cells. Biol Reprod. 2007;77:897–904.
78. Schlatt S, Ehmcke J, Jahnukainen K. Testicular stem cells for fertility preservation: preclinical studies on male germ cell transplantation and testicular grafting. Pediatr Blood Cancer. 2009;53:274–80.

# Chapter 9
# Sperm Chromatin and Environmental Factors

**Aleksander Giwercman**

During the past 20 years, a lot of attention has been given to possible time-related deterioration in the function of male reproductive organs [1]. This debate has been initiated by alarming reports on declining sperm counts – the issue that is still widely debated [2, 3]. It has also been suggested that the incidence of congenital malformations, as cryptorchidism and hypospadias, has increased, although even here some uncertainty exists [4]. On the contrary, there is no doubt that testicular cancer, has become significantly more common in the past 4–5 decades [5]. The rapidity by which this rise in the incidence of testicular cancer has occurred points towards a negative impact of environment- or lifestyle-related factors on male reproductive function. However, the deleterious effect of environment and/or lifestyle on semen parameters might not only result in declining sperm counts but even affect the quality of the spermatozoa, including the integrity of the DNA. Such an effect might not only have an impact on the fertility potential of the subject but also introduce genetic aberrations that might be transmitted to the next generation [6]. This chapter focuses on the available evidence regarding environment- and lifestyle-induced changes in the sperm DNA, and the biological and clinical implications of such effects.

A. Giwercman, MD, PhD
Reproductive Medicine Centre, Skåne University Hospital Malmö,
Lund University, Malmö, Sweden
e-mail: aleksander.giwercman@med.lu.se

A. Zini, A. Agarwal (eds.), *Sperm Chromatin for the Clinician*,
© Springer Science+Business Media New York 2013

# Biological and Clinical Relevance

The issue of the effect of environment and lifestyle has some interesting clinical and biological implications. Fist of all, it is now well established that, at least certain types of, sperm DNA damage may have a negative impact on the fertility of the subject *in vivo*, and possibly even *in vitro*. Although in many of the epidemiological studies the increase in percentage of sperms in exposed subjects is rather discrete, even such an effect may be deleterious to the fertility potential of the subject. Thus, we have recently reported that in subjects with normal standard sperm parameters the odds ratio for spontaneous pregnancy significantly decreases when the DNA Fragmentation Index (DFI), as determined by the sperm chromatin structure assay (SCSA), exceeds the level of 20% [7]. However, this decrease in fertility *in vivo* is already seen at DFI above 10%, if one of standard sperm parameters is abnormal. Since many of the environmental toxicants may affect not only sperm DNA integrity but also concentration, motility and/or morphology [8], even slight increase in percentage of sperms with abnormal DNA, combined with deterioration of some other semen characteristics, may lead to a decrease in fertility.

An intriguing, but yet unresolved, issue is the question to which degree these DNA defects are becoming repaired following the process of fertilization. Unrepaired damaged sperm DNA introduced into the embryo might, in theory, lead to poor fertilization, early or late abortion, impaired foetal growth, congenital malformations and/or diseases arising during different phases of the post-natal life. These problems might not only occur in the offspring of the man exposed to such factors but also become manifest in the subsequent generation(s) [9]. The relevance of asking the question whether sperm DNA defects are transmitted to the offspring has become even more relevant in view of the increasing use of advanced techniques of assisted reproduction, *in vitro* fertilization (IVF) and intracytoplasmatic sperm injection (ICSI). Use of this technology has made it possible to achieve pregnancies in couples in whom this has been hampered by factors as sperm DNA breaks [10]. The complexity of the question, the rather recent access to techniques for evaluation of sperm DNA integrity and the relatively short follow-up of IVF and ICSI children do not allow to answer the question, but this issue should have a high priority on the future agenda of evaluating the potential risks of assisted reproduction.

Identification of environmental- and lifestyle-related factors deleterious to sperm DNA does also have implications in relation to the possibility of prevention and treatment of male-related infertility problems. Thus, once the implications of environment and lifestyle on sperm DNA integrity are understood, proper measures aiming to prevent such effects can be taken. Furthermore, studying the mechanisms of environment/lifestyle-related changes in the genome of the male gamete will also increase our level of understanding of the mechanisms involved in impairment of testicular function. Such knowledge is crucial, not only for prevention of infertility but also for development of specific drugs for treatment of fertility problems.

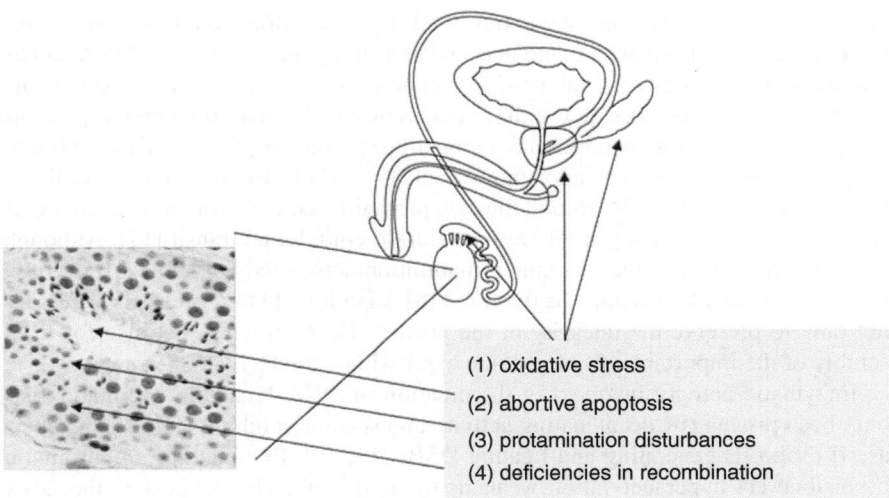

**Fig. 9.1** Examples of major mechanisms of inducing DNA damage in spermatozoa related to lifestyle and/or environmental exposure

Therefore, studying and understanding the phenomenon involved in the effects of environmental and lifestyle factors on sperm DNA may be an important step in preventing and treating infertility problems as well as other important diseases, not only in relation to the generation actually being exposed but also in their offspring and, possibly, even in the subsequent generations.

## How Can Environment/Lifestyle Affect Sperm Chromatin?

Apart from numerical and structural chromosomal changes, environmental exposure may, in principle, affect sperm DNA by introducing DNA fragmentation (or DNA strand breaks) and/or epigenetic changes in the genome of the male gamete.

Abnormal sperm chromatin/DNA structure is thought to arise from four potential sources: (1) deficiencies in recombination during spermatogenesis, (2) abnormal spermatid maturation (protamination disturbancies), (3) abortive apoptosis and (4) oxidative stress [9, 11] (Fig. 9.1).

Meiotic crossing-over is associated with the genetically programmed introduction of DNA double-strand breaks (DSBs) by specific nucleases of SPO11 family [12]. These DNA DSBs should be ligated until the end of meiosis I. Defective repair may interrupt spermatogenesis or lead to persistent sperm DNA fragmentation in ejaculated spermatozoa. Stage-specific occurrence of transient DNA strand breaks during spermiogenesis has been observed [13–15]. Both single-strand breaks (SSBs) and DSBs have been found in round and elongating spermatids. DNA breaks are necessary for transient relief of torsional stress, favouring casting off of the nucleosome histone cores, and aiding their replacement with transitional proteins and protamines during maturation of elongating spermatids [14–16]. Thus, chromatin packaging necessitates endogenous nuclease activity to both create and ligate breaks to reassemble DNA around the new protamine core. Chromatin packaging is completed and DNA integrity is restored during epididymal transit [17]. Although there is little evidence that spermatid maturation-associated DNA breaks are fully ligated, biologically this must be the case [18]. Ligation of DNA breaks is necessary not only to preserve the integrity of the primary DNA structure but also for reassembly of the important unit of genome expression – the DNA loop-domain.

Enzymatic activity involved in the creation of DNA breaks in spermatids has only been proven (by decatenating activity and specific inhibition) for topoisomerase II (Topo II) generating and ligating DSBs [14, 19]. Remodelling of chromatin by histone H4 hyperacetylation weakens the ionic interactions between the DNA and histone cores and is needed for Topo II activity to be introduced in spermatids [19]. Interestingly, Topo II activity seems to be androgen dependent [20], and since many of the environmental toxicants act as endocrine disrupters, they may, in principle, have an impact on sperm DNA integrity.

An alternative aetiology for the DNA DSBs in the spermatozoa of infertile patients can arise through an abortive apoptotic pathway. Apoptosis of testicular germ cells occurs normally throughout life, preventing their overproliferation [21, 22]. It has been suggested that an early apoptotic pathway, initiated in spermatogonia and spermatocytes, is mediated by Fas protein. Fas is a type I membrane protein that belongs to the tumour necrosis factor–nerve growth factor receptor family [23, 24]. It has been shown that Sertoli cells express Fas ligand, which by binding to Fas leads to cell    death via apoptosis [23], limiting the size of germ cell population to numbers Sertoli cells can support [22]. Ligation of Fas ligand to Fas in the cellular membrane triggers the activation of caspases; therefore, this pathway is also characterized as a caspase-induced apoptosis [25]. Men exhibiting deficiencies in their semen profile often possess a large number of spermatozoa bearing Fas. This fact prompts the suggestion that these dysfunctional cells are the product of an incomplete apoptotic cascade [26]. Also the testicular process of apoptosis seems to be under the influence of reproductive hormones, thus being a potential target for an adverse effect of chemicals interfering with the endocrine function.

Reactive oxygen species (ROS) play an important physiological role, modulating gene and protein activities vital for sperm proliferation, differentiation and function. In the semen of fertile men, the amount of ROS generation is properly controlled by seminal antioxidants. The pathogenic effects of ROS occur when they are produced in excess of the antioxidant capabilities of the male reproductive tract or seminal plasma [27]. Abnormal spermatozoa and leukocytes are the main source of excess ROS generation [27]. It seems that sperm DNA is more prone to leukocyte induced ROS damage in infertile men with abnormal semen parameters likely possessing "masked" DNA damage and/or more fragile chromatin structure, which are under the sensitivity threshold of the assays used for the sperm DNA damage assessment [28].

Processes leading to DNA damage in ejaculated sperm are interrelated. For example, a defective maturation process during spermiogenesis, resulting in diminished sperm chromatin packaging, makes sperm cells more vulnerable for ROS-induced DNA fragmentation.

Another type of potentially environmentally induced sperm chromatin alterations are *epigenetic* changes in the genome. Epigenetics refers to changes in gene expression caused by mechanisms other than changes in the underlying DNA sequence. Examples of epigentics include gene methylation or demethylation leading to their inactivation or deactivation, respectively [29].

# Epidemiological Indications of Environmentally Induced Changes in Sperm DNA

Genetic or epigenetic changes in the sperm genome introduced by environment and/or lifestyle related factors may have a serious impact on the reproductive function of an individual. Thus, such alterations may not only lead to impaired male fertility but once established, these changes may be paternally passed on to subsequent generations [30, 31].

Although there is no direct evidence of sperm DNA alterations induced by environment/lifestyle and then subsequently passed on to the offspring, there are some examples that can be considered as indirect evidence of existence of such mechanisms. The Y chromosome has been argued to be particularly vulnerable to DNA damage because it cannot correct double-stranded DNA deletions by homologous recombination [6].

Thus, paternal smoking, reported to introduce sperm DNA damage [32], has been reported to lead to an increased risk of childhood cancer in offspring [33–35], although others could not find the association [36]. Another possible consequence of sperm DNA damage might be microdeletions in the Y chromosome, which will lead to infertility in the male offspring [37].

It has been suggested, although the data seem somewhat contradictory, that increasing paternal age is associated to a higher frequency of aneuploidies, point mutations, sperm DNA breaks, loss of apoptosis, genetic imprinting and other chromosomal abnormalities, and it has even been considered as the major cause of new mutations in human populations [38]. Apart from age, paternal occupation has been linked to certain birth defects or diseases in the offspring which supposedly would act through genetic or epigenetic mechanisms [39]. Epigenetic abnormalities have been associated to imprinting diseases, for which a paternal role has been reported [40], and have been suggested to be increased in babies following conception by assisted reproduction.

A yet unresolved question being of great importance for evaluation of the risk of transmission of sperm DNA changes to the offspring is the ability of the fertilized oocyte to repair such changes. However, animal experiments might indicate that (1) sensitivity of induction of transmissible genetic damage is germ cell-stage dependent, the male post-meiotic cells being the most sensitive; (2) cytogenetic abnormalities at first metaphase after fertilization are critical intermediates between paternal exposure and abnormal reproductive outcomes and (3) the amount of sperm DNA damage that is converted into chromosomal aberrations in the zygote and that directly affect the risk for abnormal reproductive outcomes is regulated by maternal susceptibility factors [41].

## Sperm Chromatin and Environment

### Animal Experience

Animal experiments have clearly demonstrated that exposure of laboratory animals to environmental toxicants, irradiation and cytotoxic drugs may induce chromosome structural aberrations to be transmitted into the zygote [42]. However, even less dramatic negative impact of environment on sperm chromatin integrity has been reported. Such an effect has been found in different set-ups, and some examples are summarized below.

Yauk et al. [43] exposed mice in situ to ambient air near two integrated steel mills and a major highway, while the control animal breathed high-efficiency particulate air (HEPA) filtered ambient air. The animals exposed to unfiltered air presented with 1.6-fold increased rate in sperm mutation frequency and even higher levels of DNA strand breaks and hypermethylation. These results confirm findings reported earlier by Somers et al. [44].

In mice, exposure to mono-(2-ethylhexyl) phthalate (MEHP) was found to increase the germ cell apoptosis. Abortive apoptosis was suggested as one of the mechanisms leading to appearance of DNA strand breaks in ejaculated spermatozoa [45] (see above).

Another environmental toxicant, methyl tert-butyl ether, was found to exert reproductive system toxicity by increasing the oxidative stress [46], the latter also being one of the suggested causes of sperm DNA strand breaks.

Rather spectacular results were reported by Anway et al. [30]. They found that exposure of a gestating female rat during the period of gonadal sex determination to the endocrine disruptors vinclozolin (an antiandrogenic compound) or methoxychlor (an estrogenic compound) induced an adult phenotype in the F1 generation of decreased spermatogenic capacity (cell number and viability) and increased incidence of male infertility. These effects were transferred through the male germ line to nearly all males of all subsequent (F1–F4) generations examined and correlated with altered DNA methylation patterns in the germ line. These effects were also, partly, found by other groups [47], but some could not verify these findings [48, 49].

## Human Data

Several studies have addressed the issue of association between certain lifestyle and environment-related exposures and sperm DNA integrity. Generally, the results are somewhat conflicting. This may to some degree be due to use of different methods for assessment of DNA damage, large variation in sample size as well as variations in recruitment of study subjects, including men from general population, infertility patients or occupationally exposed men. Below, these results, in relation to the most extensively studied exposures, are summarized.

### Tobacco and Other Lifestyle Factors

For obvious reasons, the impact of cigarette smoking on sperm DNA integrity has been extensively studied. Some studies have shown increased level of sperm DNA damage in smoking men. Thus, Shen et al. [50] reported on a positive correlation between 8-OHdG amount and blood cotinine levels. The same was true for three studies based on the use of TUNEL [51–53] and one study using SCSA [52]. All these reports were based on relatively small sample sizes, none of them including more than 60 exposed men.

On the contrary, a number of reports could not confirm the association between tobacco smoking and sperm DNA damage [54–58]. This list includes studies based on the use of COMET, TUNEL, SCSA and 8-oxodG analyses. Interestingly, Saleh et al. [59] reported higher levels of ROS but not sperm DNA strand breaks in smokers as compared to non-smokers. Similarly, Viloria et al. [55] found lower level of sperm antioxidative enzymes in smokers as compared to non-smokers, however, without any difference in the degree of sperm DNA damage between the two groups.

One study [60] focused on the effects of prenatal exposure to cigarette smoking, and although sons of mothers smoking during pregnancy presented with lower sperm counts, no difference in regard to sperm DNA integrity was seen.

Thus, although some studies might indicate a negative effect of cigarette smoking on sperm DNA integrity, the results are rather conflicting, the largest of them finding no such effect. A list of studies dealing with effect of cigarette smoking on sperm DNA is given in Table 9.1.

Among other lifestyle related factors, one study addressed the issue of coffee drinking in relation to the sperm DNA integrity. The major finding [61] was that, using the COMET assay, men who consumed more than three cups coffee per

**Table 9.1** A list of studies dealing with the impact of cigarette smoking on sperm DNA integrity

| Smoking as a main exposure or confounding factor | Assay used | No. participants | Effect | References |
|---|---|---|---|---|
| Main exposure | 8-OHdG | 60 | [a] | [50] |
| Confounding factor | TUNEL | 113 | [a] | [51] |
| Main exposure | SCSA | 25 | [b] | [100] |
| Main exposure | SCSA | 277 | [b] | [101] |
| Main exposure | TUNEL | 70 | [a] | [52] |
| Main exposure | SCSA | 70 | [a] | [52] |
| Main exposure | TUNEL | 97 | [b] | [102] |
| Main exposure | SCSA | 65 | [b] | [59] |
| Confounding factor | COMET (alkaline) | 71 | [b] | [66] |
| Confounding factor | 8-OHdG | 225 | [b] | [58] |
| Main exposure | COMET (alkaline) | 40 | [b] | [103] |
| Main exposure | COMET (neutral) | 257 | [b] | [54] |
| Confounding factor | SCSA | 176 | [b] | [73] |
| Main exposure | TUNEL | 108 | [a] | [53] |
| Confounding factor | COMET (neutral) | 379 | [b] | [56] |
| Main exposure | OxyDNA assay | 55 | [b] | [55] |
| Confounding factor | SCSA | 279 | [b] | [104] |
| Main exposure (mother) | SCSA | 265 | [b] | [60] |

Adapted from M Spanó, unpublished data

[a] Exposure related increase in percentage of spermatozoa with DNA damage

[b] No effect found

day having approximately 20% higher percentage tail DNA under neutral but not alkaline conditions compared with men who consumed no caffeine ($P = 0.005$).

Although animal experiments have indicated that cocaine may induce increased apoptosis [62] as well as alteration of gene imprinting in germ cells [63], similar data in humans are lacking.

## Occupational Exposure

Surprisingly, few epidemiological studies have addressed the issue of occupational exposure in relation to sperm DNA integrity. Three studies dealing with impact of styrene exposure, two of them using COMET assay and one applying SCSA all found a statistically significant increase in the indices of impairment of DNA integrity in exposed workers as compared to unexposed subjects [64–66].

One study focused on occupational boron exposure reporting no significant correlations between blood and urine boron and adverse semen parameters including sperm DNA breaks and percentage apoptotic cells [67].

Hsu et al. [68] reported on the effect of lead exposure on SCSA parameters in a group of battery factory workers in Taiwan and found a positive correlation between the blood levels of the metal and the percentage of sperms with DNA fragmentation.

**Table 9.2** A list of studies dealing with impact of environmental/occupational (except pesticide and PCB) exposure on sperm DNA integrity

| Exposure | Assay used | No. participants | Effect | References |
|---|---|---|---|---|
| Air pollution | SCSA | 266 | a | [70] |
| Air pollution | SCSA | 36 | a | [71] |
| Air pollution | SCSA and CMA | 228 | b | [72] |
| Styrene (mandelic acid urinary concentration) | SCSA | 44 | a | [64] |
| Styrene (mandelic acid urinary concentration) | COMET (alkaline) | 73 | a | [66] |
| Styrene (mandelic and phenylglyoxylic acid urinary concentration) | COMET (alkaline) | 77 | a | [65] |
| Boron (blood and urine) | COMET and TUNEL | 103 | b | [67] |
| Phthalate esters | Sperm nuclear chromatin decondensation (NCD) test | 53 | a | [76] |
| Phthalate and phthalate metabolites | COMET (neutral) | 168 | a | [105] |
| Phthalate and phthalate metabolites | COMET (neutral) | 379 | a | [56] |
| Phthalate and phthalate metabolites | SCSA | 234 | b | [84] |
| Phthalate and phthalate metabolites | SCSA | 300 | a | [82] |
| Acrylonitrile | COMET (alkaline) | 60 | a | [106] |
| Lead | SCSA | 503 | At blood Pb concentration <45 μg/dl[b] | [69] |
| Lead | NCD test | 68 | a | [107] |
| Lead | SCSA | 80 | a | [68] |
| Mercury | SCSA | 195 | No synergism with PCB exposure[b] | [108] |

Adapted from M Spanó, unpublished data

[a] Exposure-related increase in percentage of spermatozoa with DNA damage

[b] No effect found

An earlier study performed by Bonde et al. [69] only partly supported these results reporting some indications of deterioration of sperm chromatin found in men with the highest concentrations of lead within spermatozoa. These data are summarized in Table 9.2. The issue of pesticide exposure is covered in a separate section below.

## Air Pollution

Animal studies (se above) have linked air pollution to the level of sperm DNA damage. Similar findings have also been done in Czech men, both in a cross-sectional [70] and a longitudinal [71] set-up. However, a recent study by Hansen et al. [72] based on a cohort of 228 fertile men could not find any association between the level of exposure to ozone and particulate matter <2.5 μm in aerodynamic diameter on sperm DNA indices as assessed by SCSA and by chromomycin A3 staining (Table 9.2).

## Persistent Organohalogen Pollutants

A number of studies have addressed the issue of the impact of exposure to persistent organohalogen pollutants (POPs) in relation to the sperm chromatin integrity. In a multi-centre European Union funded study (http://www.inuendo.dk) focus was given to association between serum levels of CB-153, a marker of exposure to polychlorinated biphenyls (PCBs) as well as concentrations of $p,p'$-DDE, a metabolite of dichlorodiphenyltrichloroethane (DDT) and sperm parameters, including DNA integrity (Tables 9.3 and 9.4). Using both SCSA and TUNEL, high levels of PCB exposure were found to be associated with increased percentage of spermatozoa with DNA damage. However, interestingly, these associations were found in Caucasian populations (Sweden, Ukraine, and Poland), but not in Greenlandic Inuits, the latter – despite very high levels of CB-153, presenting with significantly lower DFI as compared to the European men [73–75]. This finding might indicate an interaction between POP exposure and genetic (see below) and/or other lifestyle or environmental factors in relation to the integrity of sperm DNA. The Inuendo findings seem to be in agreement with an earlier study by Rozati et al. [76] showing positive correlation between seminal PCB levels and percentage of spermatozoa with single-stranded DNA.

Considering the impact of DDT exposure on sperm chromatin integrity, the results are more diverging. No correlation between $p,p'$-DDE and TUNEL as well as SCSA parameters was found in the Inuendo study – if the impact of genetic polymorphsms was not taken into consideration (see below) [74]. However, it should be kept in mind that there was a high level of correlation between serum levels of CB-153 and the $p,p'$-DDE concentration, in an epidemiological set-up [77], making it impossible to detangle the biological effects of these to compounds. Thus, in a men living in areas with endemic malaria, where due to use of DDT the plasma levels of its metabolite can reach levels 1,000-fold higher than in other populations, there was a positive correlation between SCSA DFI as well as Aniline Blue test assessing the most severe category of incomplete DNA condensation and the concentration of $p,p'$-DDE [78, 79].

## Phthalates

During the past few years, a lot of attention has been given to the potential endocrine disrupting effect of phthalate exposure; these chemicals are supposed to

**Table 9.3**   A list of studies dealing with the impact of pesticide exposure on sperm DNA integrity

| Exposure | Assay used | No. participants | Effect | References |
|---|---|---|---|---|
| $p,p'$-DDE | COMET (neutral) | 212 | [a] | [57] |
| $p,p'$-DDE | SCSA | 176 | [a] | [73] |
| $p,p'$-DDE | SCSA | 707 | [a] | [74] |
| $p,p'$-DDE | SCSA | 680 | Only in subjects with androgen receptor CAG repeat length f 21 or less [b] | [96] |
| $p,p'$-DDE/DDT | SCSA | 209 | [b] | [78] |
| $p,p'$-DDE | TUNEL | 652 | [a] | [75] |
| $p,p'$-DDE | Aniline Blue | 116 | [b] | [79] |
| Pesticides (occupation exposure) | SCSA | 251 | [a] | [85] |
| Pesticides (dietary intake) | SCSA | 256 | [a] | [86] |
| Pesticides | SCSA | 256 | [a] | [109] |
| Organophosphoric pesticides | SCSA | 66 | [b] | [88] |
| Organophosphoric pesticides | ISNT | 54 | Paraoxonase: 192RR genotype more susceptible [b] | [87] |
| Hexachlorobenzene | COMET (neutral) | 212 | [a] | [57] |
| Insecticides (fenvalerate) | COMET (alkaline) TUNEL | 63 | [b] | [90] |
| Insecticides (chlorpyrifos, carbaryl) | COMET (neutral) | 260 | [b] | [92] |
| Insecticides Pyrethroids | COMET (neutral) | 207 | [b] | [91] |
| Insecticides (carbaryl) | TUNEL | 46 | [b] | [89] |

Adapted from M Spanó, unpublished data
[a] No effect found
[b] Exposure-related increase in percentage of spermatozoa with DNA damage

**Table 9.4**   List of studies dealing with the impact of PCB exposure on sperm DNA integrity

| Exposure | Assay used | No. participants | Effect | References |
|---|---|---|---|---|
| PCB | NCD | 53 | [a] | [76] |
| PCB | COMET (neutral) | 212 | [b] | [57] |
| PCB | SCSA | 176 | [a] | [73] |
| PCB | SCSA | 707 | In Caucasians but not in Inuits [a] | [74] |
| PCB | TUNEL | 652 | In Caucasians but not in Inuits [a] | [75] |

Adapted from M Spanó, unpublished data
[a] Exposure-related increase in percentage of spermatozoa with DNA damage
[b] No effect found

interfere with the Leydig cell function [80, 81], thereby affecting the levels of intra-testicular testosterone. A recent study has shown positive correlation between the level of phthalate exposure and ROS production [82]. Therefore, these chemicals may exert a negative effect on sperm DNA integrity both by inducing high ROS levels and, through hormonal deregulation, by interfering with normal intratesticular function of DNA repair enzymes.

Three studies, based on men attending infertility clinics, found a positive association between at least some of the phthalate metabolites and indices of sperm DNA damage, assessed by COMET [56, 83] or SCSA [82]. However, no such association was found in a younger group of Swedish military conscripts [84] (Table 9.2).

### Insecticides and Pesticides Other than DDT

Within this quite heterogeneous category of environmental toxicants, the studies have focused on either occupational exposure or the one related to consumption of food containing traces of such compounds.

Generally, even within this category the results are somewhat conflicting, mainly as regards the pesticides, with no association in Danish agricultural workers and the opposite findings in Mexico [85–88]. A number of reports related to exposure to insecticides have shown positive association between the levels of these chemicals and markers of sperm DNA damage. These findings have been rather consistent when the exposure has been related to the occupation [89, 90] and when it was rather environmentally related [91, 92].

Also, the exposure to organophosphoric pesticides seems to have a negative impact on sperm DNA integrity [87, 88], whereas in two studies comparing organic and non-organic farmers [85, 86], no such effect was found (Table 9.3).

## Gene–Environment Interaction and Sperm Chromatin

Impairment of sperm chromatin integrity due to lifestyle- or environment-related factors represents a unique form of "gene–environment interaction" – namely, environmental stress having a negative impact on the genome of the gamete, those changes being potentially transmittable to the following generation(s). The results of the study by Anway et al. [30], although focusing on epigenetic changes rather than direct DNA damage, illustrate that such scenario is not unlikely. However, in traditional terms, the term "gene–environment interaction" usually refers to interindividual variation in susceptibility to environmental/lifestyle factors based on genetic differences between the subjects. There are several indications of such mechanisms operating even in relation to impairment of sperm DNA integrity.

Thus, as already mentioned, in the Inuendo study, Inuits were found to have significantly lower DFI as compared to Caucasian men [74], the association between levels of PCB exposure being seen among the latter but not in the former ethnic group. Although nutritional or other environmental factors might be the cause of such difference, genetic diversity as a causal factor is also likely.

Our research group has been focusing on polymorphisms in the androgen receptor gene (AR) as modifiers of the effect of endocrine disrupting chemicals, including POPs. One of the polymorphic regions in the *AR* is the glutamine encoding CAG repeats in the exon I of this gene [93]. It has been shown that the number of these repeats, which in a Caucasian normal population varies between 10 and 30 with a mean number of 22, has an impact on the receptor activity [93–95]. In the Inuendo study, we found that an association between *p,p'*-DDE, but not CB-153, levels and the DFI dependent on the CAG number [96]. For CAG lengths of 21 or less, those with high levels of the *p,p'*-DDE presented with 40% higher percentage of spermatozoa with impaired DNA integrity than those with low concentrations of this POP. Such an association between exposure and sperm DNA damage was not seen for other CAG lengths. These findings might, at least partly, explain the robustness of Inuits to the deleterious effects of POP exposure. The mean CAG number is on average 1.5–2 higher in Inuits as compared to Caucasians, thus a less proportion of men having the genotype encoding for higher level of susceptibility [97].

In the study of the impact of sperm pollution on sperm DNA integrity, this effect was shown to be modified by the polymorphisms in the glutathione-*S*-transferase M1 gene [98] as well as by variations in several DNA repair genes [99].

Therefore, it is to be expected that even for the other environmental and lifestyle factors shown to have an impact on sperm DNA integrity, the genetically determined susceptibility may vary between the individuals. Such gene–environment interaction might, at least partly, explain the mechanisms between the above-mentioned somewhat diverging results when different population cohorts are investigated and/or when several techniques are used for detection of sperm DNA damage.

# Conclusions

Available experimental and human data show that a number of lifestyle- and environment-related exposures may have negative effects on sperm DNA integrity. The extent of the sperm DNA damage seems to differ between different studies. Such a discrepancy may partly be due to use of several methods for assessment of sperm DNA integrity, techniques that do not measure exactly the same characteristics of sperm DNA. Another contributing factor may be the genetically determined variation in individual susceptibility.

Sperm DNA damage due to environmental and lifestyle factors may have a negative impact on fertility, and there is a potential risk of transmission to the offspring. Therefore, it is of importance to focus on the association between environment and sperm DNA integrity to prevent male subfertility and to avoid potentially serious health effects in the future generation(s).

# References

1. Giwercman A, Skakkebaek NE. The human testis–an organ at risk? Int J Androl. 1992; 15(5):373–5.
2. Carlsen E, Giwercman A, Keiding N, Skakkeb'k NE. Evidence for decreasing quality of semen during past 50 years. Br Med J. 1992;305:609–13.
3. Carlsen E, Giwercman A, Skakkeb'k NE, Keiding N. Decreasing quality of semen (letter). Br Med J. 1993;306:461.
4. Toppari J, Larsen JC, Christiansen P, et al. Male reproductive health and environmental xenoestrogens. Environ Health Perspect. 1996;104:741–803.
5. Richiardi L, Bellocco R, Adami HO, et al. Testicular cancer incidence in eight northern European countries: secular and recent trends. Cancer Epidemiol Biomark Prev. 2004; 13(12):2157–66.
6. Aitken RJ, Krausz C. Oxidative stress, DNA damage and the Y chromosome. Reproduction. 2001;122(4):497–506.
7. Giwercman A, Lindstedt L, Larsson M, et al. Sperm chromatin structure assay as an independent predictor of fertility in vivo: a case-control study. Int J Androl. 2009;33:e221–7.
8. Toft G, Rignell-Hydbom A, Tyrkiel E, et al. Semen quality and exposure to persistent organochlorine pollutants. Epidemiology. 2006;17(4):450–8.
9. Agarwal A, Agarwal A, Said TM. Role of sperm chromatin abnormalities and DNA damage in male infertility. Hum Reprod Update. 2003;9(4):331–45.
10. Bungum M, Humaidan P, Axmon A, et al. Sperm DNA integrity assessment in prediction of assisted reproduction technology outcome. Hum Reprod. 2007;22(1):174–9.
11. Sakkas D, Mariethoz E, Manicardi G, Bizzaro D, Bianchi PG, Bianchi U. Origin of DNA damage in ejaculated human spermatozoa. Rev Reprod. 1999;4(1):31–7.
12. Bannister LA, Schimenti JC. Homologous recombinational repair proteins in mouse meiosis. Cytogenet Genome Res. 2004;107(3–4):191–200.
13. Bench G, Corzett MH, De Yebra L, Oliva R, Balhorn R. Protein and DNA contents in sperm from an infertile human male possessing protamine defects that vary over time. Mol Reprod Dev. 1998;50(3):345–53.
14. de Yebra L, Ballesca JL, Vanrell JA, Bassas L, Oliva R. Complete selective absence of protamine P2 in humans. J Biol Chem. 1993;268(14):10553–7.
15. de Yebra L, Ballesca JL, Vanrell JA, Corzett M, Balhorn R, Oliva R. Detection of P2 precursors in the sperm cells of infertile patients who have reduced protamine P2 levels. Fertil Steril. 1998;69(4):755–9.
16. Carrell DT, Liu L. Altered protamine 2 expression is uncommon in donors of known fertility, but common among men with poor fertilizing capacity, and may reflect other abnormalities of spermiogenesis. J Androl. 2001;22(4):604–10.
17. Mengual L, Ballesca JL, Ascaso C, Oliva R. Marked differences in protamine content and P1/P2 ratios in sperm cells from percoll fractions between patients and controls. J Androl. 2003;24(3):438–47.
18. Nasr-Esfahani MH, Salehi M, Razavi S, et al. Effect of protamine-2 deficiency on ICSI outcome. Reprod Biomed Online. 2004;9(6):652–8.
19. Kierszenbaum AL. Transition nuclear proteins during spermiogenesis: unrepaired DNA breaks not allowed. Mol Reprod Dev. 2001;58(4):357–8.
20. Bakshi RP, Galande S, Bali P, Dighe R, Muniyappa K. Developmental and hormonal regulation of type II DNA topoisomerase in rat testis. J Mol Endocrinol. 2001;26(3):193–206.
21. Fernandez JL, Goyanes VJ, Ramiro-Diaz J, Gosalvez J. Application of FISH for in situ detection and quantification of DNA breakage. Cytogenet Cell Genet. 1998;82(3–4):251–6.
22. Yu YE, Zhang Y, Unni E, et al. Abnormal spermatogenesis and reduced fertility in transition nuclear protein 1-deficient mice. Proc Natl Acad Sci USA. 2000;97(9):4683–8.
23. Zhao M, Shirley CR, Yu YE, et al. Targeted disruption of the transition protein 2 gene affects sperm chromatin structure and reduces fertility in mice. Mol Cell Biol. 2001;21(21):7243–55.

24. Boissonneault G. Chromatin remodeling during spermiogenesis: a possible role for the transition proteins in DNA strand break repair. FEBS Lett. 2002;514(2–3):111–4.
25. Cho C, Jung-Ha H, Willis WD, et al. Protamine 2 deficiency leads to sperm DNA damage and embryo death in mice. Biol Reprod. 2003;69(1):211–7.
26. Bench GS, Friz AM, Corzett MH, Morse DH, Balhorn R. DNA and total protamine masses in individual sperm from fertile mammalian subjects. Cytometry. 1996;23(4):263–71.
27. Said TM, Paasch U, Glander HJ, Agarwal A. Role of caspases in male infertility. Hum Reprod Update. 2004;10(1):39–51.
28. Erenpreiss J, Hlevicka S, Zalkalns J, Erenpreisa J. Effect of leukocytospermia on sperm DNA integrity: a negative effect in abnormal semen samples. J Androl. 2002;23(5):717–23.
29. Trasler JM. Epigenetics in spermatogenesis. Mol Cell Endocrinol. 2009;306(1–2):33–6.
30. Anway MD, Cupp AS, Uzumcu M, Skinner MK. Epigenetic transgenerational actions of endocrine disruptors and male fertility. Science. 2005;308(5727):1466–9.
31. Cheng RY, Hockman T, Crawford E, Anderson LM, Shiao YH. Epigenetic and gene expression changes related to transgenerational carcinogenesis. Mol Carcinog. 2004;40(1):1–11.
32. Elshal MF, El-Sayed IH, Elsaied MA, El-Masry SA, Kumosani TA. Sperm head defects and disturbances in spermatozoal chromatin and DNA integrities in idiopathic infertile subjects: association with cigarette smoking. Clin Biochem. 2009;42(7–8):589–94.
33. Sorahan T, Lancashire RJ, Hulten MA, Peck I, Stewart AM. Childhood cancer and parental use of tobacco: deaths from 1953 to 1955. Br J Cancer. 1997;75(1):134–8.
34. Sorahan T, McKinney PA, Mann JR, et al. Childhood cancer and parental use of tobacco: findings from the inter-regional epidemiological study of childhood cancer (IRESCC). Br J Cancer. 2001;84(1):141–6.
35. Ji BT, Shu XO, Linet MS, et al. Paternal cigarette smoking and the risk of childhood cancer among offspring of nonsmoking mothers. J Natl Cancer Inst. 1997;89(3):238–44.
36. Schuz J, Kaatsch P, Kaletsch U, Meinert R, Michaelis J. Association of childhood cancer with factors related to pregnancy and birth. Int J Epidemiol. 1999;28(4):631–9.
37. Aitken RJ. The Amoroso Lecture. The human spermatozoon–a cell in crisis? J Reprod Fertil. 1999;115(1):1–7.
38. Sartorius GA, Nieschlag E. Paternal age and reproduction. Hum Reprod Update. 2010; 16(1):65–79.
39. Whalley LJ, Thomas BM, McGonigal G, McQuade CA, Swingler R, Black R. Epidemiology of presenile Alzheimer's disease in Scotland (1974-88) I. Non-random geographical variation. Br J Psychiatry. 1995;167(6):728–31.
40. Marques CJ, Carvalho F, Sousa M, Barros A. Genomic imprinting in disruptive spermatogenesis. Lancet. 2004;363(9422):1700–2.
41. Marchetti F, Wyrobek AJ. Mechanisms and consequences of paternally-transmitted chromosomal abnormalities. Birth Defects Res C Embryo Today. 2005;75(2):112–29.
42. Pacchierotti F, Tiveron C, Ranaldi R, et al. Reproductive toxicity of 1,3-butadiene in the mouse: cytogenetic analysis of chromosome aberrations in first-cleavage embryos and flow cytometric evaluation of spermatogonial cell killing. Mutat Res. 1998;397(1):55–66.
43. Yauk C, Polyzos A, Rowan-Carroll A, et al. Germ-line mutations, DNA damage, and global hypermethylation in mice exposed to particulate air pollution in an urban/industrial location. Proc Natl Acad Sci USA. 2008;105(2):605–10.
44. Somers CM, McCarry BE, Malek F, Quinn JS. Reduction of particulate air pollution lowers the risk of heritable mutations in mice. Science. 2004;304(5673):1008–10.
45. Giammona CJ, Sawhney P, Chandrasekaran Y, Richburg JH. Death receptor response in rodent testis after mono-(2-ethylhexyl) phthalate exposure. Toxicol Appl Pharmacol. 2002;185(2): 119–27.
46. Li D, Yuan C, Gong Y, Huang Y, Han X. The effects of methyl tert-butyl ether (MTBE) on the male rat reproductive system. Food Chem Toxicol. 2008;46(7):2402–8.
47. Stouder C, Paoloni-Giacobino A. Transgenerational effects of the endocrine disruptor vinclozolin on the methylation pattern of imprinted genes in the mouse sperm. Reproduction. 2010;139(2):373–9.

48. Schneider S, Kaufmann W, Buesen R, van Ravenzwaay B. Vinclozolin–the lack of a transgenerational effect after oral maternal exposure during organogenesis. Reprod Toxicol. 2008;25(3):352–60.
49. Inawaka K, Kawabe M, Takahashi S, et al. Maternal exposure to anti-androgenic compounds, vinclozolin, flutamide and procymidone, has no effects on spermatogenesis and DNA methylation in male rats of subsequent generations. Toxicol Appl Pharmacol. 2009;237(2):178–87.
50. Shen HM, Chia SE, Ni ZY, New AL, Lee BL, Ong CN. Detection of oxidative DNA damage in human sperm and the association with cigarette smoking. Reprod Toxicol. 1997;11(5): 675–80.
51. Sun JG et al. Detection of deoxyribomucleic acid fragmentation in human sperm: correlation with fertilization in vitro. Biol Reprod. 1997;56:602–7.
52. Potts RJ, Newbury CJ, Smith G, Notarianni LJ, Jefferies TM. Sperm chromatin damage associated with male smoking. Mutat Res. 1999;423(1–2):103–11.
53. Sepaniak S, Forges T, Gerard H, Foliguet B, Bene MC, Monnier-Barbarino P. The influence of cigarette smoking on human sperm quality and DNA fragmentation. Toxicology. 2006; 223(1–2):54–60.
54. Trisini AT, Singh NP, Duty SM, Hauser R. Relationship between human semen parameters and deoxyribonucleic acid damage assessed by the neutral comet assay. Fertil Steril. 2004;82(6):1623–32.
55. Viloria T, Meseguer M, Martinez-Conejero JA, et al. Cigarette smoking affects specific sperm oxidative defense but does not cause oxidative DNA damage in infertile men. Fertil Steril. 2009;94:631–7.
56. Hauser R, Meeker JD, Singh NP, et al. DNA damage in human sperm is related to urinary levels of phthalate monoester and oxidative metabolites. Hum Reprod. 2007;22(3):688–95.
57. Hauser R, Singh NP, Chen Z, Pothier L, Altshul L. Lack of an association between environmental exposure to polychlorinated biphenyls and p, p'-DDE and DNA damage in human sperm measured using the neutral comet assay. Hum Reprod. 2003;18(12):2525–33.
58. Loft S, Kold-Jensen T, Hjollund NH, et al. Oxidative DNA damage in human sperm influences time to pregnancy. Hum Reprod. 2003;18(6):1265–72.
59. Saleh RA, Agarwal A, Sharma RK, Nelson DR, Thomas Jr AJ. Effect of cigarette smoking on levels of seminal oxidative stress in infertile men: a prospective study. Fertil Steril. 2002; 78(3):491–9.
60. Storgaard L, Bonde JP, Ernst E, et al. Does smoking during pregnancy affect sons' sperm counts? Epidemiology. 2003;14(3):278–86.
61. Schmid TE, Eskenazi B, Baumgartner A, et al. The effects of male age on sperm DNA damage in healthy non-smokers. Hum Reprod. 2007;22(1):180–7.
62. Yang GS, Wang W, Wang YM, Chen ZD, Wang S, Fang JJ. Effect of cocaine on germ cell apoptosis in rats at different ages. Asian J Androl. 2006;8(5):569–75.
63. He F, Lidow IA, Lidow MS. Consequences of paternal cocaine exposure in mice. Neurotoxicol Teratol. 2006;28(2):198–209.
64. Kolstad HA, Bonde JP, Spano M, et al. Sperm chromatin structure and semen quality following occupational styrene exposure. Scand J Work Environ Health. 1999;25:70–3.
65. Migliore L, Colognato R, Naccarati A, Bergamaschi E. Relationship between genotoxicity biomarkers in somatic and germ cells: findings from a biomonitoring study. Mutagenesis. 2006;21(2):149–52.
66. Migliore L, Naccarati A, Zanello A, Scarpato R, Bramanti L, Mariani M. Assessment of sperm DNA integrity in workers exposed to styrene. Hum Reprod. 2002;17(11):2912–8.
67. Robbins WA, Xun L, Jia J, Kennedy N, Elashoff DA, Ping L. Chronic boron exposure and human semen parameters. Reprod Toxicol. 2010;29(2):184–90.
68. Hsu PC, Chang HY, Guo YL, Liu YC, Shih TS. Effect of smoking on blood lead levels in workers and role of reactive oxygen species in lead-induced sperm chromatin DNA damage. Fertil Steril. 2009;91(4):1096–103.
69. Bonde JP, Joffe M, Apostoli P, et al. Sperm count and chromatin structure in men exposed to inorganic lead: lowest adverse effect levels. Occup Environ Med. 2002;59(4):234–42.

70. Selevan SG, Borkovec L, Slott VL, et al. Semen quality and reproductive health of young Czech men exposed to seasonal air pollution. Environ Health Perspect. 2000;108(9):887–94.
71. Rubes J, Selevan SG, Evenson DP, et al. Episodic air pollution is associated with increased DNA fragmentation in human sperm without other changes in semen quality. Hum Reprod. 2005;20(10):2776–83.
72. Hansen C, Luben TJ, Sacks JD, et al. The effect of ambient air pollution on sperm quality. Environ Health Perspect. 2010;118(2):203–9.
73. Rignell-Hydbom A, Rylander L, Giwercman A, et al. Exposure to PCBs and p, p'-DDE and human sperm chromatin integrity. Environ Health Perspect. 2005;113(2):175–9.
74. Spano M, Toft G, Hagmar L, et al. Exposure to PCB and p, p'-DDE in European and Inuit populations: impact on human sperm chromatin integrity. Hum Reprod. 2005;20(12):3488–99.
75. Stronati A, Manicardi GC, Cecati M, et al. Relationships between sperm DNA fragmentation, sperm apoptotic markers and serum levels of CB-153 and p, p'-DDE in European and Inuit populations. Reproduction. 2006;132(6):949–58.
76. Rozati R, Reddy PP, Reddanna P, Mujtaba R. Role of environmental estrogens in the deterioration of male factor fertility. Fertil Steril. 2002;78(6):1187–94.
77. Jonsson BA, Rylander L, Lindh C, et al. Inter-population variations in concentrations, determinants of and correlations between 2,2',4,4',5,5'-hexachlorobiphenyl (CB-153) and 1,1-dichloro-2,2-bis (p-chlorophenyl)-ethylene (p, p'-DDE): a cross-sectional study of 3161 men and women from Inuit and European populations. Environ Health. 2005;4:27.
78. de Jager C, Aneck-Hahn NH, Bornman MS, et al. Sperm chromatin integrity in DDT-exposed young men living in a malaria area in the Limpopo Province, South Africa. Hum Reprod. 2009;24(10):2429–38.
79. De Jager C, Farias P, Barraza-Villarreal A, et al. Reduced seminal parameters associated with environmental DDT exposure and p, p'-DDE concentrations in men in Chiapas, Mexico: a cross-sectional study. J Androl. 2006;27(1):16–27.
80. Scott HM, Mason JI, Sharpe RM. Steroidogenesis in the fetal testis and its susceptibility to disruption by exogenous compounds. Endocr Rev. 2009;30(7):883–925.
81. Svechnikov K, Svechnikova I, Soder O. Inhibitory effects of mono-ethylhexyl phthalate on steroidogenesis in immature and adult rat Leydig cells in vitro. Reprod Toxicol. 2008;25(4):485–90.
82. Pant N, Shukla M, Kumar Patel D, et al. Correlation of phthalate exposures with semen quality. Toxicol Appl Pharmacol. 2008;231(1):112–6.
83. Duty SM, Singh NP, Silva MJ, et al. The relationship between environmental exposures to phthalates and DNA damage in human sperm using the neutral comet assay. Environ Health Perspect. 2003;111(9):1164–9.
84. Jonsson BA, Richthoff J, Rylander L, Giwercman A, Hagmar L. Urinary phthalate metabolites and biomarkers of reproductive function in young men. Epidemiology. 2005;16(4):487–93.
85. Larsen SB, Giwercman A, Spano M, Bonde JP. A longitudinal study of semen quality in pesticide spraying Danish farmers. The ASCLEPIOS Study Group. Reprod Toxicol. 1998;12(6):581–9.
86. Juhler RK, Larsen SB, Meyer O, et al. Human semen quality in relation to dietary pesticide exposure and organic food. Arch Environ Contam Toxicol. 1999;37:415–23.
87. Perez-Herrera N, Polanco-Minaya H, Salazar-Arredondo E, et al. PON1Q192R genetic polymorphism modifies organophosphorous pesticide effects on semen quality and DNA integrity in agricultural workers from southern Mexico. Toxicol Appl Pharmacol. 2008;230(2):261–8.
88. Sanchez-Pena LC, Reyes BE, Lopez-Carrillo L, et al. Organophosphorous pesticide exposure alters sperm chromatin structure in Mexican agricultural workers. Toxicol Appl Pharmacol. 2004;196(1):108–13.
89. Xia Y, Cheng S, Bian Q, et al. Genotoxic effects on spermatozoa of carbaryl-exposed workers. Toxicol Sci. 2005;85(1):615–23.
90. Bian Q, Xu LC, Wang SL, et al. Study on the relation between occupational fenvalerate exposure and spermatozoa DNA damage of pesticide factory workers. Occup Environ Med. 2004;61(12):999–1005.

91. Meeker JD, Barr DB, Hauser R. Human semen quality and sperm DNA damage in relation to urinary metabolites of pyrethroid insecticides. Hum Reprod. 2008;23(8):1932–40.
92. Meeker JD, Singh NP, Ryan L, et al. Urinary levels of insecticide metabolites and DNA damage in human sperm. Hum Reprod. 2004;19(11):2573–80.
93. Tut TG, Ghadessy FJ, Trifiro MA, Pinsky L, Young EL. Long polyglutamine tracts in the androgen receptor are associated with reduced trans-activation, impaired sperm production, and male infertility. J Clin Endocrinol Metab. 1997;82:3777–82.
94. Eckardstein SV, Schmidt A, Kamischke A, Simoni M, Gromoll J, Nieschlag E. CAG repeat length in the androgen receptor gene and gonadotrophin suppression influence the effectiveness of hormonal male contraception. Clin Endocrinol (Oxf). 2002;57(5):647–55.
95. Nenonen H, Bjork C, Skjaerpe PA, et al. CAG repeat number is not inversely associated with androgen receptor activity in vitro. Mol Hum Reprod. 2010;16(3):153–7.
96. Giwercman A, Rylander L, Rignell-Hydbom A, et al. Androgen receptor gene CAG repeat length as modifier of the association between persistent organohalogen pollutant exposure markers and semen characteristics. Pharmacogenet Genomics. 2007;17:391–401.
97. Giwercman C, Giwercman A, Pedersen HS, et al. Polymorphisms in genes regulating androgen activity among prostate cancer low-risk Inuit men and high-risk Scandinavians. Int J Androl. 2008;31(1):25–30.
98. Rubes J, Selevan SG, Sram RJ, Evenson DP, Perreault SD. GSTM1 genotype influences the susceptibility of men to sperm DNA damage associated with exposure to air pollution. Mutat Res. 2007;625(1–2):20–8.
99. Rubes J, Rybar R, Prinosilova P, et al. Genetic polymorphisms influence the susceptibility of men to sperm DNA damage associated with exposure to air pollution. Mutat Res. 2010;683(1–2):9–15.
100. Rubes J, Lowe X, Moore II D, et al. Smoking cigarettes is associated with increased sperm disomy in teenage men. Fertil Steril. 1998;70(4):715–23.
101. Spano M, Kolstad AH, Larsen SB, et al. The applicability of the flow cytometric sperm chromatin structure assay as diagnostic and prognostic tool in then human fertility clinic. Hum Reprod. 1998;13:2495–505.
102. Sergerie M, Ouhilal S, Bissonnette F, Brodeur J, Bleau G. Lack of association between smoking and DNA fragmentation in the spermatozoa of normal men. Hum Reprod. 2000;15(6):1314–21.
103. Belcheva A, Ivanova-Kicheva M, Tzvetkova P, Marinov M. Effects of cigarette smoking on sperm plasma membrane integrity and DNA fragmentation. Int J Androl. 2004;27(5): 296–300.
104. Smit M, Romijn JC, Wildhagen MF, Weber RF, Dohle GR. Sperm chromatin structure is associated with the quality of spermatogenesis in infertile patients. Fertil Steril. 2009;94: 1748–52.
105. Duty SM, Calafat AM, Silva MJ, Ryan L, Hauser R. Phthalate exposure and reproductive hormones in adult men. Hum Reprod. 2005;20:604–10.
106. Xu DX, Zhu QX, Zheng LK, et al. Exposure to acrylonitrile induced DNA strand breakage and sex chromosome aneuploidy in human spermatozoa. Mutat Res. 2003;537(1):93–100.
107. Hernandez-Ochoa I, Garcia-Vargas G, Lopez-Carrillo L, et al. Low lead environmental exposure alters semen quality and sperm chromatin condensation in northern Mexico. Reprod Toxicol. 2005;20(2):221–8.
108. Rignell-Hydbom A, Axmon A, Lundh T, Jonsson BA, Tiido T, Spano M. Dietary exposure to methyl mercury and PCB and the associations with semen parameters among Swedish fishermen. Environ Health. 2007;6:14.
109. Larsen SB, Spano M, Giwercman A, Bonde JP. Semen quality and sex hormones among organic and traditional Danish farmers. ASCLEPIOS Study Group. Occup Environ Med. 1999;56(2):139–44.

# Chapter 10
# Effects of Male Accessory Gland Infection on Sperm Parameters

**Aldo E. Calogero, Sandro La Vignera, Rosita A. Condorelli, Rosario D'Agata, and Enzo Vicari**

## Male Accessory Glands Infection

Male accessory gland infection (MAGI) has been identified among diagnostic categories having a negative impact on male reproductive function and fertility [1]. According to the WHO [1], MAGI is diagnosed when a patient has oligo-, astheno-, and/or teratozoospermia associated with at least one factor A plus one factor B, one factor A plus one factor C, one factor B plus one factor C or two factors C (Table 10.1).

MAGI is an umbrella term that includes the following different clinical categories: prostatitis, prostatovesiculitis, and prostatovesiculoepididymitis (PVE). They share some characteristics: they are common diseases, have mainly a chronic course, rarely cause obstruction of the seminal pathways, can have an unpredictable intracanicular spread to one or more sexual accessory glands of the reproductive tract, as well as to one or both sides. Therefore, ultrasound evaluation of epididymis, prostate, and seminal vesicles is an important diagnostic tool that helps to define MAGI extension to the various accessory glands. Thus, we have developed the following ultrasonographic criteria to evaluate the inflammatory involvement of each male accessory gland [2–4] (Table 10.2).

A.E. Calogero, MD (✉)
Section of Endocrinology, Andrology and Internal Medicine,
and Master in Andrological, Human Reproduction and Biotechnology Sciences,
Department of Internal Medicine and Systemic Diseases, University of Catania,
Policlinico "G. Rodolico", Via S. Sofia, 78, Building 4, Catania 95123, Italy
e-mail: acaloger@unict.it

S. La Vignera, MD • R.A. Condorelli, MD • R. D'Agata, MD
Section of Endocrinology, Andrology and Internal Medicine,
Human Reproduction and Biotechnology Sciences, Department of Biomedical Sciences,
University of Catania, Catania, Italy

E. Vicari, MD
Department of Internal Medicine and Systemic Diseases, University of Catania, Catania, Italy

A. Zini, A. Agarwal (eds.), *Sperm Chromatin for the Clinician*,                    185
© Springer Science+Business Media New York 2013

**Table 10.1** WHO diagnosis of male accessory gland infection

| Factors | Description |
| --- | --- |
| A | *History*: positive for urinary infection, epididymitis, and/or sexually transmitted disease |
| | *Physical signs*: thickened or tender epididymis, tender vas deferens, and/or abnormal digital rectal examination |
| B | *Prostatic fluid*: abnormal prostate fluid expression and/or abnormal urine after prostatic massage |
| C | *Ejaculate signs*: leucocyte >1 mil/mL, culture with significant growth of pathogenic bacteria, abnormal appearance, increased viscosity, increased pH, and/or abnormal biochemistry of the seminal plasma |

According to the WHO [1], MAGI is diagnosed when a patient has oligo-, astheno-, and/or teratozoospermia associated with at least one factor A plus one factor B, one factor A plus one factor C, one factor B plus one factor C or two factors C

From World Health Organization [1], with permission of Cambridge University Press

**Table 10.2** Ultrasonographic criteria to evaluate the inflammatory involvement of each male accessory gland

| Gland | Ultrasonograhic abnormalities (presence of at least two of the following) |
| --- | --- |
| Prostatitis | Asymmetry of the gland volume |
| | Areas of ipoechogenicity |
| | Areas of iperechogenicity |
| | Dilatation of periprostatic venous plexus |
| Vesiculitis | Mono- or bilateral increased (>14 mm) anteroposterior diameter |
| | Asymmetry >2.5 mm (normal 7–14 mm) compared with the contralateral vesicle |
| | Mono- or bilateral reduced (<7 mm) anteroposterior diameter |
| | Thickened and/or calcified glandular epithelium |
| | Polycyclic areas separated by hyperechoic septa in one or both vesicles |
| Epididymitis | Increased size of the head (craniocaudal diameter >12 mm) and/or of the tail (craniocaudal diameter >6 mm) present mono- or bilaterally |
| | Presence of multiple microcystis in the head and/or tail present mono- or bilaterally |
| | Mono or bilateral hypo- or hyperechogenicity |
| | Large mono- or bilateral hydrocele |

Using scrotal and transrectal prostate-vesicular ultrasound scans, MAGI may be classified into (a) uncomplicated form, which includes prostatitis alone and (b) complicated forms, which encounter the inflammatory involvement of both prostate and seminal vesicles (prostatovesiculitis) or the involvement of all the three glands (i.e., PVE). This categorization of MAGI is of clinical importance because of the different impact it has on male fertility. Indeed, the negative impact of the inflammatory process on the sperm quality and, consequently, on fertility is more profound in patients with PVE compared to patients with prostatovesiculitis or prostatitis alone [2, 5]. More recently, we have also reported that the ultrasonographic evaluation of patients with PVE allows for discriminating whether there is a unilateral or bilateral involvement of the accessory glands. As expected, patients with bilateral PVE have poorer sperm parameters compared to those with a unilateral involvement [4].

The presence of a significant number of the above-reported ultrasound abnormalities found in one or more male accessory glands, found associated with elevated bacteriospermia and radical oxygen species (ROS) production [2], likely depicts the following peculiar anatomopathology hallmarks of chronic inflammation occurring simultaneously: (1) inflammation processes primarily mediated by monocytes, long-lived macrophages, and lymphocytes. Macrophages engulf and digest microorganisms, foreign invaders, and senescent cells. Macrophages release several different chemical mediators, including IL-1, TNFα, and prostaglandins, that perpetuate the proinflammatory response; (2) destruction of the inflamed tissue through macrophages and other leukocytes release of ROS, resulting in an "oxidative burst" from neutrophils/macrophages as a first-line defense mechanism, and of proteases; (3) repair of the damaged tissue by replacement with cells of the same type or with fibrous connective tissue. An important part of the inflammatory process involves local angiogenesis, resulting in the development of new blood vessels. In some instances, the host is unable to repair the damaged tissue and the (chronic) inflammatory cascade continues.

In this chapter, we show that all components of the inflammatory response (from the agents that first trigger it to each component of the inflammatory response dynamic) can deteriorate conventional and/or nonconventional sperm parameters arising from one or more of the following mechanisms: (a) altered secretory function of the epididymis, seminal vesicles, and prostate, which reduces the antioxidant properties or scavenging role of the seminal plasma, (b) deterioration of spermatogenesis, and (c) (unilateral or bilateral) organic or functional subobstruction of the seminal tract.

## Effects of MAGI on Sperm Parameters

Over the years, a debate has been going on to establish the effects, if any, of MAGI on sperm parameters. A large body of literature suggests that MAGI may negatively interfere with sperm quality in many ways. Indeed, sperm output and quality is the final product of (a) microorganisms/viruses intrinsic properties (degree of virulence, bacterial/viral load, etc.), (b) time of interaction between the microorganism and the germ cells, and (c) the involvement of one or more male accessory glands.

The inflammatory response of one or more glands contributes to the negative impact on sperm function, since many inflammatory mediators released in higher amounts during MAGI have a detrimental effect on germ cells [6, 7]. These include ROS and cytokines [3, 8–12]. These bioactive substances may persist even after successful treatment with antimicrobials because the antioxidant capacity of the seminal plasma is progressively exhausted and cannot be restored because of often dysfunctional male accessory glands. Indeed, ultrasound abnormalities have been found in the accessory glands (prostate, seminal vesicles, and/or epididymis) of infertile patients with MAGI and elevated bacteriospermia ($\geq 10^5$ CFU/mL) or with *Chlamydia trachomatis* or *Ureaplasma urealyticum* infection (in urethral swabs after prostate massage) [2, 4]. These patients have also an increased inflammatory response and an impaired semen quality directly related to the extension of MAGI being progressively worst in patients with prostatitis alone, prostatovesiculitis, or PVE [2, 5].

Conventional sperm parameters, biofunctional markers, and chromatin/DNA integrity have been reported to be altered in patients with MAGI. Three main different mechanisms have been hypothesized as a cause of sperm DNA damage. These include abortive apoptosis, abnormal chromatin packaging, or increased oxidative stress, which is often present in patients with MAGI [13]. Infections acting at the testicular level cause sperm death very likely due to necrosis by itself or necrosis that occurs as a final step of apoptosis [14]. Interestingly, these authors reported that the recovery from infections does not seem to coincide with improved sperm quality, probably because of a persistent inflammatory state, suggested by a high percentage of sperm necrosis sometimes associated with leukocytospermia. The effects of inflammation could progress even in the absence of germs due to the hyperproduction of proinflammatory mediators. Therefore, the results of this study suggest that the presence of necrosis, sometimes associated with apoptosis, may be regarded as an indicator of male genital tract inflammation [15].

In summary, germ cells are the target of many possible pathophysiological mechanisms that may contribute to the onset of infertility in the course of MAGI. We briefly review the effects of (a) microorganisms and viruses, (b) ROS hyperproduction, and (c) the main proinflammatory cytokines.

## Effects of Various Microorganisms and Viruses

Some Gram-negative Enterobacteriaceae, such as *Escherichia coli*, *Klebsiella* sp., *Proteus*, *Serratia*, *Pseudomonas* sp., etc., have been recognized as known prostate pathogens (category II, NIH classification), since they have a strong association with a clear positive clinical history (prior and/or recurrent urinary tract infection, sexually transmitted disease, congenital urogenital abnormalities) and some urogenital abnormalities during physical examination. On the contrary, the only presence of some microorganisms is interpreted by some investigators as "probable" (when Gram-positive pathogens, such as *Enterococcus* sp. and *Staphylococcus aureus*, are present) or "possible" (when coagulase-negative anaerobic pathogens, such as *Staphylococcus*, *C. trachomatis*, *U. urealyticum*, are present) prostate infection. The major difficulty in interpreting microbiological findings is the presence of contaminating, indigenous microbiota, or of inhibitory substances known to be present in the prostatic secretions, as well as previous courses of antibiotics. Thus, the diagnosis of bacterial prostatitis may be confirmed by quantitative bacteriological cultures in the semen (growth of $>10^3$ pathogenic bacteria or $>10^4$ nonpathogenic bacteria in seminal plasma diluted 1:2 with saline solution) [16] or segmented cultures, i.e., four [17] and/or two [18] glass test.

Various germs and viruses have been shown able to alter sperm function. Indeed, they may damage conventional sperm parameters, particularly motility, as well as sperm mitochondrial function and/or chromatin/DNA integrity. Paradoxically, literature has focused more toward experimental infection mediated by "possible" microbiota responsible for urogenital infection, reporting in vitro models and impaired effects on conventional and nonconventional sperm parameters, whereas a lower attention has been devoted to evaluate the effects of "known prostate pathogens."

## *Escherichia coli*

Many studies have explored the effects of *E. coli* on sperm function mainly using an in vitro approach. Diemer et al. evaluated the effect of the uropathogenic *E. coli* serotype 06 on normal spermatozoa separated by swim-up and found a significant inhibition of sperm progressive motility. The inhibitory effect was achieved at a sperm–bacteria ratio of 1, and it was prevented by chloramphenicol. On the contrary, no effect on sperm motility was observed after incubation with *E. coli* culture filtrates. Electron microscopy analysis revealed multiple adhesions of *E. coli* to spermatozoa [19]. An inhibitory effect of *E. coli*, but not of the enterococcus, on sperm motility was subsequently confirmed by the same group of researchers [20]. The coincubation of normal spermatozoa with *E. coli* and polymorphonuclear (PMN) has been reported to reduce sperm motility evaluated by computer-assisted sperm analysis (CASA) more profoundly than when spermatozoa were incubated with PMN alone, suggesting that *E. coli* is the primary agent that interferes with sperm motility [21].

Normal spermatozoa incubated with *E. coli* resulted in an increased percentage of spermatozoa with phosphatidylserine (PS) externalization (early apoptosis event) and with apoptosis/necrosis (annexin V-FITC-positive/propidium iodide-positive), whereas incubation with PMN activated by phorbol-12-myristate-13-acetate showed only a small increase in apoptosis/necrosis [22]. These results suggest that *E. coli* is directly able to alter ejaculated sperm function without involving any of the molecular mechanisms that alter their motility, vitality, and DNA integrity. Accordingly, incubation with *E. coli* decreased the percentage of spermatozoa with elevated mitochondrial membrane potential (MMP); this was found associated with decreased sperm motility and viability. Reactive oxygen species (ROS) production and PS externalization did not change significantly. Interestingly, a similar effect was observed incubating spermatozoa with the supernatant from *E. coli* culture, suggesting the soluble factors damage sperm function [23]. Very recently, in an attempt to understand the mechanism by which *E. coli* inhibits sperm motility, Prabha et al. have isolated and purified the factor responsible for such an effect which they named sperm immobilization factor (SIF). SIF is a 56-kDa molecule that causes instant immobilization without agglutination of human spermatozoa at a concentration of about 1 mg/mL and death at a concentration of about 2 mg/mL. Spermatozoa incubated with SIF revealed multiple and profound alterations involving all superficial structures of spermatozoa as observed by electron microscopy [24].

## Neisseria gonorrhoeae

Few studies have explored the effects of *Neisseria gonorrhoeae* on sperm parameters. Liu et al. evaluated the effects of this microorganism on the motility parameters of normal spermatozoa by CASA at a ratio of 1:50. They did not found any effect after 2 and 4 h of incubation, whereas using the same experimental model, *S. aureus* significantly decreased sperm motility and viability [25]. Interestingly, it has been shown that *N. gonorrhoeae* is able to upregulate several host antiapoptotic mechanisms on urethral epithelium and that the gonococcal infection protects host cells from subsequent in vitro staurosporine exposure-induced death. The upregulation of antiapoptotic mechanisms in the urethral epithelium by the gonococcus may represent a mechanism employed by this pathogen to survive and proliferate in host epithelium [26]. It is not known whether a similar mechanism is also exerted on germ cells.

## Chlamydia trachomatis

*C. trachomatis* infection may cause sperm apoptosis because the rate of cells with fragmented DNA has been reported to be higher in patients with chlamydial infection compared with controls [27]. Asymptomatic men with ejaculates positive for chlamydial infection, diagnosed by nested plasmid polymerase chain reaction (PCR), have a significantly higher number of leukocytes and a higher ejaculate volume than those whose ejaculates resulted PCR negative for chlamydial infection. No significant differences were observed for all the other parameters [28]. By contrast, sperm concentration, motility, and morphology were significantly worse in men with both chlamydial and/or mycoplasma infection, whereas sperm viability was not significantly affected. Interestingly, these patients had also an increased percentage of spermatozoa with DNA fragmentation, which decreased after antibiotic administration [29]. Ultrastructural examination suggested that the presence of abnormal spermatozoa during chlamydial infection may relate to the microorganism per se or to the host immune/inflammatory response. In addition, bacteria were detected within the leukocytes of these semen samples. This intracellular persistence of germs may be responsible for the establishment of a latent or chronic infection that may circumvent bactericidal immune mechanisms, impair the efficacy of the antimicrobial treatment, and favor the spreading of the infection in the female genital tract [30]. More recently, chlamydial infection has been found associated with significantly higher pH and seminal leukocyte number as well as a significantly lower percentage of progressive motile spermatozoa in infertile patients compared to fertile men with chlamydial infection. This was associated with higher semen plasma IL-8 and IL-6 levels [31].

Some studies have tried to elucidate the mechanism(s) by which *C. trachomatis* alters sperm function. An in vitro model showed that elementary bodies (EB) of *C. trachomatis* serovar E, incubated with spermatozoa of normal men for 1–6 h, reduced significantly sperm motility and viability, whereas serovar LGV reduced only sperm viability. No effect was reported on the rate of the acrosome reaction. The coincubation with dead EB did not have any effect, suggesting that the detrimental effects on sperm motility and viability are due to live microorganisms and not due to their soluble components [32]. A subsequent study showed that the lipopolysaccharide (LPS) extracted from *C. trachomatis* EB decreased sperm motility and increased the number of dead spermatozoa by the same extent as serovar E EBs, suggesting that LPS mediate the spermicidal effects of *C. trachomatis* [33]. In addition, LPS has been shown to cause sperm apoptosis when incubated in vitro with normal spermatozoa. This effect is caspase 3-mediated, as shown by the inhibition of DNA fragmentation in presence of a pancaspase or caspase-3 inhibitor. These data suggest that sperm death is, at least in part, due to apoptosis [34]. We have investigated the effects of *C. trachomatis* on sperm apoptosis by incubating spermatozoa from normozoospermic healthy men with increasing concentrations of *C. trachomatis* serovar E EBs for 6 and 24 h. After 6 h of incubation, *C. trachomatis* did not have any effect on the percentage of spermatozoa with PS externalization, whereas a significant effect on this parameter was observed after 24 h of incubation. Sperm DNA fragmentation increased significantly after 6 and 24 h of incubation. These findings support the contention that *C. trachomatis* alters directly sperm fertilizing capability [35]. To further evaluate the role of the various LPS molecules on sperm function, Hakimi et al. showed that the lipid A and the 3-deosxy-D-manno-octulosonic acid, toxic components of the *C. trachomatis* LPS, have spermicidal effects similar to LPS. In addition, both molecules were shown to induce sperm apoptosis with a mechanism caspase-mediated [36].

## *Ureaplasma urealyticum*

*U. urealyticum* is the most common microorganism found in infertile men with a prevalence ranging between 10 and 40% (for review see Dieterle [37]). The presence of *U. urealyticum* in the human male genital tract has been found associated with a significantly lower sperm concentration, whereas no effect has been reported on semen volume and sperm motility, viability, or morphology. Seminal biochemical parameters (zinc, magnesium, acid phosphatase, and fructose) were not affected by *U. urealyticum* [38]. A more profound effect on sperm parameters was subsequently reported. Indeed, infertile men with genital tract infection caused by various microorganisms including *U. urealyticum* have decreased semen volume, sperm concentration, motility, morphology, and viability. However, this study does not allow for identifying specifically the effects of *U. urealyticum* on sperm parameters because these end points have been reported regardless of the etiology of the infection [39]. In patients with isolated *U. urealyticum* infection, Wang et al. found an altered semen viscosity, pH value and sperm concentration, whereas all the other parameters were not affected significantly [40]. Altogether these findings suggest that *U. urealyticum* affects negatively sperm concentration, but does not seem to have a relevant effect on the other conventional sperm parameters. However, a study conducted in Chinese infertile men who have an elevated prevalence of *U. urealyticum* infection (about 34%), showed that, in addition to sperm concentration, sperm motility and viability were also significantly lower compared with patients without *U. urealyticum* infection. Computerized sperm analysis showed that several sperm motility parameters were significantly lower in the patients with the infection. These effects on motility were associated to a decreased seminal plasma α-glucosidase levels, whereas seminal plasma acid phosphatase and fructose were unchanged, suggesting a possible epididymal site of action [41].

In vitro overnight incubation with *U. urealyticum*, as well as with *Mycoplasma hominis*, decreased significantly sperm motility and the percentage of spermatozoa with normal form, hyperactivation, and calcium ionophore-induced acrosome reaction [42]. A reduction of sperm acrosome reaction inducibility has also been reported in vivo in men with *U. urealyticum* infection. This alteration normalized after antimicrobial treatment in about two thirds of the patients treated. The effect on the acrosome reaction seems specific to *U. urealyticum*, since *M. hominis* affected sperm functions in vitro, but had no effects in vivo [43]. *U. urealyticum* has been shown to bind spermatozoa, to reduce sperm motility, and to alter sperm membrane after a long-term incubation (4 h or overnight) in vitro, whereas it increases sperm velocity after a short time (45 min) [44]. To explain these opposite effects of *U. urealyticum*, the authors hypothesized that when sperm activity depends on mitochondrial oxidative phosphorylation, usually at low pH, *U. urealyticum* competes with mitochondrial energy production with a consequent decline of sperm motility and viability, whereas when sperm energy metabolism depends on glycolysis, usually at higher pH, *U. urealyticum* stimulates glycolysis and, therefore, sperm activity [45].

*U. urealyticum* serotype 4 was most effective in reducing the Hamster's oocyte sperm penetration rate compared with other mycoplasmas. Since the number of spermatozoa adsorbed to Hamster's oocytes was not influenced by mycoplasma preincubation. This suggests that the inhibition of penetration is not due to a masking of sperm membrane sites [46, 47].

Pyospermia was reported in patients with the simultaneous presence of *U. urealyticum* and *Gardnerella vaginalis* [48]. Examination of specimens from infertile patients and fertile men showed the adhesion of *U. urealyticum* to the membrane of spermatozoa, mainly in the midpiece and the postacrosomial region, and exfoliated germ cells. To further study the effects of *U. urealyticum* on fertility, the authors infected artificially male rats with *U. urealyticum*, serotype 8 (T960). A drastic spermatogenesis impairment was found in about a quarter of the rats and infertility in a similar percentage of animals after mating experiments. In addition, the offspring of the infected rats were significantly smaller than those of controls in terms of prenatal and birth weights, suggesting a profound impact on the reproductive function [49].

Shi et al. showed that *U. urealyticum* has antigens (UreG) which cross-react with human sperm membrane proteins and in particular with the nuclear autoantigenic sperm protein [50]. Because of the cross-reaction between NASP and UreG, some men infected with *U. urealyticum* display positive antisperm antibodies in their serum and/or semen, which may cause infertility with an autoimmune mechanism, as reported in an experimental mouse model.

Interestingly, the infection with *U. urealyticum* has also been reported to be able to alter the concentration of microelements in the seminal fluid of infertile patients. In fact, patients with *U. urealyticum* infection had an increased ratios Cu/Zn and Cd/Zn and of the concentrations of As and Mg in the seminal fluid [51]. These abnormalities may contribute to the sperm quality decline found by some authors.

It is noteworthy to recall that mycoplasma infection may alter glycolipid metabolism in the early primary spermatocytes. Particularly, these microorganisms may desulfate sulfogalactosylglycerolipid (SGG), an important molecule for the sperm–egg binding. Therefore, this mechanism may contribute to the negative impact of *U. urealyticum* infection on human fertility [52]. Furthermore, the presence of *U. urealyticum* may affect negatively the implantation of the embryo [37].

To gain further insight into the effects of *U. urealyticum* on sperm function, nonconventional sperm parameters have also been studied. Shang et al. found that patients with *U. urealyticum* infection have an increased number of spermatozoa with fragmented DNA, evaluated by TUNEL assay, compared to controls [53]. This has been confirmed by a subsequent study, which also reported an increased percentage of spermatozoa with less stable chromatin. After treatment with doxycyclin, a significant improvement of both parameters was observed. The authors replicated these in vivo findings in an in vitro model. Spermatozoa incubated with *U. urealyticum* showed a significant dose- and time-dependent chromatin decondensation and DNA damage. The percentage of human spermatozoa with denatured DNA increased by almost 50% after 30 min of incubation with the serotypes 3 and 8, at a concentration of 100 ureaplasmas/spermatozoon compared with uninfected control spermatozoa [54]. A study in male rats experimentally infected with *U. urealyticum* (serotype 8) showed an increased number of TUNEL-positive cells and areas in the testis and a Fas-FasL overexpression in germinal and Sertoli cells. These findings suggest that *U. urealyticum* increases germ cell apoptosis [55].

Despite these evidences, other studies have reported no effect of *U. urealyticum* infection on sperm parameters. *U. urealyticum* infection had no effect on sperm function as assessed by seminal fluid analysis, in vitro sperm penetration of bovine cervical mucus, and the Hamster's oocyte sperm penetration assay [56]. In vitro, *U. urealyticum* experimental infection did not alter sperm motility or penetration capability when spermatozoa were incubated with the germ for 45 min at very high *U. urealyticum*–spermatozoa ratios (up to 100:1) [57]. In vivo studies showed no statistically significant difference between sperm parameters in subfertile patients with or without *U. urealyticum* infection [58], and no correlation was found between abnormal sperm parameters and the presence of *U. urealyticum* in 86 unselected asymptomatic men [59]. Similarly, infertile patients with *U. urealyticum* infection, diagnosed by PCR analysis in their semen sample, did not have any significant difference in seminal volume, sperm concentration, viability, motility, morphology, and leukocyte count [60]. The same authors confirmed these findings in a group of asymptomatic male partners of infertile Tunisian couples who had the concomitant presence of *Mycoplasma* and *U. urealyticum* DNA in their semen samples [61].

## Mycoplasma hominis and Others

The effects of *M. hominis* on sperm parameters have often been evaluated in the presence of other germs [29, 61–64]. These studies reported a detrimental effect on sperm motility [29, 62, 64], morphology [29, 61, 63], and concentration [29, 61]. Agbakoba et al. reported that many patients infected with various strains of mycoplasmas were oligozoospermics [65]. The presence of *M. hominis* DNA in semen samples is associated with low sperm concentration and abnormal sperm morphology; a negative correlation between sperm concentration and the detection of *Mycoplasma genitalium* in semen samples of infertile men has also been reported [60].

A direct in vitro interaction between *M. hominis* and spermatozoa has also been evaluated. An overnight incubation with mycoplasma species decreased significantly sperm motility and the percentage of normally shaped and the proportion of acrosome-reacted spermatozoa after incubation with the calcium ionophore [42]. Confocal microscopy showed that *M. hominis* binds sperm heads, tails and, to a lower extent, the midpiece 10 min after coincubation. Moreover, infected spermatozoa had the germ within the head and the midpiece in cytosolic space. Only a subtle sperm damage was observed after a short-term *M. hominis* interaction with spermatozoa [66]. Interestingly, experimentally *M. genitalium* attaches to motile spermatozoa, and thus, the microorganism may be carried along with the spermatozoa to the female genital tract [67].

Spermatozoa preincubated with various strains of mycoplasmas had lower penetration rate using the sperm–Hamster egg fertilization test compared to controls. A lower penetration rate has been reported in Percoll-washed spermatozoa, which resulted positive for the presence of mycoplasma DNA compared to those without infection. The similarities of hypoosmotic swelling and kinematic parameters between the two groups suggest that the reduced sperm–oocyte penetration rate is not due to the latter two parameters [68].

By contrast, a number of studies failed to show any effect of mycoplasmas on sperm parameters both in vivo and in vitro. The presence of *M. hominis* and/or *U. urealyticum* in semen was not associated with any significant difference in sperm parameters in men attending an IVF unit [69]. Eggert-Kruse et al. reported no difference on conventional sperm parameters following antimicrobial treatment in patients with *C. trachomatis*, *M. hominis*, *U. urealyticum*, and *N. gonorrhoeae* infections [70]. Similar results were reported examining semen samples for routine analysis. Despite the high prevalence of mycoplasmas in these samples, conventional sperm parameters of the men infected resulted similar to those of the uninfected men [71]. On this account, a systematic search for mycoplasmas infection has not been suggested [72].

## *Candida albicans*

Studies suggest that *Candida albicans* infection has a negative effect on sperm function and spermatozoon fertilizing ability. Experimentally induced *C. albicans* infection has been reported to inhibit sperm motility in a time-dependent manner [73]. A significant inhibitory effect of *C. albicans* was only detected in the samples with the initial bacterial concentration of 20 million microorganisms/mL [20]. A significant degree of sperm nonspecific agglutination, detected after 2 and 4 h of incubation, was also reported, as well as a clear head-to-head sperm agglutination with *C. albicans* interposition [74], suggesting the formation of a mechanical barrier that hampers sperm motility [20]. Subsequent studies showed, however, that mitochondrial and tail alterations may contribute to the sperm motility decline. In addition, spermatozoa in contact with *C. albicans* undergo acrosomal swelling, vesiculation (outer membrane), and rupture [74], which may impair sperm fertilization capability. In this regard, a case report showed that in the presence of *C. albicans* no fertilization occurred after IVF and ICSI [75]. Subsequently, we reported that spermatozoa isolated from normozoospermic healthy men and incubated with increasing concentrations *C. albicans* had a significantly sperm motility decline associated with an increased percentage of spermatozoa with low MMP or PS externalization. *C. albicans* did not seem to have any significant effect on sperm DNA fragmentation or chromatin integrity, at least under these experimental conditions [76]. Indeed, we found an increased sperm chromatin packaging damage and apoptosis in a patient with *C. albicans* infection [75]. This suggests that the adverse effects of *C. albicans* on sperm chromatin/DNA integrity require the presence of other factors (leukocyte, etc.) that are present in vivo. Recently, it has been shown that farnesol, a sesquiterpene alcohol produced by many organisms, which acts as a quorum sensing molecule and as a virulence factor of *C. albicans*, reduces sperm motility and causes sperm apoptosis and necrosis. Moreover, sublethal doses of this signaling molecule induce premature acrosome loss [77].

## *Trichomonas vaginalis*

*Trichomonas vaginalis* is a flagellated parasite often found as an occult resident of the genital tract of sexually active women and men. Its presence in the seminal samples of asymptomatic men resulted in a significant increase of viscosity and number of particulate debris, decreased sperm motility, number of normal forms, and viability (evaluated by the hypoosmotic swelling test). After a single course of treatment with metronidazole (400 mg × 3/day for 10 days), a significant improvement of the semen characteristics was observed in about half of the patients treated [78]. These findings suggest that *T. vaginalis* may cause infertility.

In vitro, this protozoan has been shown to be capable of reducing sperm motility after 2, 4, and 6 h of incubation without causing any sperm agglutination [79]. Subsequent studies confirmed a detrimental effect of *T. vaginalis* on sperm motility and have attempted to establish the mechanism(s) by which this happens [80–83]. Jarecki-Black et al. reported that spent medium of *T. vaginalis* culture caused complete cessation of sperm motility after 15 min of incubation. Trophozoite soluble fraction or formalin-killed trophozoites caused a 50% reduction in sperm motility, compared to 25% reduction caused by the trophozoite particulate fraction or the sterile medium and 3% by saline (control). The *T. vaginalis* spermicidal activity was heat-stable, trypsin-sensitive, and had a molecular weight of 12–15 kDa by gel filtration. This proteinaceous substance was present in and secreted by *T. vaginalis* trophozoites during normal growth in axenic culture [80]. An inhibitory role of *T. vaginalis* metabolites [81] or of a soluble extract [82] of this protozoan on sperm motility was further reported. The incubation with a *T. vaginalis* soluble factor resulted also in an increased viscosity, number of debris, and sperm membrane damage in vitro [82]. Benchimol et al. reported that *T. vaginalis* is also able to bind sperm head and flagella and that the reduction of sperm motility was associated with an intense agglutination. In this regard, *T. vaginalis* appeared to be much more virulent than *T. foetus* whose effects were evaluated in the same study on bull spermatozoa [83].

By contrast, Daly et al. did not report any effect of *T. vaginalis* on sperm motility up to 24 h of incubation, though protozoa survived well in the semen samples [84]. The lack of effect may relate to low number of *T. vaginalis* (about 2,500/mL semen) used in this study compared to the higher range used ($10^4$–$10^7$ protozoa/mL) in other studies [79].

## Hepatitis B Virus and Hepatitis C Virus

Various studies have explored the effects of Hepatitis B virus (HBV) or Hepatitis C virus (HCV) infection on sperm parameters. Garrido et al., in an attempt to determine the predictive value of sperm parameters, sperm washing procedure, and the infection status for the postwash viral positivity, found that sperm parameters of HCV-affected patients did not differ from those of noninfected men [85]. We evaluated the sperm parameters of infertile patients in Child–Pugh classification A with HBV or HCV infection, compared with those of a group of 30 patients with primary infertility due to causes different from liver diseases. HBV patients (median HBV-DNA load of $6 \times 10^5$ copies/mL, range: $1 \times 10^5$–$1 \times 10^7$ copies/mL) had sperm density, total number, forward motility, morphology, and viability significantly worse than those found in patients with HCV (median HCV-RNA load of $2.3 \times 10^6$ copies/mL, range: $2 \times 10^5$–$1.2 \times 10^7$ copies/mL). No significant correlation between sperm parameters and the duration of viral infection or the viral HBV-DNA load was found with the exception of sperm morphology, which exhibited a trend for a negative correlation with the viral HBV-DNA load [86]. HCV-infected patients had a significantly lower sperm motility and percentage of normal forms than controls. Combined antiviral treatment with interferon and ribavirin worsened sperm morphology, while it did not have any effect on the other sperm parameters [87]. A negative effect on sperm motility [88, 89] and morphology [89] has been confirmed in HCV- and HBV-positive patients. However, Moretti et al. did not find any significant effect on sperm concentration [88], whereas Lorusso et al. found lower sperm concentration and viability in both HBV and HCV seropositive men compared with controls [89].

Very little is known about the mechanism by which HBV affects sperm function. A recent study, evaluating the role of the HBV S protein (HBs), the main component of HBV envelop protein, has reported that HBs reduces sperm motility in a dose- and time-dependent fashion and increases the number of spermatozoa with low MMP. The fertilization rate in HBs-treated group was significantly lower than that of the control group [90].

Electronic microscopy revealed significantly higher values of sperm apoptosis and necrosis in patients with HBV- or HCV-infection compared with controls, whereas the disomy and diploidy rates for chromosomes 18, X, and Y did not differ significantly from controls [88]. By contrast, a significantly higher total sperm chromosome abnormalities, evaluated after zona-free Hamster oocyte penetration, were found in patients with HBV infection compared with healthy men. In addition, sperm chromosomes in HBV patients present stickiness, clumping, failure to staining, etc. These findings suggest that HBV infection may cause sperm chromosome aberrations [91].

The possibility that the HBV may integrate into sperm chromosomes has been evaluated in patients with HBV infection. Specific fluorescent spots for HBV DNA have been detected in sperm chromosomes, although with a different intensity. These results suggest the possibility of vertical transmission of HBV via the germ line to the next generation [91, 92].

## Human Immunodeficiency Virus Type 1

The effect of human immunodeficiency virus (HIV) type 1 infection on sperm parameters was evaluated in asymptomatic or minimally symptomatic HIV-seropositive men and in men with AIDS. All the men with AIDS had leukocytospermia and grossly abnormal spermatozoa. By contrast, sperm parameters of seropositive men did not differ significantly from those of healthy seronegative donors. Zidovudine therapy did not affect sperm morphology or seminal characteristics [93]. No sperm parameters alteration was subsequently confirmed in HIV seropositive men [94]. However, this study showed that HIV seropositive men had a significantly higher percentage of (a) spermatozoa with cytoplasmic droplet, (b) immature germ cells, and (c) spermiophages. In addition, HIV seropositive men showed a significant positive correlation between blood CD4+ and sperm motility, as well as a significant inverse correlation between CD4+ and sperm abnormalities [94].

In contrast to seropositive men, HIV type 1 men have a significantly lower ejaculate volume, sperm concentration, total count, progressive motility, and normal morphology compared with controls. A significant positive correlation was observed between CD4 count and sperm concentration, total count, motility, progressive motility (type a and b) [95]. These data demonstrate that sperm parameters are significantly impaired by the presence of HIV infection. Men with HIV have been reported to have low sperm motility compared to HIV negative men and leucocytospermia irrespective of a previous history of sexual transmitted diseases. These findings suggest that sperm motility impairment in HIV positive men may relate to an increase oxidative stress leukocyte-mediated [96]. However, Garrido et al. did not find any significant alteration of the sperm parameters in HIV-affected patients compared with noninfected men [85]. Because of this inconsistency in the results on sperm parameters in HIV-infected men, Bujan et al. investigated sperm parameters in 190 HIV type 1-infected patients and compared them with those of a control group of fertile, noninfected men ($n = 218$). They found that semen volume, percentages of progressive motile spermatozoa, total sperm counts, and seminal leukocytes were lower, while pH values and spermatozoa multiple anomaly indices were higher in HIV-infected patients [97]. Abnormal sperm parameters have been found in the 83% of HIV-infected and in 42% HIV-uninfected ($n = 83$) male partners of 130 HIV-infected women seeking fertility with an Odds ratio of 7 (95% CI = 2.1–23) [98]. Principal component analysis method showed that HIV-positive men have worst sperm parameters, whereas the distribution of mannose receptors and cytokine levels in HIV-1-positive men were similar to uninfected individuals. The similar distribution of mannose receptors suggests that spermatozoa from infected individuals interact normally with oocytes [99]. Recently, a study conducted in HCV-HIV seropositive men has showed that the only sperm parameter affected was progressive motility (grade a+b), which was significantly lower compared to that of controls [89]. TUNEL analysis revealed an increased percentage of DNA-fragmented ejaculated spermatozoa in semen of HIV-infected men [100].

A prolonged exposure to asymptomatic, untreated HIV-1 infection does not seem to affect sperm parameters. Indeed, no significant variation was observed in 55 men with HIV-1 infection whose sperm parameters were evaluated biannually for a mean follow-up period of 77 weeks. These findings should be reassuring for untreated men infected with HIV-1 who wish to father a child [101].

Aside HIV, many drugs used for the treatment of HIV-infected men have profound spermotoxic effect. Nucleoside analogs reverse transcriptase inhibitors (NRTI), used for the treatment of HIV-infected patients, have important adverse effects that are linked with a common mechanism: alteration of mitochondrial activity. Given the relevant role played by these organelles on sperm function, the effects of these drugs have been evaluated on sperm function. Studies suggest that NRTI exposure alters mitochondrial energy-generating ability in spermatozoa. NRTI are known to increase ROS production, which results in a decreased MMP. The reduced MMP leads to the release some specific apoptotic factors, such as cytochrome C, that initiate programmed cell death [102]. The effects of antiretroviral therapy on semen quality were longitudinally evaluated in a cohort of male patients with different estimated duration of HIV-1 infection. The median period of follow-up was 48 weeks. Five patients underwent thymidine analog-containing treatment, 23 used tenofovir-based treatment, and 6 used other regimens. At all time points, the percentage of progressively motile spermatozoa was low, and it decreased significantly from 28 to 17% during follow-up. All other semen parameters were in the normal range and remained stable [103].

**Papillomavirus**

Over the years, the role of papillomavirures (HPV) on sperm parameters and/or function has been examined with contrasting results. The presence of HPV gene sequences have been shown in the 64% of Percoll-separated spermatozoa. The HPV type 16 was detected about twice as often as the type 18 [104]. Lai et al. reported that not only HPV types 16 and 18 are able to infect human spermatozoa but also some of their genes are actively transcribed in the infected germ cells [105]. Following experimental infection, the viral DNA appears tenaciously bound to spermatozoa, suggesting an internalization into the sperm. Indeed, sperm washing (centrifuge, two-layer Isolate colloid wash, or test-yolk buffer procedures) was not capable of removing exogenous HPV DNA [106]. In an attempt to clarify the mechanism(s) by which HPV binds to spermatozoa, Pèrez-Andino et al. reported that the capsids of HPV type 16 specifically interact with spermatozoa. Purified HPV16 virions directly adsorb to live spermatozoa in native semen and in conditions that resemble the female genital tract. In particular, the authors found that HPV16 capsids bind to two distinct sites at the equatorial region of the sperm head surface [107]. More recently, the presence of HPV DNA has been shown in about the 25% of the sperm head of infected young (18 years old) adults who had unprotected sexual intercourse. However, the authors could not clarify whether the virus was integrated in the nucleus or not [108]. The presence of the virus makes spermatozoa carriers for the sexual transmission of HPV to sexual partners.

The evaluation of the effects of the in vivo HPV infection on sperm parameters suggests a detrimental role of HPV on sperm motility. Indeed, the incidence of asthenozoospermia has been reported to be higher among patients HPV (type 16 and 18)-positive compared with those without infection (75 vs. 8%). Nevertheless, many sperm kinematic parameters did not differ significantly between the two groups [109]. A reduction of sperm motility has been, recently, reported in infertile patients and subjects with risk factors, in particular when the infection was present in spermatozoa [110], and in young adults [108]. By contrast, no effects on semen quality and assisted reproductive technique (ART) variables (pregnancy and abortion rates) have been reported in men and women HPV type 16-positive [111]. The lack of effect on the HPV infection on sperm parameters has also been confirmed by Rintala et al. Indeed, the presence of HPV DNA did not affect semen volume, sperm concentration, motility, and vitality. Neither oligozoospermia nor asthenozoospermia was associated with the presence of seminal HPV DNA [112].

Using an experimental in vitro model of infection, HPV DNA seems to increase sperm motility. HPV DNA increased sperm total motility and progression, evaluated by computer-assisted sperm analysis. This suggests that HPV DNA increases sperm metabolism or enhances the calcium-regulated motility mechanism. Although an artifact of PCR products cannot be ruled out [106], Connelly et al. confirmed that normal spermatozoa had higher motility after incubation with HPV types 16, 18, 31, and 33, but not 6/11, and increased linearity after incubation with all HPV types tested with the exception of the type 18 [113]. An opposite effect of HPV types 6b/11, 16, 18, 31, and 33 exposure has been reported on motility (decreased) and hyperactivation (increased), which suggests that HPV-exposed spermatozoa retain some fertilizing capacity [114].

Normal motile spermatozoa incubated with E6-E7 HPV DNA fragments had increased DNA fragmentation after exposure to DNA of the HPV types 16 and 31, whereas the types 18, 33, and 6/11 did not alter sperm DNA integrity [113]. Lee et al., in the attempt to further evaluate the role, if any, of HPV on sperm DNA of specific gene regions, examined the effects of HPV exposure on the integrity of exons 5 and 8 of the p53 gene. Fragmentation of exon 5 occurred after exposure to HPV DNA type 18. By contrast, only exon 8 was affected by HPV type 16. HPV DNA from type 31 or 33 was without effect on the p53 exons [114].

## Effects of Oxidative Stress

An increased production of ROS and/or a decrease of the antioxidant defenses cause sperm abnormalities. These include decreased sperm motility, acrosine activity, and sperm–oocyte fusion capability (see Lanzafame et al. [115] for review). Indeed, a sperm–oocyte penetration rate <25% is associated with an increased ROS production in an elevated number of oligozoospermic patients with this abnormality of sperm function [116]. Sperm motility inhibition caused by ROS has been reported to negatively correlate with MDA seminal plasma levels [117], whereas a decrement of MDA is associated with an increased pregnancy rate [118]. An increased oxidative stress has been suggested to cause seminal plasma hyperviscosity in infertile males [119].

An increased oxidative stress damages sperm chromatin/DNA integrity also. Indeed, ROS exposure increases DNA fragmentation in normal spermatozoa [116], causes DNA protein cross-linking in chromatin [120], increases the frequency of DNA single and double-strand breaks [121], and oxidates DNA base changes in asthenozoospermic and normozoospermic infertile patients compared with fertile men [122]. Sperm DNA fragmentation does not correlate with the fertilization rate, but is associated with a significant reduction of the pregnancy rate in ART programs when TUNEL-positive spermatozoa are used [123]. Therefore, spermatozoa with damaged DNA are able to fertilize oocytes, but at the time when the paternal genome is switched on, further development stops [124]. DNA damage seems to lead to an amplified risk of miscarriage and chromosomal abnormalities [125].

## Effects of Proinflammatory Cytokines

Cytokines are a group of soluble mediators produced by lymphoid and nonlymphoid cells that play a key role in the afferent and efferent phases of immune responses of both the innate and acquired immune systems. In the dynamic of the inflammatory response, cytokines have pleiotropic and redundant effects, being the same cytokines present in more moments of the inflammatory response. For example, tumor necrosis factor-α (TNFα) is present in the initial inflammatory trigger, but it is also an inductor of chemokines, contributes to the neutrophil chemotaxis, enhances the toxic final effect, and induces apoptosis; IL-6 contributes to the initial inflammatory trigger, but it also causes activation and differentiation of leukocytes, as well as it contributes to the toxic final effect through ROS hyperproduction; IL-8 contributess to the phase of chemoattraction of neutrophils to the site of inflammation, and to the activation of neutrophils toward phagocytosis. Thus, cytokines have a multitasking role that reverberates negatively on male accessory gland function.

## Interleukin 1

The seminal plasma concentration of interleukin 1 (IL-1) has been reported to be higher in infertile patients than in normal controls. However, no difference was found different subgroups of patients divided on the basis of progressive motility or percentage of sperm with abnormal forms [126]. IL-1 has been reported to have no effect on both spontaneous or calcium ionophore-induced acrosome reaction in normal spermatozoa [127] as well as sperm MDA production in vitro when used alone or in combination with leukocytes [128].

## Interleukin 6

Interleukin 6 (IL-6) seminal plasma levels have been reported to be higher in infertile patients than in normal fertile men and to negatively correlate with sperm MDA formation, suggesting a ROS-mediated lipoperoxidation process [129]. An inhibitory dose- and time-dependent effect of IL-6 on sperm motility has been reported in vitro, which seems to relate to hyperproduction of nitric oxide [130]. In addition, IL-6 has been shown to decrease both spontaneous and calcium ionophore- or progesterone-induced acrosome reaction of normal spermatozoa separated by swim-up procedure. This inhibitory effect was, however, of lower intensity compared with that obtained by incubating spermatozoa with TNF-α in the same experimental model [131].

## Interleukin 8

Fedder and Ellerman-Eriksen showed that interleukin 8 (IL-8) had no effect on sperm motility and on the ionophore-induced acrosome reaction in vitro [132]. By contrast, in subfertile patients, IL-8 seminal plasma concentrations have been shown to negatively correlate with the total number of motile spermatozoa or with the number of motile spermatozoa harvested after swim-up technique. A significant positive correlation was found between seminal plasma IL-8 concentration and leukocyte counts [133]. An increasing effect of IL-8 has also been reported on normal spermatozoa in vitro, both after physiological or infection–inflammation concentrations [134].

## Interferon Gamma

A significant inhibitory effect of interferon-γ (IFNγ) on sperm motility has been reported in vitro [69, 132]. Such an effect has been confirmed in experiments using both TNFα and IFNγ [135]. Sperm motility inhibition was associated with a significantly reduced capacity of spermatozoa to penetrate Hamster oocytes [136]. At physiological concentration, IFNγ increased sperm membrane lipoperoxidation, but no further increment of MDA production was observed when this cytokine was used at higher concentrations, such as those measured during infection/inflammation [134]. IFNγ has been reported to have both no significant effect on calcium ionophore-induced acrosome reaction [132] and a suppressive effect on spontaneous acrosome reaction and acrosine activity [137]. A marked reduction of $Na^+/K^+$-ATPase, $Ca^{2+}$-ATPase and superoxide dismutase activities and an increased production of nitric oxide have been reported in normal spermatozoa incubated with IFNγ [137]. These latter effects may explain the detrimental effects of IFNγ on sperm acrosine activity and acrosome reaction. It is noteworthy that IFNγ did not alter motility and viability of normal spermatozoa following incubation with this cytokine for up to 3 h [138].

## Macrophage Migration Inhibitory Factor

Macrophage migration inhibitory factor (MIF), a proinflammatory cytokine, is a constituent of the seminal plasma. It is expressed in the epididymis and has been shown to be an important factor in sperm maturation [139]. Sperm-associated, but not seminal plasma, MIF negatively correlates with sperm motility [140]. We have shown a negative correlation between MIF levels in human seminal fluid and fertility status. In addition, MIF added to normal spermatozoa decreased sperm total and progressive motility and increased the percentage of spermatozoa with PS externalization or with DNA fragmentation [141]. A deleterious effect on sperm motility was also reported by Carli et al. but only at high concentrations, whereas MIF may play a physiological role in sperm capacitation process at lower concentrations [142].

## Tumor Necrosis Factor-α

Several studies have shown that TNFα is present in the seminal plasma of normal men at a concentration similar to that found in the seminal plasma of patients with bacterial infection [143]. Other studies have instead shown that the seminal plasma concentrations of TNFα are higher in patients with bacterial or mycoplasma infections than in normal controls [144]. In addition, it has been shown that leuko-cytospermia [145, 146] and/or bacteriospermia [145] are associated with a higher release of TNFα.

Though several studies have explored the effect of TNFα on sperm parameters, no clear conclusion can be drawn. Wincek et al. showed that sperm motility and Hamster oocyte penetration were not affected by the incubation with TNFα [147]. Haney et al. reported that motile spermatozoa obtained from fertile men and sepa-rated by the swim-up technique did not show any decreased motility after of expo-sure to TNFα, IL-1α, and IFNγ alone or in combination even at doses higher than those observed in vivo [148]. Accordingly, no relationship between seminal plasma TNFα concentration and sperm parameters has been reported in normal men [143]. Fedder and Ellerman-Eriksen showed that TNFα had no effect on sperm motility and on the ionophore-induced acrosome reaction [132]. Lewis et al. did not report any effect of TNF-α on sperm viability [149].

On the contrary, a significant in vitro negative effects of TNFα on sperm motility and sperm fertilizing ability of Hamster oocytes have been reported [69, 136]. Similarly, Gruschwitz et al. showed that seminal plasma TNFα concentrations in patients with bacterial or mycoplasma infections correlated negatively with the number of progressively motile spermatozoa [144]. Kocak et al. reported that TNFα levels correlate negatively with sperm motility and morphology, but not with total sperm counts [150]. Estrada et al. showed that although the inflammatory cytokines TNFα plus IFNγ have only partial detrimental effects on sperm motility, viability, membrane integrity, and lateral head displacement, they may contribute to the poor fertilizing potential of human spermatozoa during inflammatory conditions [135]. Accordingly, the peritoneal fluid of women with endometriosis which contains ele-vated concentrations of TNFα caused a significant reduction in both total and pro-gressive sperm motility after 4 and 21 h incubation compared with spermatozoa incubated with peritoneal fluid which did contain TNFα. The ability of TNFα to hamper sperm motility in vitro suggests that this may be a mechanism for the infer-tility observed in women with minimal endometriosis [151]. We found that TNFα inhibits total and progressive sperm motility in a concentration- and time-dependent manner [152]. This detrimental effect may relate to a reduced sperm mitochondrial function, as shown by an increased number of spermatozoa with low MMP [152, 153], as well as an increased nitric oxide production [130].

Divergent results have been reported about the effects of TNFα on lipid sperm mem-brane peroxidation, evaluated by the production of malondialdehyde. In fact, TNFα has been reported both to increase MDA production at physiological concentrations and, to a greater extent, at infection–inflammation concentrations [134] and to have no effect on MDA production from spermatozoa isolated by swim-up technique [128].

TNFα has also been reported to inhibit spontaneous and induced (by calcium ion-ophore or progesterone) acrosome reaction in normal spermatozoa [127, 131, 137].

In keeping with previous observation showing TNFα capable of inducing apop-tosis, we found that this proinflammatory cytokine causes sperm apoptosis also. Indeed, TNFα increased both the percentage the PS externalization, an early molec-ular event of apoptosis, and DNA fragmentation, a late sign of apoptosis. Similar

TNFα toxic effects were reported on sperm motility, functional integrity of the sperm membrane, and DNA fragmentation. These effects were reversed by coincubation with infliximab, a selective TNF-α antibody [154]. More recently, a positive correlation has been reported between seminal plasma TNFα levels and apoptotic spermatozoa as shown by an increased percentage of spermatozoa with PS externalization [155].

# Conclusions

Though an open debate on pros and cons of the role of MAGI in male infertility is going on, andrologists should at least consider MAGI as a risk factor of male infertility [5]. In fact, MAGI may impair sperm function and cause male infertility through the above-reported multiple pathophysiological mechanisms.

# References

1. World Health Organization. In: Rowe P, Comhaire F, Hargreave TB, Mellows HJ, editors. World Health Organization manual for the standardised investigation and diagnosis of the infertile couple. Cambridge: Cambridge University Press; 1993.
2. Vicari E. Seminal leukocyte concentration and related specific reactive oxygen species production in patients with male accessory gland infections. Hum Reprod. 1999;14:2025–30.
3. Vicari E. Effectiveness and limits of antimicrobial treatment on seminal leukocyte concentration and related reactive oxygen species production in patients with male accessory gland infection. Hum Reprod. 2000;15:2536–44.
4. Vicari E, La Vignera S, Castiglione R, et al. Sperm parameters abnormalities, low seminal fructose and reactive oxygen species overproduction do not discriminate patients with unilateral or bilateral post-infectious inflammatory prostato-vesiculo-epididymitis. J Endocrinol Invest. 2006;29:18–25.
5. Bayasgalan G, Naranbat D, Radnaabazar J, et al. Male infertility: risk factors in Mongolian men. Asian J Androl. 2004;6:305–11.
6. Agarwal A, Saleh RA, Bedaiwy MA. Role of reactive oxygen species in the pathophysiology of human reproduction. Fertil Steril. 2003;79:829–43.
7. Sanocka D, Jedrzejczak P, Szumała-Kaekol A, et al. Male genital tract inflammation: the role of selected interleukins in regulation of pro-oxidant and antioxidant enzymatic substances in seminal plasma. J Androl. 2003;24:448–55.
8. Ochsendorf FR. Infections in the male genital tract and reactive oxygen species. Hum Reprod Update. 1999;5:399–420.
9. Vicari E, Calogero AE. Effects of treatment with carnitines in infertile patients with prostato-vesiculo-epididymitis. Hum Reprod. 2001;16:2338–42.
10. Vicari E, La Vignera S, Calogero AE. Antioxidant treatment with carnitines is effective in infertile patients with prostatovesiculoepididymitis and elevated seminal leukocyte concentrations after treatment with nonsteroidal anti-inflammatory compounds. Fertil Steril. 2002;78:1203–8.
11. Weidner W, Colpi GM, Hargreave TB, et al. EAU guidelines on male infertility. Eur Urol. 2002;42:313–22.
12. Diemer T, Hales DB, Weidner W. Immune-endocrine interactions and Leydig cell function: the role of cytokines. Andrologia. 2003;35:55–63.

13. Aitken RJ, De Iuliis GN. Origins and consequences of DNA damage in male germ cells. Reprod Biomed Online. 2007;14:727–33.
14. Collodel G, Baccetti B, Capitani S. Necrosis in human spermatozoa. I. Ultrastructural features and FISH study in semen from patients with uro-genital infections. J Submicrosc Cytol Pathol. 2005;37:93–8.
15. Moretti E, Baccetti B, Capitani S, et al. Necrosis in human spermatozoa. II. Ultrastructural features and FISH study in semen from patients with uro-genital infections. J Submicrosc Cytol Pathol. 2005;37:93–8.
16. Comhaire F, Verschraegen G, Vermeulen L. Diagnosis of accessory gland infection and its possible role in male infertility. Int J Androl. 1980;3:32–45.
17. Meares EM, Stamey TA. Bacteriologic localization patterns in bacterial prostatitis and urethritis. Invest Urol. 1968;5:492–518.
18. Nickel JC. The pre and post massage test (PPMT): a simple screen for prostatitis. Tech Urol. 1997;3:38–43.
19. Diemer T, Weidner W, Michelmann HW, et al. Influence of *Escherichia coli* on motility parameters of human spermatozoa in vitro. Int J Androl. 1996;19:271–7.
20. Huwe P, Diemer T, Ludwig M, et al. Influence of different uropathogenic microorganisms on human sperm motility parameters in an in vitro experiment. Andrologia. 1998;30 Suppl 1:55–9.
21. Diemer T, Huwe P, Ludwig M, et al. Influence of autogenous leucocytes and *Escherichia coli* on sperm motility parameters in vitro. Andrologia. 2003;35:100–5.
22. Villegas J, Schulz M, Soto L, et al. Bacteria induce expression of apoptosis in human spermatozoa. Apoptosis. 2005;10:105–10.
23. Schulz M, Sànchez R, Soto L, et al. Effect of *Escherichia coli* and its soluble factors on mitochondrial membrane potential, phosphatidylserine translocation, viability and motility of human spermatozoa. Fertil Steril. 2010;94:619–23.
24. Prabha V, Sandhu R, Kaur S, et al. Mechanism of sperm immobilization by *Escherichia coli*. Adv Urol. 2010;2010:240–68.
25. Liu JH, Li HY, Cao ZG, et al. Influence of several uropathogenic microorganisms on human sperm motility parameters in vitro. Asian J Androl. 2002;4:179–82.
26. Binnicker MJ, Williams RD, Apicella MA. Infection of human urethral epithelium with *Neisseria gonorrhoeae* factors and protects cells from staurosporine-induced apoptosis. Cell Microbiol. 2003;5:549–60.
27. Wan CC, Wang H, Hao BJ, et al. Infection of *Chlamydia trachomatis* and apoptosis of spermatogenic cells. Zhonghua Nan Ke Xue. 2003;9:350–1.
28. Hosseinzadeh S, Eley A, Pacey AA. Semen quality of men with asymptomatic chlamydial infection. J Androl. 2004;25:104–9.
29. Gallegos G, Ramos B, Santiso R, et al. Sperm DNA fragmentation in infertile men with genitourinary infection by *Chlamydia trachomatis* and mycoplasma. Fertil Steril. 2008;90: 328–34.
30. Gallegos-Avila G, Ortega-Martínez M, Ramos-González B, et al. Ultrastructural findings in semen samples of infertile men infected with *Chlamydia trachomatis* and mycoplasmas. Fertil Steril. 2009;91:915–9.
31. Kokab A, Akhondi MM, Sadeghi MR, et al. Raised inflammatory markers in semen from men with asymptomatic chlamydial infection. J Androl. 2010;31:114–20.
32. Hosseinzadeh S, Brewis IA, Eley A, et al. Co-incubation of human spermatozoa with *Chlamydia trachomatis* serovar E causes premature sperm death. Hum Reprod. 2001;16:293–9.
33. Hosseinzadeh S, Pacey AA, Eley A. *Chlamydia trachomatis*-induced death of human spermatozoa is caused primarily by lipopolysaccharide. J Med Microbiol. 2003;52(Pt 3):193–200.
34. Eley A, Pacey AA, Galdiero M, et al. Can *Chlamydia trachomatis* directly damage your sperm? Lancet Infect Dis. 2005;5:53–7.
35. Satta A, Stivala A, Garozzo A, et al. Experimental *Chlamydia trachomatis* infection causes apoptosis in human sperm. Hum Reprod. 2006;21:134–7.
36. Hakimi H, Geary I, Pacey A, et al. Spermicidal activity of bacterial lipopolysaccharide is only partly due to lipid A. J Androl. 2006;27:774–9.
37. Dieterle S. Urogenital infections in reproductive medicine. Andrologia. 2008;40:117–9.

38. Upadhyaya M, Hibbard BM, Walker SM. The effect of *Ureaplasma urealyticum* on semen characteristics. Fertil Steril. 1984;41:304–8.
39. Sanocka-Maciejewska D, Ciupińska M, Kurpisz M. Bacterial infection and semen quality. J Reprod Immunol. 2005;67:51–6.
40. Wang Y, Liang CL, Wu JQ, et al. Do *Ureaplasma urealyticum* infections in the genital tract affect semen quality? Asian J Androl. 2006;8:562–8.
41. Zheng J, Yu SY, Jia DS, et al. *Ureaplasma urealyticum* infection in the genital tract reduces seminal quality in infertile men. Zhonghua Nan Ke Xue. 2008;14:507–12.
42. Rose BI, Scott B. Sperm motility, morphology, hyperactivation, and ionophore-induced acrosome reactions after overnight incubation with mycoplasmas. Fertil Steril. 1994;61:341–8.
43. Köhn FM, Erdmann I, Oeda T, et al. Influence of urogenital infections on sperm functions. Andrologia. 1998;30 Suppl 1:73–80.
44. Núñez-Calonge R, Caballero P, Redondo C, et al. *Ureaplasma urealyticum* reduces motility and induces membrane alterations in human spermatozoa. Hum Reprod. 1998;13:2756–61.
45. Reichart M, Levi H, Kahane I, et al. Dual energy metabolism-dependent effect of *Ureaplasma urealyticum* infection on sperm activity. J Androl. 2001;22:404–12.
46. Busolo F, Zanchetta R. Do mycoplasmas inhibit the human sperm fertilizing ability in vitro? Isr J Med Sci. 1984;20:902–4.
47. Soffer Y, Ron-El R, Golan A, et al. Male genital mycoplasmas and *Chlamydia trachomatis* culture: its relationship with accessory gland function, sperm quality, and autoimmunity. Fertil Steril. 1990;53:331–6.
48. Kjaergaard N, Kristensen B, Hansen ES, et al. Microbiology of semen specimens from males attending a fertility clinic. APMIS. 1997;105:566–70.
49. Xu C, Sun GF, Zhu YF, et al. The correlation of *Ureaplasma urealyticum* infection with infertility. Andrologia. 1997;29:219–26.
50. Shi J, Yang Z, Wang M, et al. Screening of an antigen target for immunocontraceptives from cross-reactive antigens between human sperm and *Ureaplasma urealyticum*. Infect Immun. 2007;75:2004–11.
51. Wang Y, Kang L, Hou Y, et al. Microelements in seminal plasma of infertile men infected with *Ureaplasma urealyticum*. Biol Trace Elem Res. 2005;105:11–8.
52. Ma J, Xu C. Relationship between mycoplasma infection and germ cell sulfogalactosylglycerolipid. Zhonghua Nan Ke Xue. 2004;10:215–7.
53. Shang XJ, Huang YF, Xiong CL, et al. *Ureaplasma urealyticum* infection and apoptosis of spermatogenic cells. Asian J Androl. 1999;1:127–9.
54. Reichart M, Kahane I, Bartoov B. In vivo and in vitro impairment of human and ram sperm nuclear chromatin integrity by sexually transmitted *Ureaplasma urealyticum* infection. Biol Reprod. 2000;63:1041–8.
55. Xu C, Lu MG, Feng JS, et al. Germ cell apoptosis induced by *Ureaplasma urealyticum* infection. Asian J Androl. 2001;3:199–204.
56. Shalhoub D, Abdel-Latif A, Fredericks CM, et al. Physiological integrity of human sperm in the presence of *Ureaplasma urealyticum*. Arch Androl. 1986;16:75–80.
57. Talkington DF, Davis JK, Canupp KC, et al. The effects of three serotypes of *Ureaplasma urealyticum* on spermatozoal motility and penetration in vitro. Fertil Steril. 1991;55:170–6.
58. Cintron RD, Wortham Jr JW, et al. The association of semen factors with the recovery of *Ureaplasma urealyticum*. Fertil Steril. 1981;36:648–52.
59. Gregoriou O, Botsis D, Papadias K, et al. Culture of seminal fluid in infertile men and relationship to semen evaluation. Int J Gynaecol Obstet. 1989;28:149–53.
60. Gdoura R, Kchaou W, Chaari C, et al. *Ureaplasma urealyticum, Ureaplasma parvum, Mycoplasma hominis* and *Mycoplasma genitalium* infections and semen quality of infertile men. BMC Infect Dis. 2007;7:129.
61. Gdoura R, Kchaou W, Ammar-Keskes L, et al. Assessment of *Chlamydia trachomatis, Ureaplasma urealyticum, Ureaplasma parvum, Mycoplasma hominis,* and *Mycoplasma genitalium* in semen and first void urine specimens of asymptomatic male partners of infertile couples. J Androl. 2008;29:198–206.

62. Hofstetter A, Schmiedt E, Schill WB, et al. Genital mycoplasma strains as a cause of male infertility. Helv Chir Acta. 1978;45:329–33.
63. Bornman MS, Mahomed MF, Boomker D, et al. Microbial flora in semen of infertile African men at Garankuwa hospital. Andrologia. 1990;22:118–21.
64. Corradi G, Molnàr G, Pànovics J. Andrologic significance of genital mycoplasma. Orv Hetil. 1992;133:3085–8.
65. Agbakoba NR, Adetosoye AI, Ikechebelu JI. Genital mycoplasmas in semen samples of males attending a tertiary care hospital in Nigeria: any role in sperm count reduction? Niger J Clin Pract. 2007;10:169–73.
66. Dìaz-Garcìa FJ, Herrera-Mendoza AP, Giono-Cerezo S, et al. *Mycoplasma hominis* attaches to and locates intracellularly in human spermatozoa. Hum Reprod. 2006;21:1591–8.
67. Svenstrup HF, Fedder J, Abraham-Peskir J, et al. *Mycoplasma genitalium* attaches to human spermatozoa. Hum Reprod. 2003;18:2103–9.
68. Kalugdan T, Chan PJ, Seraj IM, et al. Polymerase chain reaction enzyme-linked immunosorbent assay detection of mycoplasma consensus gene in sperm with low oocyte penetration capacity. Fertil Steril. 1996;66:793–7.
69. Hill JA, Haimovici F, Politch JA, et al. Effects of soluble products of activated lymphocytes and macrophages (lymphokines and monokines) on human sperm motion parameters. Fertil Steril. 1987;47:460–5.
70. Eggert-Kruse W, Hofmann H, Gerhard I, et al. Effects of antimicrobial therapy on sperm-mucus interaction. Hum Reprod. 1988;3:861–9.
71. Andrade-Rocha FT. *Ureaplasma urealyticum* and *Mycoplasma hominis* in men attending for routine semen analysis. Prevalence, incidence by age and clinical settings, influence on sperm characteristics, relationship with the leukocyte count and clinical value. Urol Int. 2003;71:377–81.
72. Rosemond A, Lanotte P, Watt S, et al. Systematic screening tests for *Chlamydia trachomatis*, *Mycoplasma hominis* and *Ureaplasma urealyticum* in urogenital specimens of infertile couples. Pathol Biol (Paris). 2006;54:125–9.
73. Tuttle Jr JP, Bannister ER, Derrick FC. Interference of human spermatozoal motility and spermatozoal agglutination by *Candida albicans*. J Urol. 1997;118:797–9.
74. Tian Y-H, Xiong JW, Hu L, et al. *Candida albicans* and filtrates interfere with human spermatozoal motility and alter the ultrastructure of spermatozoa: an in vitro study. Int J Androl. 2007;30:421–9.
75. Burrello N, Calogero AE, Perdichizzi A, et al. Inhibition of oocyte fertilization by assisted reproductive techniques and increased sperm DNA fragmentation in the presence of *Candida albicans*: a case report. Reprod Biomed Online. 2004;8:569–73.
76. Burrello N, Salmeri M, Perdichizzi A, et al. *Candida albicans* experimental infection: effects on human sperm motility, mitochondrial membrane potential and apoptosis. Reprod Biomed Online. 2009;18:496–501.
77. Rennemeier C, Frambach T, Hennicke F. Microbial quorum-sensing molecules induce acrosome loss and cell death in human spermatozoa. Infect Immun. 2009;77:4990–7.
78. Gopalkrishnan K, Hinduja IN, Kumar TC. Semen characteristics of asymptomatic males affected by *Trichomonas vaginalis*. J In Vitro Fert Embryo Transf. 1990;7:165–7.
79. Tuttle Jr JP, Holbrook TW, Derrick FC. Interference of human spermatozoal motility by *Trichomonas vaginalis*. J Urol. 1977;118:1024–5.
80. Jarecki-Black JC, Lushbaugh WB, Golosov L. *Trichomonas vaginalis*: preliminary characterization of a sperm motility inhibiting factor. Ann Clin Lab Sci. 1988;18:484–9.
81. Han Q, Liu J, Wang T. Influence of the metabolite produced by *Trichomonas vaginalis* on human sperm motility in vitro. Zhonghua Nan Ke Xue. 2004;10:272–4.
82. Kranjcić-Zec I, Dzamić A, Mitrović S, et al. The role of parasites and fungi in secondary infertility. Med Pregl. 2004;57:30–2.
83. Benchimol M, de Andrade Rosa I, da Silva Fontes R, et al. Trichomonas adhere and phagocytose sperm cells: adhesion seems to be a prominent stage during interaction. Parasitol Res. 2008;102:597–604.

84. Daly JJ, Sherman JK, Green L, et al. Survival of *Trichomonas vaginalis* in human semen. Genitourin Med. 1989;65:106–8.
85. Garrido N, Meseguer M, Remohí J, et al. Semen characteristics in human immunodeficiency virus (HIV)- and hepatitis C (HCV)-seropositive males: predictors of the success of viral removal after sperm washing. Hum Reprod. 2005;20:1028–34.
86. Vicari E, Arcoria D, Di Mauro C, et al. Sperm output in patients with primary infertility and hepatitis B or C virus; negative influence of HBV infection during concomitant varicocele. Minerva Med. 2006;97:65–77.
87. Durazzo M, Premoli A, Di Bisceglie C, et al. Alterations of seminal and hormonal parameters: an extrahepatic manifestation of HCV infection? World J Gastroenterol. 2006;12:3073–6.
88. Moretti E, Federico MG, Giannerini V, et al. Sperm ultrastructure and meiotic segregation in a group of patients with chronic hepatitis B and C. Andrologia. 2008;40:286–91.
89. Lorusso F, Palmisano M, Chironna M, et al. Impact of chronic viral diseases on semen parameters. Andrologia. 2010;42:121–6.
90. Zhou XL, Sun PN, Huang TH, et al. Effects of hepatitis B virus S protein on human sperm function. Hum Reprod. 2009;24:1575–83.
91. Huang JM, Huang TH, Qiu HY, et al. Effects of hepatitis B virus infection on human sperm chromosomes. World J Gastroenterol. 2003;9:736–40.
92. Huang JM, Huang TH, Qiu HY, et al. Studies on the integration of hepatitis B virus DNA sequence in human sperm chromosomes. Asian J Androl. 2002;4:209–12.
93. Krieger JN, Coombs RW, Collier AC, et al. Fertility parameters in men infected with human immunodeficiency virus. J Infect Dis. 1991;164:464–9.
94. Dondero F, Rossi T, D'Offizi G, et al. Semen analysis in HIV seropositive men and in subjects at high risk for HIV infection. Hum Reprod. 1996;11:765–8.
95. Nicopoullos JDM, Almeida PA, Ramsay JWA, et al. The effect of human immunodeficiency virus on sperm parameters and the outcome of intrauterine insemination following sperm washing. Hum Reprod. 2004;19:2289–97.
96. Umapathy E. STD/HIV association: effects on semen characteristics. Arch Androl. 2005;51:361–5.
97. Bujan L, Sergerie M, Moinard N, et al. Decreased semen volume and spermatozoa motility in HIV-1-infected patients under antiretroviral treatment. J Androl. 2007;28:444–52.
98. Coll O, Lopez M, Vidal R, et al. Fertility assessment in non-infertile HIV-infected women and their partners. Reprod Biomed Online. 2007;14:488–94.
99. Cardona-Maya W, Velilla P, Montoya CJ, et al. Presence of HIV-1 DNA in spermatozoa from HIV-positive patients: changes in the semen parameters. Curr HIV Res. 2009;7:418–24.
100. Muciaccia B, Corallini S, Vicini E, et al. HIV-1 viral DNA is present in ejaculated abnormal spermatozoa of seropositive subjects. Hum Reprod. 2007;22:2868–78.
101. van Leeuwen E, Wit FW, Prins JM, et al. Semen quality remains stable during 96 weeks of untreated human immunodeficiency virus-1 infection. Fertil Steril. 2008;90:636–41.
102. Sergerie M, Martinet S, Kiffer N, et al. Impact of reverse transcriptase inhibitors on sperm mitochondrial genomic DNA in assisted reproduction techniques. Gynecol Obstet Fertil. 2004;32:841–9.
103. van Leeuwen E, Wit FW, Repping S, et al. Effects of antiretroviral therapy on semen quality. AIDS. 2008;22:637–42.
104. Chan PJ, Su BC, Kalugdan T, et al. Human papillomavirus gene sequences in washed human sperm deoxyribonucleic acid. Fertil Steril. 1994;61:982–5.
105. Lai YM, Yang FP, Pao CC. Human papillomavirus deoxyribonucleic acid and ribonucleic acid in seminal plasma and sperm cells. Fertil Steril. 1996;65:1026–30.
106. Brossfield JE, Chan PJ, Patton WC, et al. Tenacity of exogenous human papillomavirus DNA in sperm washing. Int J STD AIDS. 1999;15:740–3.
107. Pèrez-Andino J, Buck CB, Ribbeck K. Adsorption of human papillomavirus 16 to live human sperm. PLoS ONE. 2009;4:e5847.
108. Foresta C, Garolla A, Zuccarello D, et al. Human papillomavirus found in sperm head of young adult males affects the progressive motility. Fertil Steril. 2010;93:802–6.

109. Lai YM, Lee JF, Huang HY, et al. The effect of human papillomavirus infection on sperm cell motility. Fertil Steril. 1997;67:1152–5.
110. Foresta C, Pizzol D, Moretti A, et al. Clinical and prognostic significance of human papillomavirus DNA in the sperm or exfoliated cells of infertile patients and subject with risk factors. Fertil Steril. 2010;94:1723–7.
111. Tanaka H, Karube A, Kodama H, et al. Mass screening for human papillomavirus type 16 infection in infertile couples. J Reprod Med. 2000;45:907–11.
112. Rintala MA, Grènman SE, Pöllänen PP, et al. Detection of high-risk HPV DNA in semen and its association with the quality of semen. Int J STD AIDS. 2004;15:740–3.
113. Connelly DA, Chan PJ, Patton WC, et al. Human sperm deoxyribonucleic acid fragmentation by specific types of papillomavirus. J Assist Reprod Genet. 2001;184:1068–70.
114. Lee CA, Huang CT, King A, et al. Differential effects of human papillomavirus DNA types on p53 tumor-suppressor gene apoptosis in sperm. Gynecol Oncol. 2002;85:511–6.
115. Lanzafame F, La Vignera S, Vicari E, et al. Oxidative stress and antioxidant medical treatment in male infertility. Reprod Biomed Online. 2009;19:638–59.
116. Aitken RJ, Clarkson JS, Hargreave TB, et al. Analysis of the relationship between defective sperm function and the generation of reactive oxygen species in cases of oligozoospermia. J Androl. 1989;10:214–20.
117. Saraniya A, Koner BC, Doureradjou P, et al. Altered malondialdehyde, protein carbonyl and sialic acid levels in seminal plasma of microscopically abnormal semen. Andrologia. 2008;40:56–7.
118. Suleiman SA, Ali ME, Zaki ZM, et al. Lipid peroxidation and human sperm motility: protective role of vitamin E. J Androl. 1996;17:530–7.
119. Aydemir B, Onaran I, Kiziler AR, et al. The influence of oxidative damage on viscosity of seminal fluid in infertile men. J Androl. 2008;29:41–6.
120. Twigg JP, Irvine DS, Aitken RJ. Oxidative damage to DNA in human spermatozoa does not preclude pronucleus formation at intracytoplasmic sperm injection. Hum Reprod. 1998;13:1864–71.
121. Barroso G, Morshedi M, Oehringer S. Analysis of DNA fragmentation, plasma membrane translocation of phosphatidylserine and oxidative stress in human spermatozoa. Hum Reprod. 2000;15:1338–44.
122. Kodama H, Yamaguchi R, Fukuda J, et al. Increased deoxyribonucleic acid damage in the spermatozoa of infertile male patients. Fertil Steril. 1997;65:519–24.
123. Henkel R, Kierspel E, Hajimohammad M, et al. DNA fragmentation of spermatozoa and assisted reproduction technology. Reprod Biomed Online. 2003;7:477–84.
124. Evenson DP, Larson KL, Jost LK. Sperm chromatin structure assay: its clinical use for detecting sperm DNA fragmentation in male infertility and comparisons with the other techniques. J Androl. 2002;23:25–43.
125. Griveau JF, Le Lannou D. Reactive oxygen species and human spermatozoa: physiology and pathology. Int J Androl. 1997;20:61–9.
126. Dousset B, Hussenet F, Daudin M, et al. Seminal cytokine concentrations (IL-1beta, IL-2, IL-6, sR IL-2, sR IL-6), semen parameters and blood hormonal status in male infertility. Hum Reprod. 1997;12:1476–9.
127. Dimitrov DG, Petrovská M. Effects of products of activated immune cells and recombinant cytokines on spontaneous and ionophore-induced acrosome reaction. Am J Reprod Immunol. 1996;36:150–6.
128. Fraczek M, Sanocka D, Kamieniczna M, et al. Proinflammatory cytokines as an intermediate factor enhancing lipid sperm membrane peroxidation in in vitro conditions. J Androl. 2008;29:85–92.
129. Camejo MI, Segnini A, Proverbio F. Interleukin-6 (IL-6) in seminal plasma of infertile men, and lipid peroxidation of their sperm. Arch Androl. 2001;47:97–101.
130. Lampiao F, du Plessis SS. TNF-alpha and IL-6 affect human sperm function by elevating nitric oxide production. Reprod Biomed Online. 2008;17:628–31.
131. Lampiao F, du Plessis SS. Effects of tumour necrosis factor alpha and interleukin-6 on progesterone and calcium ionophore-induced acrosome reaction. Int J Androl. 2009;32:274–7.

132. Fedder J, Ellerman-Eriksen S. Effect of cytokines on sperm motility and ionophore-stimulated acrosome reaction. Arch Androl. 1995;35:173–85.

133. Eggert-Kruse W, Boit R, Rohr G, et al. Relationship of seminal plasma interleukin (IL) -8 and IL-6 with semen quality. Hum Reprod. 2001;16:517–28.

134. Martínez P, Proverbio F, Camejo MI. Sperm lipid peroxidation and pro-inflammatory cytokines. Asian J Androl. 2007;9:102–7.

135. Estrada LS, Champion HC, Wang R, et al. Effect of tumour necrosis factor-alpha (TNF-alpha) and interferon-gamma (IFN-gamma) on human sperm motility, viability and motion parameters. Int J Androl. 1997;20:237–42.

136. Hill JA, Cohen J, Anderson DJ. The effects of lymphokines and monokines on human sperm fertilizing ability in the zona-free hamster egg penetration test. Am J Obstet Gynecol. 1989;160(5 Pt 1):1154–9.

137. Bian SL, Jin HB, Wang SZ, et al. Effects of interferon-gamma and tumor necrosis factor-alpha on the fertilizing capacity of human sperm and their mechanisms. Zhonghua Nan Ke Xue. 2007;13:681–4.

138. Sikka SC, Champion HC, Bivalacqua TJ, et al. Role of genitourinary inflammation in infertility: synergistic effects of lipopolysaccharide and interferon-gamma on human spermatozoa. Int J Androl. 2001;24:136–41.

139. Eickhoff R, Baldauf C, Koyro HW, et al. Influence of macrophage migration inhibitory factor (MIF) on the zinc content and redox state of protein-bound sulphydryl groups in rat sperm: indications for a new role of MIF in sperm maturation. Mol Hum Reprod. 2004;10:605–11.

140. Frenette G, Légaré C, Saez F, et al. Macrophage migration inhibitory factor in the human epididymis and semen. Mol Hum Reprod. 2005;11:575–82.

141. Aljabari B, Calogero AE, Perdichizzi A, et al. Imbalance in seminal fluid MIF indicates male infertility. Mol Med. 2007;13:199–202.

142. Carli C, Leclerc P, Metz CN, et al. Direct effect of macrophage migration inhibitory factor on sperm function: possible involvement in endometriosis-associated infertility. Fertil Steril. 2007;88(4 Suppl):1240–7.

143. Hussenet F, Dousset B, Cordonnier JL, et al. Tumour necrosis factor alpha and interleukin 2 in normal and infected human seminal fluid. Hum Reprod. 1993;8:409–11.

144. Gruschwitz MS, Brezinschek R, Brezinschek HP. Cytokine levels in the seminal plasma of infertile males. J Androl. 1996;17:158–63.

145. Omu AE, Al-Qattan F, Al-Abdul-Hadi FM, et al. Seminal immune response in infertile men with leukocytospermia: effect on antioxidant activity. Eur J Obstet Gynecol Reprod Biol. 1999;86:195–202.

146. Sikorski R, Kapec E, Krzeminski A, et al. Levels of proinflammatory cytokines (Il-1 alpha, Il-6, TNF-alpha) in the semen plasma of male partners of infertile couples. Ginekol Pol. 2001;72:1325–8.

147. Wincek TJ, Meyer TK, Meyer MR, et al. Absence of a direct effect of recombinant tumor necrosis factor-alpha on human sperm function and murine preimplantation development. Fertil Steril. 1991;56:332–9.

148. Haney AF, Hughes SF, Weinberg JB. The lack of effect of tumor necrosis factor-alpha, interleukin-1-alpha, and interferon-gamma on human sperm motility in vitro. J Androl. 1992;13:249–53.

149. Lewis SE, Donnelly ET, Sterling ES, et al. Nitric oxide synthase and nitrite production in human spermatozoa: evidence that endogenous nitric oxide is beneficial to sperm motility. Mol Hum Reprod. 1996;2:873–8.

150. Kocak I, Yenisey C, Dundar M, et al. Relationship between seminal plasma interleukin-6 and tumor necrosis factor alpha levels with semen parameters in fertile and infertile men. Urol Res. 2002;30:263–7.

151. Eisermann J, Register KB, Strickler RC, et al. The effect of tumor necrosis factor on human sperm motility in vitro. J Androl. 1989;10:270–4.

152. Perdichizzi A, Nicoletti F, La Vignera S, et al. Effects of tumour necrosis factor-alpha on human sperm motility and apoptosis. J Clin Immunol. 2007;27:152–62.

153. Bian J, Guo X, Xiong C, et al. Experimental study of the effect of rhTNF-alpha on human sperm mitochondrial function and motility in vitro. Zhonghua Nan Ke Xue. 2004;10:415–9.
154. Said TM, Agarwal A, Falcone T, et al. Infliximab may reverse the toxic effects induced by tumor necrosis factor alpha in human spermatozoa: an in vitro model. Fertil Steril. 2005;83:1665–73.
155. Allam JP, Fronhoffs F, Fathy A, et al. High percentage of apoptotic spermatozoa in ejaculates from men with chronic genital tract inflammation. Andrologia. 2008;40:329–34.

# Chapter 11
# Antioxidants and Sperm DNA Damage

**Armand Zini and Maria San Gabriel**

Infertile men have higher levels of sperm DNA damage than do fertile men, and this damage may reduce male fertility potential and may impact on reproductive capacity. This is particularly important in the context of assisted reproductive technologies (ARTs), as there is a mounting concern regarding the safety of utilizing DNA-damaged spermatozoa in this setting. A better understanding of the etiology of sperm DNA damage may help identify strategies to reduce sperm DNA damage. In this chapter, we will discuss the rationale for antioxidant therapy, examine the relationship between oxidative stress and sperm DNA damage, and evaluate the studies on dietary and in vitro antioxidants on sperm DNA damage. The review focuses primarily on clinical (human) studies with some examples taken from experimental (animal) data.

## Etiology of Sperm DNA Damage

The etiology of sperm DNA damage in humans is multifactorial. Several clinical conditions have been associated with sperm DNA damage (e.g., chemotherapy, smoking, genital tract infection, varicocele) [1–9]. These conditions can be categorized as primary defects in spermatogenesis (e.g., genetic or developmental abnormalities) and secondary or extrinsic factors (e.g., gonadotoxins, hyperthermia, oxidants, endocrine disruption).

A number of theories have been proposed to explain the DNA damage in human spermatozoa at the cellular level. Studies have suggested that protamine deficiency (with aberrant chromatin remodeling), reactive oxygen species (ROS), and abortive

A. Zini, MD (✉) • M.S. Gabriel, BS
Department of Surgery, Division of Urology, McGill University,
St. Mary's Hospital Center, Montreal, QC, Canada
e-mail: ziniarmand@yahoo.com

A. Zini, A. Agarwal (eds.), *Sperm Chromatin for the Clinician,*
© Springer Science+Business Media New York 2013

213

apoptosis may be responsible for sperm DNA damage [10–13]. Recently, De Iuliis et al. [12] have proposed a two-step hypothesis to explain the generation of sperm DNA damage. Based on their model, sperm DNA damage is sustained as a result of an oxidative injury (second step) to poorly protaminated cells (i.e., cells with incomplete replacement of histones by protamines) that are generated by defective spermiogenesis (first step).

## Relationship Between Oxidative Stress and Sperm DNA Damage

Several studies have reported that sperm DNA damage is associated with oxidative stress, and this represents the basis for the use of antioxidants in the treatment of sperm DNA damage [14–23]. Moreover, both exogenous and endogenous ROS can induce sperm DNA damage in vitro, indicating that ROS can cause sperm DNA damage [15, 23, 24]. Approximately 25% of infertile men have high levels of semen ROS [25, 26], and the levels of sperm DNA oxidation are higher in infertile men compared to fertile men [27, 28]. Semen ROS are generated by spermatozoa (especially, defective or immature) and semen leukocytes [29–33]. While the controlled release of low levels of ROS is necessary for normal sperm function, high levels of ROS can cause sperm dysfunction [29]. The levels of sperm-derived ROS have been associated with sperm DNA damage, although there is no established ROS threshold level above which sperm DNA damage is detected [8, 17, 30].

The susceptibility of human spermatozoa to oxidative stress stems primarily from the characteristics of the sperm plasma membrane. The human sperm plasma membrane contains an abundance of unsaturated fatty acids, and these fatty acids provide fluidity that is necessary for sperm motility and membrane fusion events, such as the acrosome reaction and sperm–egg interaction. However, this characteristic of the membrane predisposes spermatozoa to free radical attack and peroxidation of the plasma membrane lipids. Once this process has been initiated, accumulation of lipid peroxides occurs on the sperm surface and oxidative damage to DNA can ensue [23, 34]. It has been shown that ROS can cause damage to the sperm DNA directly or indirectly via production and subsequent translocation of lipid peroxides [35–38].

## Seminal Antioxidant Capacity and Sperm DNA Damage

Seminal fluid is a rich source of enzymatic and nonenzymatic antioxidants (ROS scavengers), and this fluid protects spermatozoa from oxidative injury [20, 26, 39–41]. The antioxidant properties of seminal plasma are vital to the survival of spermatozoa because these cells have minimal antioxidant capacity (spermatozoa have little cytoplasmic fluid and no capacity for protein synthesis) [26]. The endogenous ROS scavenging enzymes in the male reproductive tract include superoxide dismutase (SOD), catalase, and glutathione peroxidase (GPX) [26, 40, 42–46]. Experimental studies have shown that a deficiency in any of these enzymes can increase oxidative stress and lead to male infertility [47, 48]. These antioxidant enzymes (SOD, catalase, and GPX) are also found in semen [35]. Additionally, there are several nonenzymatic antioxidants (e.g., vitamins C and E, hypotaurine, taurine, L-carnitine, lycopene) that are found in semen, and these nonenzymatic antioxidants are believed to account for much of the total seminal antioxidant activity [26, 49].

A number of investigators have proposed that oxidative sperm DNA damage may be secondary to reduced semen antioxidant capacity; however, clinical studies have reported conflicting results in this respect. Several studies have, indeed, demonstrated that a deficiency in semen antioxidants is associated with sperm DNA damage, whereas other studies have not observed the same relationship [50–53]. Similarly, several studies have shown that seminal antioxidant activity is lower in infertile men with high levels of seminal ROS (relative to those with normal levels of ROS), whereas others have not shown this to be the case [26, 54–56].

Although a relationship between male infertility and systemic antioxidant deficiency has not been reported to date, it is possible that a subset of infertile men may be at risk for antioxidant deficiency, particularly, vitamin C deficiency [57]. We suspect that infertile men with specific lifestyles (e.g., smoking, increased alcohol intake, dieting) may be at high risk for antioxidant or vitamin deficiency but this remains to be tested [58, 59]. Recently, investigators have evaluated dietary antioxidant intake (vitamins C, E, or β-carotene) and sperm DNA damage in a cohort of fertile men but failed to identify any relationships between these parameters [60].

# Clinical Studies

## *Effect of Dietary Antioxidants on Sperm DNA Damage*

An effective dietary antioxidant should be readily absorbed and concentrated in reproductive tract tissues. ideally, the antioxidant preparation must also replete a deficiency (in the testis, epididymis or semen) and be a vital element of reproductive function. The antioxidant must either improve testicular function and spermatogenesis and/or epididymal function, resulting in improved sperm function and chromatin compaction and integrity. Additionally, the antioxidant preparation should enhance semen antioxidant capacity and reduce seminal oxidative stress.

There are few reports on the role of dietary antioxidant supplements and sperm DNA integrity. Most of the studies are small with no evaluation of the mechanism of action of antioxidants and the only outcomes measured are the integrity of the sperm DNA and/or the pregnancy rate. Moreover, all of the studies evaluate the effects of a short treatment course (with no long-term follow-up), and most are not randomized and fail to include a placebo-control group. Additionally, there may be an inherent bias because many studies select men with high levels of sperm DNA damage or oxidative stress at baseline, and in these studies, treatment is generally associated with an improvement in sperm DNA integrity and fertility potential (Table 11.1) [51, 61–67].

Fraga et al. [51] provided the most convincing demonstration that antioxidants can protect sperm DNA from oxidative damage. In their experiments, they demonstrated that oral vitamin C intake increases semen vitamin C levels and improves sperm DNA integrity (lowers DNA oxidation levels) in men on a vitamin C-depleted diet (with vitamin C deficiency). As stated earlier, several studies of infertile men with high levels of sperm DNA damage or oxidative stress (two were randomized controlled studies and four uncontrolled trials) have shown that antioxidant therapy is effective in improving sperm DNA integrity or pregnancy rates (Table 11.1). In men with idiopathic infertility, the effect of dietary antioxidants on sperm DNA integrity is equivocal with one of two controlled trials showing a benefit of antioxidants on sperm DNA integrity (Table 11.1) [27, 68]. However, in these eight recent studies of antioxidants and sperm DNA damage, there has been no evaluation of systemic or semen vitamin levels and no estimation of seminal oxidative stress. As such, the precise mechanism of action of these antioxidant supplements on sperm DNA quality is unknown.

## Effect of In Vitro Antioxidants on Sperm DNA Damage

Several studies have evaluated the potential benefit of adding antioxidants to in vitro preparations so as to protect the sperm DNA from oxidative damage. This has important clinical relevance because sperm collection and subsequent in vitro processing is routinely performed prior to the application of ARTs (e.g., intrauterine insemination and in vitro fertilization). Oxidative injury to the sperm DNA may result particularly from sperm processing techniques (e.g., centrifugation, aerobic incubation), as spermatozoa are vulnerable to oxidants because seminal plasma (rich in antioxidants) has been removed in the process [41].

There is good evidence to show that subpopulations of spermatozoa will exhibit differing susceptibility to oxidative stress: the DNA of normal spermatozoa is less susceptible to gentle processing techniques than is the DNA of abnormal or immature spermatozoa [33, 69]. Experimental studies suggest that the susceptibility of the sperm DNA to oxidative injury is related to the degree of sperm chromatin compaction (i.e., level of protamination) [12, 70]. We have recently shown that the spermatozoa of FSH-receptor knock-out mice are more susceptible to oxidative DNA injury but also benefit more so from antioxidant treatment than do spermatozoa of

**Table 11.1** Effect of dietary antioxidant supplements on sperm DNA integrity

| Study | Patients/test | Treatment(s) | $n$ | Results |
|---|---|---|---|---|
| Infertile men with high sperm DNA fragmentation levels or oxidative stress | | | | |
| Greco et al. [63] | 1 Failed ICSI TUNEL >15% | Vits C 1 g, E 1 g | 38 | Rx (2 months): ↓DD in 76%, 48% ICSI pregnancy No control group |
| Greco et al. [62] | Infertility TUNEL >15% | Vits C 1 g, E 1 g | 32 32 | Rx (2 months): ↓DD (22 → 9%) Placebo group: no effect on DD (22 → 22%) |
| Menezo et al. [64] | 2 Failed ICSI DFI >15% Decond >15% | Vits C, E (400 mg), zinc, Se, β-carotene | 57 | Rx (90 days):↓sperm %DFI (32 → 26%: by 19%), but ↑ sperm %HDS (17.5 → 25.5%: by 23%) No control group |
| Tremellen et al. [65] | Male Infert TUNEL >25% | Menevit (lyco-pene, vits C, E, zinc, Se, folate, garlic) | 36 16 | Rx (3 months): 39% ICSI pregnancy rate, but no ↑ in embryo quality, no post-Rx DD Placebo group: 16% ICSI pregnancy rate |
| Gil-Villa et al. [61] | Pregnancy loss ↑LPO or DFI | Vits C, E, zinc, β-carotene | 9 | Rx (3 months): six (of nine) couples got pregnancy No control group |
| Tunc et al. [66] | Male Infert ↑Semen OS | Menevit (lyco-pene, vits C, E, zinc, Se, folate, garlic) | 45 | Rx (3 months): ↓DD (22 → 18%) ↓ROS production and ↑sperm protamination No control group |
| Unselected infertile men | | | | |
| Piomboni et al. [68] | Asthenosp. AO stain | Vits C, E, β-glucan, papaya, lactoferrin | 36 15 | Rx (90 days): ↑motility and morph but not DD Control group: no effect |
| Kodama et al. [27] | Male infert 8-OHdG | Vits C, E (200 mg) Glutathione (400 mg) | 14 7 | Rx (2 months): ↓in 8-OHdG (1.5 → 1.1/10$^5$ dG) Control group: no change in 8-OHdG levels |

*8-OHdG* 8-hydroxy-2-deoxyguanosine; *AO* acridine orange; *DD* DNA damage; *Decond* decondensation; *DFI* DNA fragmentation index; *LPO* lipid peroxidation; *OS* oxidative stress; *Rx* Treatment; *ROS* reactive oxygen species; *Se* selenium; *TUNEL* terminal nucleotidyl transferase dUTP nick-end labeling; *vit* vitamin

wild-type animals [71]. These data suggest that the spermatozoa of infertile men may be more susceptible to oxidative injury yet may be afforded greater protection by antioxidants.

Studies on in vitro antioxidant supplementation have evaluated the capacity of antioxidants to protect spermatozoa from exogenous and endogenous ROS and from the effects of semen processing and cryopreservation. It is quite clear from

**Table 11.2** Role of in vitro antioxidant supplements in protecting sperm DNA from exogenous ROS

| Study | Assay | Exogenous ROS | Antioxidant supplement and results |
|---|---|---|---|
| Lopes et al. [18] | TUNEL | X + XO | GSH + hypotaurine protect spz from X + XO-induced DD<br>Catalase protects spz from X+XO-induced DD<br>n-Acetylcysteine protects spz from X + XO-induced DD |
| Potts et al. [20] | TUNEL | $H_2O_2$ + Fe + ADP | S. plasma (>60%v/v) lowers oxidative spz damage ($\downarrow$DD, LPO) |
| Sierens et al. [73] | Comet | $H_2O_2$ | Isoflavones, vitamin C and E protect spz from $H_2O_2$-induced DD (Isoflavones: genistein, equol). Dose effect noted |
| Russo et al. [72] | Comet | $H_2O_2$<br>Benzopyrene<br>$H_2O_2$+Fe+ADP | Propolis lowers oxidative spz damage ($\downarrow$LPO, DD, LDH) (Propolis – a natural resinous hive product) |

*ADP* adenosine diphosphate; *Comet* single-cell gel electrophoresis; *DD* DNA damage; *Fe* iron; *GSH* glutathione; *LDH* lactate dehydrogenase; *LPO* lipid peroxidation; *S. plasma* seminal plasma; *spz* sperm; *TUNEL* terminal nucleotidyl transferase dUTP nick-end labeling; *X* xanthine; *XO* xanthine oxidase

**Table 11.3** Role of in vitro antioxidant supplements in protecting sperm DNA from stimulated endogenous reactive oxygen species (ROS) generation

| Study | Assay | ROS stimulant | Antioxidant supplement and results |
|---|---|---|---|
| Twigg et al. [23] | ISNTL | NADPH | Vit E, SOD, catalase, hypotaurine, albumin all ineffective in protecting spz DNA from endogenous ROS |
| Cemeli et al. [76] | Comet | Estrogens (1 h 37°C) | Flavonoid (Kaempferol) protects sperm from estrogen-induced oxidative DD |
| Dobrzynska et al. [77] | Comet | DES, T3, T4, NA (1 h 37°C) | Flavonoids and catalase protect spz from stimulant-induced oxidative DD (Flavonoids: Kaempferol, Quercetin) |
| Anderson et al. [75] | Comet | Estrogens | Catalase protects spz from estrogen-induced oxidative DD, SOD and vit C less effective (Estrogens: equol, daidzein, genistein, DES, E2) |

*Comet* alkaline single-cell gel electrophoresis; *DD* DNA damage; *ISNTL* in situ nick translation assay; *NA* noradrenaline; *ROS* reactive oxygen species; *SOD* superoxide dismutase; *spz* sperm; *T3* triiodothyronine; *T4* thyroxine; *vit* vitamin

several studies that antioxidants (e.g., vitamins C and E, catalase, glutathione) can effectively protect sperm DNA from the effects of exogenous ROS (see Table 11.2) [18, 20, 72, 73]. This is clinically relevant because many semen samples contain leukocytes and the sperm processing (with removal of seminal plasma) can cause these cells to generate high levels of unchecked exogenous ROS (e.g., centrifugation) [74]. By contrast, a number of studies have shown that

**Table 11.4** Role of in vitro antioxidant supplements in protecting sperm DNA from semen processing

| Study | Assay | Semen processing | Antioxidant supplement and results |
|---|---|---|---|
| Hughes et al. [81] | Comet | Percoll DGC | Vitamins C, E or urate lower sperm DD after DGC |
| | | | Vitamins C + E or AC increase sperm DD after DGC |
| Donnelly et al. [79] | Comet | Percoll DGC | Vit C or E do not lower baseline sperm ROS and DD |
| | | | Vit C or E protect sperm from $H_2O_2$ induced ROS and DD |
| | | | Vits C + E induce sperm DD and increase $H_2O_2$-induced DD |
| Donnelly et al. [80] | Comet | Percoll DGC ±$H_2O_2$ | GSH, hypotaurine or both do not alter baseline sperm DD |
| | | | GSH, hypotaurine or both do not alter sperm motility at 4 h |
| | | | GSH and/or hypotaurine lower $H_2O_2$-induced sperm DD |
| Chi et al. [78] | Comet | Centrifugation (1,000 rpm ×2) + 1 h incubation | EDTA or catalase lower centrifugation-induced sperm ROS |
| | | | EDTA or catalase lower centrifugation-induced sperm DD |
| | | | EDTA or datalase have no protective effect on LPO |

*AC* Acetyl cysteine; *Comet* alkaline single-cell gel electrophoresis; *DD* DNA damage; *DGC* density-gradient centrifugation; *GSH* glutathione; *LPO* lipid peroxidation; *ROS* reactive oxygen species; *vit* vitamin

antioxidants are of limited value in protecting the DNA of normal spermatozoa (with normal chromatin compaction) from endogenous ROS production (for example, ROS may be generated by incubating spermatozoa with NADPH or by centrifugation) (Table 11.3) [23, 75–77]. Although there are few data to support this, some studies suggest that in those samples with poor morphology and poor sperm chromatin compaction, antioxidants may protect the sperm DNA from endogenous ROS production, as these samples are inherently more vulnerable to oxidative stress [33, 69].

Antioxidants appear to be of minimal value in terms of protecting sperm DNA from gentle semen processing (e.g., incubation or density-gradient centrifugation) (Table 11.4) [78–81], and in some cases, these antioxidants (e.g., combination of vitamins C and E) may increase the levels of sperm DNA damage [80, 81]. Five clinical studies have evaluated the potential protective effect(s) of antioxidants on sperm DNA integrity during cryopreservation. Although Taylor et al. [82] reported that the antioxidant vitamin E does not protect sperm DNA during cryopreservation, four other studies have shown that antioxidants (vitamin C, catalase, resveratrol, genistein) can protect the sperm DNA from oxidative injury during cryopreservation and subsequent thawing [82–86] (Table 11.5).

**Table 11.5** The role of in vitro antioxidants in protecting human sperm DNA from injury caused by cryopreservation and thawing

| Study | Assay | Antioxidant | Effect of antioxidant on cryopreservation and thawing |
|---|---|---|---|
| Taylor et al. [82] | TUNEL | Vitamin E | No effect on sperm DNA integrity<br>Improved post-thaw motility |
| Li et al. [84] | Comet | Catalase<br>Ascorbic acid | Improved sperm DNA integrity<br>Reduced ROS production |
| Branco et al. [83] | Comet | Resveratol or<br>Ascorbic acid | Improved sperm DNA integrity |
| Martinez-Soto et al. [85] | TUNEL | Genistein | Improved sperm DNA integrity<br>Reduced ROS production, improved post-thaw motility |
| Thomson et al. [86] | 8-OHdG<br>TUNEL | Genistein | Improved sperm DNA integrity<br>(reduced oxidative damage) |

*8-OHdG* 8-Hydroxy-2-deoxyguanosine; *COMET* alkaline single-cell gel electrophoresis; *ROS* reactive oxygen species; *TUNEL* terminal nucleotidyl transferase dUTP nick-end labeling

## Summary

In vitro studies have demonstrated a beneficial effect of antioxidant supplements in protecting normal sperm DNA from exogenous oxidants, but the effect of these antioxidants in protecting normal spermatozoa from endogenous ROS and gentle sperm processing has not been established. By contrast, when evaluating spermatozoa from infertile men, clinical and experimental studies indicate a beneficial effect of antioxidant supplements in protecting the DNA from exogenous and endogenous oxidants and from gentle sperm processing. The limited data on the protective effect(s) of antioxidants on sperm DNA integrity during cryopreservation and thawing suggest that antioxidants are useful in this context. Dietary antioxidants may be beneficial in reducing sperm DNA damage, particularly in men with high levels of DNA fragmentation. However, the exact mechanism of action of dietary antioxidants has not been established and most of studies on this subject are small.

## Expert Commentary

The biological basis for the use of antioxidants in male infertility is sound and is based on the body of literature showing that sperm dysfunction (including DNA damage) is strongly related to oxidative stress. Clinical studies of dietary antioxidants demonstrate a promising positive effect of these antioxidants on the integrity of the sperm DNA; however, most studies are small and mechanistic studies are lacking. Moreover, the optimal antioxidant complement has not been defined, but most studies report on one or more of the following: vitamins C and E, folic acid, and zinc. Clinical studies of in vitro antioxidants support the use of antioxidants in protecting spermatozoa (particularly abnormal spermatozoa) from oxidative stress. However, the optimal antioxidant and its concentration have not been established yet.

## Five-Year View

In order to see a real advance in the field of dietary antioxidants for male infertility, we need to undertake larger studies with a longer treatment course and some evaluation of the mechanism of action of these agents. Additional in vitro antioxidant studies are needed to better define the differences in treatment response between normal (fertile) and subnormal (infertile) semen samples and identify the optimal protocol (type and concentration of antioxidant).

## References

1. Banks S, King SA, Irvine DS, Saunders PT. Impact of a mild scrotal heat stress on DNA integrity in murine spermatozoa. Reproduction. 2005;129:505–14.
2. Bungum M, Humaidan P, Axmon A, Spano M, Bungum L, Erenpreiss J, et al. Sperm DNA integrity assessment in prediction of assisted reproduction technology outcome. Hum Reprod. 2007;22:174–9.
3. Erenpreiss J, Hlevicka S, Zalkalns J, Erenpreisa J. Effect of leukocytospermia on sperm DNA integrity: a negative effect in abnormal semen samples. J Androl. 2002;23:717–23.
4. Fossa SD, De Angelis P, Kraggerud SM, Evenson D, Theodorsen L, Clausen OP. Prediction of posttreatment spermatogenesis in patients with testicular cancer by flow cytometric sperm chromatin structure assay. Cytometry. 1997;30:192–6.
5. O'Flaherty C, Vaisheva F, Hales BF, Chan P, Robaire B. Characterization of sperm chromatin quality in testicular cancer and Hodgkin's lymphoma patients prior to chemotherapy. Hum Reprod. 2008;23:1044–52.
6. Potts RJ, Newbury CJ, Smith G, Notarianni LJ, Jefferies TM. Sperm chromatin damage associated with male smoking. Mutat Res. 1999;423:103–11.
7. Sailer BL, Sarkar LJ, Bjordahl JA, Jost LK, Evenson DP. Effects of heat stress on mouse testicular cells and sperm chromatin structure. J Androl. 1997;18:294–301.
8. Saleh RA, Agarwal A, Sharma RK, Said TM, Sikka SC, Thomas Jr AJ. Evaluation of nuclear DNA damage in spermatozoa from infertile men with varicocele. Fertil Steril. 2003; 80:1431–6.
9. Zini A, Sigman M. Are tests of sperm DNA damage clinically useful? Pros and cons. J Androl. 2009;30:219–29.
10. Aoki VW, Emery BR, Liu L, Carrell DT. Protamine levels vary between individual sperm cells of infertile human males and correlate with viability and DNA integrity. J Androl. 2006;27:890–8.
11. Aoki VW, Moskovtsev SI, Willis J, Liu L, Mullen JB, Carrell DT. DNA integrity is compromised in protamine-deficient human sperm. J Androl. 2005;26:741–8.
12. De Iuliis GN, Thomson LK, Mitchell LA, Finnie JM, Koppers AJ, Hedges A, et al. DNA damage in human spermatozoa is highly correlated with the efficiency of chromatin remodeling and the formation of 8-hydroxy-2'-deoxyguanosine, a marker of oxidative stress. Biol Reprod. 2009;81:517–24.

13. Sakkas D, Seli E, Bizzaro D, Tarozzi N, Manicardi GC. Abnormal spermatozoa in the ejaculate: abortive apoptosis and faulty nuclear remodelling during spermatogenesis. Reprod Biomed Online. 2003;7:428–32.
14. Agarwal A, Said TM. Oxidative stress, DNA damage and apoptosis in male infertility: a clinical approach. BJU Int. 2005;95:503–7.
15. Aitken RJ, Gordon E, Harkiss D, Twigg JP, Milne P, Jennings Z, et al. Relative impact of oxidative stress on the functional competence and genomic integrity of human spermatozoa. Biol Reprod. 1998;59:1037–46.
16. Aitken RJ, Krausz C. Oxidative stress, DNA damage and the Y chromosome. Reproduction. 2001;122:497–506.
17. Irvine DS, Twigg JP, Gordon EL, Fulton N, Milne PA, Aitken RJ. DNA integrity in human spermatozoa: relationships with semen quality. J Androl. 2000;21:33–44.
18. Lopes S, Jurisicova A, Sun JG, Casper RF. Reactive oxygen species: potential cause for DNA fragmentation in human spermatozoa. Hum Reprod. 1998;13:896–900.
19. Oger I, Da Cruz C, Panteix G, Menezo Y. Evaluating human sperm DNA integrity: relationship between 8-hydroxydeoxyguanosine quantification and the sperm chromatin structure assay. Zygote. 2003;11:367–71.
20. Potts RJ, Notarianni LJ, Jefferies TM. Seminal plasma reduces exogenous oxidative damage to human sperm, determined by the measurement of DNA strand breaks and lipid peroxidation. Mutat Res. 2000;447:249–56.
21. Said TM, Aziz N, Sharma RK, Lewis-Jones I, Thomas Jr AJ, Agarwal A. Novel association between sperm deformity index and oxidative stress-induced DNA damage in infertile male patients. Asian J Androl. 2005;7:121–6.
22. Saleh RA, Agarwal A, Nada EA, El-Tonsy MH, Sharma RK, Meyer A, et al. Negative effects of increased sperm DNA damage in relation to seminal oxidative stress in men with idiopathic and male factor infertility. Fertil Steril. 2003;79 Suppl 3:1597–605.
23. Twigg J, Fulton N, Gomez E, Irvine DS, Aitken RJ. Analysis of the impact of intracellular reactive oxygen species generation on the structural and functional integrity of human spermatozoa: lipid peroxidation, DNA fragmentation and effectiveness of antioxidants. Hum Reprod. 1998;13:1429–36.
24. Sawyer DE, Mercer BG, Wiklendt AM, Aitken RJ. Quantitative analysis of gene-specific DNA damage in human spermatozoa. Mutat Res. 2003;529:21–34.
25. Iwasaki A, Gagnon C. Formation of reactive oxygen species in spermatozoa of infertile patients. Fertil Steril. 1992;57:409–16.
26. Zini A, de Lamirande E, Gagnon C. Reactive oxygen species in semen of infertile patients: levels of superoxide dismutase- and catalase-like activities in seminal plasma and spermatozoa. Int J Androl. 1993;16:183–8.
27. Kodama H, Yamaguchi R, Fukuda J, Kasai H, Tanaka T. Increased oxidative deoxyribonucleic acid damage in the spermatozoa of infertile male patients. Fertil Steril. 1997;68:519–24.
28. Shen HM, Chia SE, Ong CN. Evaluation of oxidative DNA damage in human sperm and its association with male infertility. J Androl. 1999;20:718–23.
29. Aitken RJ, West K, Buckingham D. Leukocytic infiltration into the human ejaculate and its association with semen quality, oxidative stress, and sperm function. J Androl. 1994;15:343–52.
30. Barroso G, Morshedi M, Oehninger S. Analysis of DNA fragmentation, plasma membrane translocation of phosphatidylserine and oxidative stress in human spermatozoa. Hum Reprod. 2000;15:1338–44.
31. de Lamirande E, Jiang H, Zini A, Kodama H, Gagnon C. Reactive oxygen species and sperm physiology. Rev Reprod. 1997;2:48–54.
32. Gomez E, Buckingham DW, Brindle J, Lanzafame F, Irvine DS, Aitken RJ. Development of an image analysis system to monitor the retention of residual cytoplasm by human spermatozoa: correlation with biochemical markers of the cytoplasmic space, oxidative stress, and sperm function. J Androl. 1996;17:276–87.
33. Muratori M, Piomboni P, Baldi E, Filimberti E, Pecchioli P, Moretti E, et al. Functional and ultrastructural features of DNA-fragmented human sperm. J Androl. 2000;21:903–12.

34. Alvarez JG, Touchstone JC, Blasco L, Storey BT. Spontaneous lipid peroxidation and production of hydrogen peroxide and superoxide in human spermatozoa. Superoxide dismutase as major enzyme protectant against oxygen toxicity. J Androl. 1987;8:338–48.
35. Aitken RJ, Clarkson JS. Cellular basis of defective sperm function and its association with the genesis of reactive oxygen species by human spermatozoa. J Reprod Fertil. 1987; 81:459–69.
36. de Lamirande E, Gagnon C. Reactive oxygen species and human spermatozoa. I. Effects on the motility of intact spermatozoa and on sperm axonemes. J Androl. 1992;13:368–78.
37. Lewis SE, Aitken RJ. DNA damage to spermatozoa has impacts on fertilization and pregnancy. Cell Tissue Res. 2005;322:33–41.
38. Yang MH, Schaich KM. Factors affecting DNA damage caused by lipid hydroperoxides and aldehydes. Free Radic Biol Med. 1996;20:225–36.
39. Gagnon C, Iwasaki A, De Lamirande E, Kovalski N. Reactive oxygen species and human spermatozoa. Ann N Y Acad Sci. 1991;637:436–44.
40. Jeulin C, Soufir JC, Weber P, Laval-Martin D, Calvayrac R. Catalase activity in human spermatozoa and seminal plasma. Gamete Res. 1989;24:185–96.
41. Twigg J, Irvine DS, Houston P, Fulton N, Michael L, Aitken RJ. Iatrogenic DNA damage induced in human spermatozoa during sperm preparation: protective significance of seminal plasma. Mol Hum Reprod. 1998;4:439–45.
42. Jow WW, Schlegel PN, Cichon Z, Phillips D, Goldstein M, Bardin CW. IDentification and localization of copper-zinc superoxide dismutase gene expression in rat testicular development. J Androl. 1993;14:439–47.
43. Watanabe S. Frequent structural chromosome aberrations in immotile human sperm exposed to culture media. Hum Reprod. 2004;19:940–7.
44. Zini A, Schlegel PN. Catalase mRNA expression in the male rat reproductive tract. J Androl. 1996;17:473–80.
45. Zini A, Schlegel PN. Expression of glutathione peroxidases in the adult male rat reproductive tract. Fertil Steril. 1997;68:689–95.
46. Zini A, Schlegel PN. IDentification and characterization of antioxidant enzyme mRNAs in the rat epididymis. Int J Androl. 1997;20:86–91.
47. Chabory E, Damon C, Lenoir A, Kauselmann G, Kern H, Zevnik B, et al. Epididymis seleno-independent glutathione peroxidase 5 maintains sperm DNA integrity in mice. J Clin Invest. 2009;119:2074–85.
48. Weir CP, Robaire B. Spermatozoa have decreased antioxidant enzymatic capacity and increased reactive oxygen species production during aging in the Brown Norway rat. J Androl. 2007;28:229–40.
49. Holmes RP, Goodman HO, Shihabi ZK, Jarow JP. The taurine and hypotaurine content of human semen. J Androl. 1992;13:289–92.
50. Appasamy M, Muttukrishna S, Pizzey AR, Ozturk O, Groome NP, Serhal P, et al. Relationship between male reproductive hormones, sperm DNA damage and markers of oxidative stress in infertility. Reprod Biomed Online. 2007;14:159–65.
51. Fraga CG, Motchnik PA, Shigenaga MK, Helbock HJ, Jacob RA, Ames BN. Ascorbic acid protects against endogenous oxidative DNA damage in human sperm. Proc Natl Acad Sci USA. 1991;88:11003–6.
52. Song GJ, Lewis V. Mitochondrial DNA integrity and copy number in sperm from infertile men. Fertil Steril. 2008;90:2238–44.
53. Verit FF, Verit A, Kocyigit A, Ciftci H, Celik H, Koksal M. No increase in sperm DNA damage and seminal oxidative stress in patients with idiopathic infertility. Arch Gynecol Obstet. 2006;274:339–44.
54. Lewis SE, Boyle PM, McKinney KA, Young IS, Thompson W. Total antioxidant capacity of seminal plasma is different in fertile and infertile men. Fertil Steril. 1995;64:868–70.
55. Sanocka D, Miesel R, Jedrzejczak P, Kurpisz MK. Oxidative stress and male infertility. J Androl. 1996;17:449–54.
56. Smith R, Vantman D, Ponce J, Escobar J, Lissi E. Total antioxidant capacity of human seminal plasma. Hum Reprod. 1996;11:1655–60.

57. Hampl JS, Taylor CA, Johnston CS. Vitamin C deficiency and depletion in the United States: the Third National Health and Nutrition Examination Survey, 1988 to 1994. Am J Public Health. 2004;94:870–5.
58. Jacob RA. Assessment of human vitamin C status. J Nutr. 1990;120 Suppl 11:1480–5.
59. Ryle PR, Thomson AD. Nutrition and vitamins in alcoholism. Contemp Issues Clin Biochem. 1984;1:188–224.
60. Silver EW, Eskenazi B, Evenson DP, Block G, Young S, Wyrobek AJ. Effect of antioxidant intake on sperm chromatin stability in healthy nonsmoking men. J Androl. 2005;26:550–6.
61. Gil-Villa AM, Cardona-Maya W, Agarwal A, Sharma R, Cadavid A. Role of male factor in early recurrent embryo loss: do antioxidants have any effect? Fertil Steril. 2009;92:565–71.
62. Greco E, Iacobelli M, Rienzi L, Ubaldi F, Ferrero S, Tesarik J. Reduction of the incidence of sperm DNA fragmentation by oral antioxidant treatment. J Androl. 2005;26:349–53.
63. Greco E, Romano S, Iacobelli M, Ferrero S, Baroni E, Minasi MG, et al. ICSI in cases of sperm DNA damage: beneficial effect of oral antioxidant treatment. Hum Reprod. 2005;20:2590–4.
64. Menezo YJ, Hazout A, Panteix G, Robert F, Rollet J, Cohen-Bacrie P, et al. Antioxidants to reduce sperm DNA fragmentation: an unexpected adverse effect. Reprod Biomed Online. 2007;14:418–21.
65. Tremellen K, Miari G, Froiland D, Thompson J. A randomised control trial examining the effect of an antioxidant (Menevit) on pregnancy outcome during IVF-ICSI treatment. Aust N Z J Obstet Gynaecol. 2007;47:216–21.
66. Tunc O, Thompson J, Tremellen K. Improvement in sperm DNA quality using an oral antioxidant therapy. Reprod Biomed Online. 2009;18:761–8.
67. Tunc O, Tremellen K. Oxidative DNA damage impairs global sperm DNA methylation in infertile men. J Assist Reprod Genet. 2009;26:537–44.
68. Piomboni P, Gambera L, Serafini F, Campanella G, Morgante G, De Leo V. Sperm quality improvement after natural anti-oxidant treatment of asthenoteratospermic men with leukocytospermia. Asian J Androl. 2008;10:201–6.
69. Said TM, Agarwal A, Sharma RK, Thomas Jr AJ, Sikka SC. Impact of sperm morphology on DNA damage caused by oxidative stress induced by beta-nicotinamide adenine dinucleotide phosphate. Fertil Steril. 2005;83:95–103.
70. Cho C, Willis WD, Goulding EH, Jung-Ha H, Choi YC, Hecht NB, et al. Haploinsufficiency of protamine-1 or -2 causes infertility in mice. Nat Genet. 2001;28:82–6.
71. Libman J, Gabriel MS, Sairam MR, Zini A. Catalase can protect spermatozoa of FSH receptor knock-out mice against oxidant-induced DNA damage in vitro. Int J Androl. 2010;33(6):818–22.
72. Russo A, Troncoso N, Sanchez F, Garbarino JA, Vanella A. Propolis protects human spermatozoa from DNA damage caused by benzo[a]pyrene and exogenous reactive oxygen species. Life Sci. 2006;78:1401–6.
73. Sierens J, Hartley JA, Campbell MJ, Leathem AJ, Woodside JV. In vitro isoflavone supplementation reduces hydrogen peroxide-induced DNA damage in sperm. Teratog Carcinog Mutagen. 2002;22:227–34.
74. Aitken RJ, Buckingham DW, Brindle J, Gomez E, Baker HW, Irvine DS. Analysis of sperm movement in relation to the oxidative stress created by leukocytes in washed sperm preparations and seminal plasma. Hum Reprod. 1995;10:2061–71.
75. Anderson D, Schmid TE, Baumgartner A, Cemeli-Carratala E, Brinkworth MH, Wood JM. Oestrogenic compounds and oxidative stress (in human sperm and lymphocytes in the Comet assay). Mutat Res. 2003;544:173–8.
76. Cemeli E, Schmid TE, Anderson D. Modulation by flavonoids of DNA damage induced by estrogen-like compounds. Environ Mol Mutagen. 2004;44:420–6.
77. Dobrzynska MM, Baumgartner A, Anderson D. Antioxidants modulate thyroid hormone- and noradrenaline-induced DNA damage in human sperm. Mutagenesis. 2004;19:325–30.

78. Chi HJ, Kim JH, Ryu CS, Lee JY, Park JS, Chung DY, et al. Protective effect of antioxidant supplementation in sperm-preparation medium against oxidative stress in human spermatozoa. Hum Reprod. 2008;23:1023–8.
79. Donnelly ET, McClure N, Lewis SE. The effect of ascorbate and alpha-tocopherol supplementation in vitro on DNA integrity and hydrogen peroxide-induced DNA damage in human spermatozoa. Mutagenesis. 1999;14:505–12.
80. Donnelly ET, McClure N, Lewis SE. Glutathione and hypotaurine in vitro: effects on human sperm motility, DNA integrity and production of reactive oxygen species. Mutagenesis. 2000;15:61–8.
81. Hughes CM, Lewis SE, McKelvey-Martin VJ, Thompson W. The effects of antioxidant supplementation during Percoll preparation on human sperm DNA integrity. Hum Reprod. 1998;13:1240–7.
82. Taylor K, Roberts P, Sanders K, Burton P. Effect of antioxidant supplementation of cryopreservation medium on post-thaw integrity of human spermatozoa. Reprod Biomed Online. 2009;18:184–9.
83. Branco CS, Garcez ME, Pasqualotto FF, Erdtman B, Salvador M. Resveratrol and ascorbic acid prevent DNA damage induced by cryopreservation in human semen. Cryobiology. 2010;60(2):235–7.
84. Li Z, Lin Q, Liu R, Xiao W, Liu W. Protective effects of ascorbate and catalase on human spermatozoa during cryopreservation. J Androl. 2010;31(5):437–44.
85. Martinez-Soto JC, de Dioshourcade J, Gutierrez-Adan A, Landeras JL, Gadea J. Effect of genistein supplementation of thawing medium on characteristics of frozen human spermatozoa. Asian J Androl. 2010;12(3):431–41.
86. Thomson LK, Fleming SD, Aitken RJ, De Iuliis GN, Zieschang JA, Clark AM. Cryopreservation-induced human sperm DNA damage is predominantly mediated by oxidative stress rather than apoptosis. Hum Reprod. 2009;24:2061–70.

# Part III
# Sperm Chromatin and Assisted
# Reproductive Technologies (ART)

# Chapter 12
# The Impact of Sperm Processing and Cryopreservation on Sperm DNA Integrity

**Dan Yu, Luke Simon, and Sheena E.M. Lewis**

## The Clinical Need for Sperm Processing

To maintain their fertility, sperm must be separated from seminal plasma as soon as possible after ejaculation, as it has been shown that long exposure to seminal plasma results in reduced motility and vitality [1]. There are also a number of seminal plasma components that inhibit acrosome reactions, capacitation and, thus, the fertilization potential of the sperm. For clinical use, sperm should be separated from seminal plasma as soon as possible after liquefaction. The most common method is by discontinuous two-step density-gradient centrifugation (DCG) that isolates the subpopulation of sperm with the best motility, morphology [2], superior nuclear and mitochondrial DNA quality [3] and without endogenous nicks [4]. The importance and efficacy of DCG in selecting out a population of sperm where most are of high quality are reflected in terms of higher assisted conception rates [5, 6]. However, centrifugation of a semen sample prior to its use in assisted reproductive techniques (ART) can exacerbate sperm oxidative stress. Since sperm do not have any repair mechanisms, as they are transcriptionally silent and lack functional repair enzymes [7–9], this can cause irreversible damage. This can be limited by reducing the time of centrifugation in the preparation of sperm for ART [10, 11]. Furthermore, culturing sperm under low oxygen tension (5%$O_2$/95% $CO_2$ vs. 20% atmospheric $O_2$ content) has been shown to significantly improve sperm quality by reducing seminal leukocyte reactive oxygen species (ROS) production [12, 13].

D. Yu, MD • L. Simon, MSc, PhD • S.E.M. Lewis, PhD (✉)
Centre for Public Health, Queen's University of Belfast,
Room 208, Institute of Clinical Science, Belfast,
Northern Ireland, UK
e-mail: s.e.lewis@qub.ac.uk

A. Zini, A. Agarwal (eds.), *Sperm Chromatin for the Clinician,*
© Springer Science+Business Media New York 2013

229

## The Hazards of Seminal Plasma Removal During DCG

Although DGC facilitates the isolation of high-quality sperm, most suitable for use in ART, the removal of the seminal plasma's protective antioxidants makes sperm DNA more vulnerable to oxidative insult through generation of ROS by adjacent damaged sperm [14, 15]. Furthermore, the semen from infertile men is often associated with higher levels of ROS than that of fertile men, and numerous studies have shown the association between male infertility and raised ROS in semen [14, 16, 17]. Negative associations have been reported between ROS and quantitative velocity parameters, sperm DNA integrity and also lower total antioxidant levels (TAC) in sperm of men with male infertility attending a tertiary centre [18]. Increased ROS levels and reduced antioxidants have also been reported in semen of infertile men with varicocele [19].

When these men's sperm are then exposed to sperm processing for ART, they are at further risk of oxidative damage. Previous studies from our group have shown that depriving sperm of seminal antioxidant protection during DCG preparation for ART leads to DNA damage [20].

All sperm are particularly vulnerable to damage from ROS because of their high polyunsaturated fatty acid content and limited ability to repair damage. In contrast to somatic cells, which contain protective antioxidants within their cytoplasm, sperm lose most of their cytoplasm during the maturation process and, therefore, lack the endogenous repair mechanisms and enzymatic defences observed in other cell types. This leaves them at a significant disadvantage especially since the absence of RNA transcription and DNA repair mechanisms means that any damage induced to sperm will be permanent. ROS are also among the most powerful instigators of sperm DNA damage [21, 22].

## Antioxidants: Physiological and Therapeutic Uses

Antioxidants act to remove damaging ROS such as $O_2$ and $H_2O_2$, and scavengers such as albumin and taurine [23]. Metal chelators can also be useful in reducing ROS generation and preventing lipid peroxidation of sperm membranes, thereby protecting sperm nuclear DNA (reviewed by Agarwal and Said [24]). Paradoxically, the addition of combinations of antioxidants such as vitamins C and E can have damaging effects to DNA in vitro [25] and in vivo where DNA decondensation can increase [26] or they can be ineffective [27]. Ascorbate and catalase, which are both found naturally in seminal plasma, reduce the level of ROS that induce sperm nuclear DNA damage, improving the quality of sperm following cryopreservation prior to ART [28]. Mature ejaculated sperm are protected from oxidative insult by the surrounding seminal plasma, which contains enzymes such as superoxide dismutase, catalase and chain breaking antioxidants such as ascorbate, which is ten times more concentrated than in blood plasma [29], emphasizing the physiological importance of antioxidants. Alpha tocopherol and acetyl cysteine have also been found [30, 31] to be of benefit in protecting motility against ROS impairment and enhancing sperm zona binding. Our group has shown that protection from the DNA damage that can occur during DCG can be provided by supplementing media with antioxidants [3, 20]. Ascorbic acid, alpha tocopherol and urate separately significantly decreased the level of sperm DNA fragmentation.

Recently the human endogenous cannabinoid system (ECS) has been strongly implicated in various aspects of female and male fertility (reviewed by Battista et al. [32]). Some members of the ECS (*N*-acylethanolamide, oleoylethanolamide and Cannabidiol) are potent antioxidants in somatic cells, which may also exert protective effects on sperm DNA, if supplemented during assisted conception processes. Further research is urgently needed to find the most effective antioxidant therapy and dosage for sperm nuclear DNA protection during ART.

## The Heightened Vulnerability of Testicular Sperm

Testicular sperm, retrieved for ART via testicular biopsy, are especially vulnerable to oxidative assault and resultant DNA damage in comparison to mature ejaculated sperm, as chromatin packaging is not completed until SH bonds are oxidized during transit through the epididymis. All sperm naturally produce low levels of ROS as by-products of the electron transfer chain, which are essential for normal sperm maturation and function. However, testicular sperm retain a significant proportion of cytoplasm that may facilitate excess ROS generation, and unlike ejaculated sperm, testicular sperm have no seminal plasma to confer antioxidant protection. This presents a significant clinical problem, since the use of testicular sperm for assisted conception is an increasingly used avenue of treatment for males with problems such as obstructive azoospermia and ejaculatory dysfunction.

## The Clinical Need for Sperm Cryopreservation

A second inadvertent cause of damage in the laboratory is through cryopreservation. Semen cryopreservation is a core technique in the process of preservation and storage of male gametes prior to ART, or before cytotoxic chemotherapy [33], radiotherapy or surgical treatment, whichmay lead to testicular damage or ejaculatory dysfunction. The process of freezing sperm before beginning the treatment, which may affect fertility potential, enables many patients to father their own children post treatment through the use of IVF or intracytoplasmic sperm injection (ICSI). In addition, sperm cryopreservation is mandatory in donor-insemination programmes, as the use of frozen semen allows screening of sperm donors for infections such as HIV and hepatitis B prior to release for insemination [34]. The technique is also widely used for storage of sperm retrieved from azoospermic patients who have undergone testicular sperm biopsy or percutaneous epididymal sperm aspiration, avoiding the need for repeat biopsies or aspiration on the day of ART. Despite many refinements in methodology (reviewed by Anger et al. [35]), the procedure is not without risk and adverse affects. The quality of post-thaw samples remains suboptimal, and IUI and IVF success rates are lower with frozen sperm than with fresh samples [36].

## The Impact of Cryopreservation on Conventional Sperm Parameters

Sperm motility is the function most vulnerable to cryoinjury [37]. Post-thaw motilities are routinely only 50% of pre-freeze values (reviewed by Nijs and Ombelet [38]; Anger et al. [35]). Quantitative motility assessments show reductions in straight line and curvilinear velocities of 25–75% [39]. This functional impairment is due to structural damage in the flagella caused by alterations in permeability and membrane fluidity [40], and conformation of phospholipid bilayers [41, 42]. Pentoxifylline and 2-deoxyadenosine have been utilized to optimize flagging energy levels by inhibiting the breakdown of cAMP and cGMP [42–45] but the adverse effects of phosphodiesterase inhibitors on fertilization rates and early embryo cleavage [46, 47] demand caution in their clinical usage. Reduced sperm penetration of the cervical mucus has also been reported [48].

Organelle damage is also observed in mitochondrial distortion [49]. Alterations in plasma and mitochondrial membrane potentials, observed by reduced R123 uptake [47] leads to reductions in $[Ca^{2+}]_i$. This, in turn, impairs the cell's response to progesterone and ability to progress into capacitative motility [50]. Further damage has been reported as a reduction in intact acrosomal caps and in acrosin activity. There is also an increase in gross morphological abnormalities; particularly in amorphous sperm heads, midpiece anomalies and, cytoplasmic vacuolation [49, 51]. The ultimate cryoinjury, which occurs in up to 30% of sperm, is the fatal loss of membrane integrity [35].

## The Impact of Cryopreservation on Human Sperm DNA

All previous semen freezing suitability criteria have been based on concentration, motility and morphology [24, 52]. However, these have now been largely rejected as fertility biomarkers. In their place, sperm DNA integrity is recognized as a more robust measure of male fertility potential. As a result the scientific community has been readdressing the impact of numerous clinical procedures, including cryopreservation, on sperm DNA integrity.

For the past decade there was a general belief that sperm DNA was impervious to cryodamage [53]. This was largely based on a small study by Duru et al. [54] comparing sperm DNA fragmentation measured by the TUNEL of freeze-thawed sperm from 5 donors and 10 men undergoing infertility investigations and finding no significant differences. This study was supported by several groups using the sperm chromatin structure assay [55–57] where semen samples are frozen in liquid Nitrogen without cryoprotectant and transported by dry shipper to a central lab for SCSA testing. By contrast, studies from our group reported that sperm DNA was fragmented by cryopreservation. Recently interest in sperm DNA cryoinjury has revived and a quite a number of interesting papers have been published [58–63]. In the study by de Paula et al. [59] of men with oligozoospermia, higher DNA damage, by TUNEL, was observed before and after freezing in comparison with a group of normozoospermic men attending for infertility treatment because of female problems. In this study, the increase in post-thaw damage in both groups was similar.

## The Greater Susceptibility of Infertile Mens' Sperm to Cryoinjury

The degree of DNA damage in sperm from infertile men has been reported to be significantly higher than in sperm from fertile donors [39, 64]. This was even true of infertile men with normozoospermic profiles susceptibility to cryoinjury so our groups has suggested that resistance to cryoinjury might be used as an additional diagnostic test to semen analysis. In another study of men with abnormal semen profiles; in this case teratozoospermia, a threefold increase on DNA fragmentation, by Comet and acridine orange binding, was reported in the teratozoospermic samples compared with a normozoospermic group. This adds to the literature confirming greater vulnerability of "infertile" sperm. It also suggests a relationship between abnormal morphology and DNA damage. Teratospermic semen samples have increased levels of ROS [65]. Since many of these abnormal sperm have retained cytoplasm, major source of free radicals, the amount of ROS produced during cryopreservation of such sperm may be higher than that of morphologically normal sperm, which may be the cause of the increased levels of DNA damage in these teratospermic samples [61].

## *Mechanisms of Cryoinjury*

Cryopreservation can result in cryodamage at different levels and functions of the cell, such as thermal shock, formation of intracellular ice crystals, cellular dehydration, increased concentration of salts and osmotic shock [66]. Such processes can lead to alterations of the acrosomal structure, decrease of acrosome activity, swelling or shrinkage of nuclei and cytoplasmic membranes and loss of plasma membrane integrity [40, 41, 67, 68].

Some of the cellular damage that human sperm encounter in cryopreservation has been attributed to the formation of intracellular ice. Clinical cryopreservation usually uses high and very high cooling rates [69, 70]. Supercooling can lead to intracellular ice formation, which can be fatal to the cell. However, no direct evidence of intracellular ice damage in sperm has been presented. Morris et al. [71] carried out a study to examine whether intracellular ice formation during rapid cooling causes the observed damage. Their results suggested that sperm damage at least for cooling rates up to 3,000°C/min is not caused by intracellular ice formation. Further, there was no evidence for intracellular ice, even upon warming and refreezing samples; conditions that would be expected to result in the recrystallization of any ice present within cells.

If intracellular ice formation is not the reason of cell damage at rapid rates of cooling, other physical factors, such as extracellular ice formation in the cryosolution surrounding the spermatozoa, must be responsible. During freezing of cell suspensions, the water outside the cells forms ice first in the extracellular space, which sets up an osmotic gradient between the intracellular isomotic solution and the freeze-concentrated extracellular solution. Morris et al. [72] demonstrated that the viscosity of the freeze-concentrated material can be increased rapidly by freezing an aqueous solution of the glycerol. Following ice nucleation, water from the adjacent solution migrates to the ice crystal, which causes the growth of ice crystal. During the thawing process of rapidly cooled glycerol solutions, a number of recrystallization patterns have been observed [73]. It is believed that either the crystallization during freezing or recrystallization during thawing could be a major cause of sperm cryoinjury.

The efflux of water from the cell can cause extracellular ice formation and, more damagingly, cellular dehydration. Various transport pathways in cell membranes for substrates, fluids, ions and gases preserve optimal osmotic balance between the intracellular and the extracellular environments [74, 75]. Cell transport machinery associated with cryopreservation involves water and permeable solutes [76, 77]. At the freezing temperature, the extracellular solution almost always freezes first. The extracellular solutes are concentrated in the remaining unfrozen extracellular water, so all solutes and suspended materials, including the cells, get localized in freeze-concentrated compartments [78]. During the further reduction in temperature, the cells are exposed to increasingly concentrated solutions. The hypertonic conditions that the cells encounter lead to an osmotic loss of water, which dehydrates the cells by osmosis as water diffuses from the cytoplasm into the more concentrated external solution [72].

The exposure of sperm to hypotonic solutions and the subsequent changes are termed osmotic shock. Osmotic damage caused by the exposure of frozen–thawed spermatozoa to isotonic conditions after a period of hypertonic exposure, is lethal due to extensive cell shrinkage. Subsequent rewarming and thawing of the cells can further deteriorate their viability through possible excessive osmotic swelling [53, 79, 80].

Cryosurvival of human sperm is also associated with cryoprotectants, as they were confirmed to lower the water freezing point and prevent the formation of ice crystals during freezing and, therefore, avoid structural damage and motility loss after cryopreservation [81].

## Is Apoptosis a Cause of DNA Cryodamage?

In studies by Baumber et al. [82] the percentage of apoptotic sperm significantly increased after cryopreservation. Apoptosis is physiologically programmed cell death and an underlying mechanism for normal spermatogenesis [83, 84]. "Abortive apoptosis" is a theory proposed by Sakkas et al. [85, 86], in which the correct clearance of sperm via apoptosis is failed. Therefore, spermatozoa showing abnormal morphological forms, irregular biochemical function [87] or DNA damage fails to be eliminated. Abortive apoptosis may play a role in cryoinjury to sperm DNA because cryopreservation of spermatozoa resulted in activation of caspase, which has been reported in both human [88, 89] and bull sperm [90]. Caspases are particular aspartic acid-directed cysteine proteases, which are shown to play a key role in the cellular apoptotic and eventual cell death [91]. Although a correlation between the presence of activated caspases and sperm DNA fragmentation are reported [92, 93], the results are far from compelling. The total amount of DNA damage in spermatozoa cannot be explained by apoptosis alone. DNA damage can also occur due to oxidative stress [94, 95]. Furthermore, there is no any strong evidence to suggest a caspase/apoptosis-related increase in sperm DNA fragmentation during cryopreservation [90, 96]. Thomson et al. [63] carried out a study on the mechanisms of sperm DNA fragmentation increase following cryopreservation and measured caspase activation as an indicator of apoptosis, but this did not affect damage levels; so, this led them to conclude that cryopreservation causes damage via oxidative stress and not by apoptosis.

## Is Sperm DNA Damage a Result of Oxidation?

The effects of cryopreservation on sperm DNA have recently been assessed using novel tests. Zribi et al. [62] determined DNA fragmentation by TUNEL supplemented with a measure of sperm DNA oxidation b using oxy-DNA test. They found an increase in fragmentation after thawing but just an insignificant trend towards increased DNA oxidation and therefore no relationship between DNA fragmentation and oxidation. However, this study was small ($n = 15$) and perhaps larger numbers would show differences. In contrast to this study, in a larger group ($n = 60$), Thomson et al. [97] cryopreservation caused a marked increase in sperm DNA fragmentation, by TUNEL and DNA oxidation by 8-OHdG using the oxyDNA test with a positive correlation before ($r = 0.756, p < 0.001$) and after treatment ($r = 0.528, p < 0.017$).

## Why Freeze Neat Semen?

To prevent the damage to healthy sperm by weaker ROS releasing sperm during cryo-preservation, the solution may be to prepare sperm before freezing and freeze only the DCG population. Perez-Sanchez et al. [98] reported an improvement in post-thaw sperm quality if sperm were prepared beforehand. Freezing prepared sperm has been shown to have no adverse effects on fertilization as indicated by sperm zona binding [99]. However, in studies by Donnelly et al. [39] and Thomson et al. [97], DCG sperm frozen without seminal plasma protection showed marked damage. The removal of seminal plasma protection, evidently necessary to resist cryoinjury, was probably from antioxidants, as cryoprotectants without antioxidants were not sufficient. Thomson et al. [97] demonstrated the percentage of sperm DNA fragmentation post-DCG significantly increase after cryopreservation both with and without the addition of cryoprotectant. The observed increase of DNA fragmentation in DGC-prepared spermatozoa might due to the removal of seminal fluid via DCG and the stresses of centrifugation. Centrifugation is also known to exacerbate oxidative stress within a semen sample [10, 22], which could lead to further damage to sperm.

When DGC sperm were frozen with seminal plasma and cryoprotectant added, post-thaw DNA fragmentation was the same as pre-freeze levels showing the efficacy of this combination of removing damaging sperm together with adding physiological protection [39]. The disadvantage of this method is the reduced numbers of sperm, but this may be outweighed by their quality and preservation of structure and function.

## Recent Advances in Cryopreservation

### The Efficacy of Different Cryoprotectants

In an attempt to reduce chilling injury and improve the optimal survival and fertility capacity of human sperm following cryopreservation, many different cryoprotectant media have been developed. Currently, the most widely used cryoprotectant is the permeating agent glycerol, as it has been confirmed the most effective in lowering the freezing point of intracellular water [100]. Other compounds are added to glycerol-containing media as buffers to yield optimal cryosurvival rates [101], In spite of these advances, a gold-standard method of cryopreserving human semen with an optimal cryoprotectant is yet to be determined.

Cryoprotectants themselves can pose a threat to cellular survival and cellular structures by causing the cell to shrink and swell beyond viable limits, thereby inducing osmotic shock and spermolysis [102, 103]. Commonly used cryoprotectants include glycerol and buffers. Higher glycerol concentrations have also been linked to increased activation of caspases via direct toxic effects to mitochondria during cryopreservation of spermatozoa [89].

This third paper by Thomson et al. [97] has contributed appreciably to our knowledge of the usefulness of cryoprotectants. In it, seven of the most commonly used cryoprotectant media were compared in how they protected sperm from 320 men from DNA damage. Neither the presence nor the type of cryoprotectant protected sperm DNA from cryoinjury followed by DCG. This conclusion was disappointing, but not surprising. The medium called SpermCryo gave least protection against DNA damage compared to Medicult Sperm Freezing Medium and FertiPro Sperm Freeze. This is the medium with the highest proportion of glycerol (68% glycerol compared with the others <25%). The authors explain this by highlighting a study showing high levels of glycerol cause cell death [42]. With their high proportion of membrane lipids, sperm, in particular, are sensitive to osmotic changes and vulnerable to lethal injury in hyper-osmotic conditions [104] through inappropriate re aggregation post-thawing [105]. How these processes impair DNA specifically needs elucidation.

There were, however, surprising results for men with low levels of DNA damage before freezing in that their sperm appeared to undergo a higher degree of cryoinjury than those who had higher levels of damage in their fresh samples. One explanation for this may be that these samples with high DNA damage were suboptimal in other parameters too as seen by O'Connell et al. [49] and so they also lose their motility through cryoinjury. So that only the sperm with better DNA are isolated in the DGC fraction.

## *Effects of Repeated Freezing and Thawing*

There are many reasons for freezing sperm in small numbers. Oligozoospermia is a very common problem in men attending for ART. Further, 10% of male infertility cases are azoospermic and of those more than half have obstructive azoospermia so spermatogenesis may be relatively normal and testicular sperm may be extracted. As this is an invasive procedure, it would be useful to store sperm surplus to one ART cycle so that repeated biopsies are unnecessary. Third, cancer patients often wish to have sperm stored before treatment with spermotoxic drugs. Often when they present to have sperm stored, they are unwell and sperm concentration and/or quality is reduced [106–108]. However, techniques for cryopreservation of individual or small numbers of sperm have not been optimized and very small numbers of pregnancies have been reported using any of the techniques available. This being the case, it is of interest to examine the effects of repeated freezing and thawing on sperm DNA. In ART clinics, as donor sperm is expensive and increasingly scarce, it is routine to offer patients a repeated cryocycle to maximize the use of sperm. For example, couples may wish to have siblings from the same donor's sample.

There is overall agreement that, following each freeze–thaw cycle, the number of recovered motile and viable sperm decrease steadily [109–111] and the standard semen parameters of overall motility and vitality drop steadily [109–111]. A study carried by Thomson et al. [63] shows that the percentage of motile sperm and vital sperm dropped by half following the first cycle of freezing and thawing, and continued to drop by half following each subsequent cycle.

In the same study, the effects of repeated freeze thawing on sperm DNA fragmentation by TUNEL were also assessed. They found that repeated freezing and thawing increases the percentage of sperm exhibiting DNA fragmentation in raw, non-separated semen samples. Furthermore, when the samples were washed and fresh cryoprotectant added after each thaw, the percentage of sperm DNA fragmentation increased significantly. However, when the sample was refrozen in the original cryoprotectant without and further treatment or wash, the percentage of sperm DNA fragmentation only increased slightly after the second and third thaw. Therefore, Thomson et al. [97] recommended to avoid washing steps and the addition of fresh cryoprotectant in between each freeze–thaw cycle. Samples are refrozen in their original cryoprotectant and not washed or altered in any way in between, and separated by DGC or swim-up before use in ART. By this protocol, the increase of percentage of sperm DNA fragmentation will be terminated in up to three cycles of freezing and thawing, even though it is still higher than the fresh sample.

Thus, preparing sperm by DCG for ART with the concomitant removal of seminal protection before freezing increased DNA damage and reduced vitality. If samples are frozen in their original cryoprotectant without further processing but are subjected to DGC after thawing, the "risk" (described as the relative chance of fertilization with a cell containing fragmented DNA) of three F–T cycles is equivalent to one cycle. This study again highlights the necessity of seminal plasma and the adverse effects of laboratory processing.


## The Benefits of Antioxidant Supplements to Cryoprotectant Media

As described previously, sperm DNA damage has been associated with high levels of ROS in fresh and cryopreserved semen [28, 112, 113]. A study by Li et al. [28] shows that the addition of ascorbate or catalase in human semen samples reduces ROS levels and sperm nuclear DNA damage, and improves the human sperm quality in the process of freezing and thawing. In addition, Gadea et al. [114] reported that the addition of glutathione (L-gamma-glutamyl-L-cysteinylglycine) to the thawing medium resulted in a similar result in frozen bull spermatozoa.

The work of Bilodeau et al. [115] and Peris et al. [116] have confirmed the belief that DNA instability is increased during cryopreservation as a result of reduced sperm antioxidant defence mechanisms. Specific factors such as alpha – tocopherol and ascorbate have been shown to increase post-thaw viability. Further studies have reported the addition of superoxide dismutase and catalase an increase in hamster egg penetration, increased embryo numbers [117] and increased implantation in bovine studies [118].

Freezing has been shown to reduce gluthathione (GSH) and superoxide dismutase levels [119], whereas post-thaw addition of thiols (GSH, Cysteine, N acetyl cysteine) and pyruvate, metal chelators or oviductal catalase prevented $H_2O_2$ prevented a $H_2O_2$ mediated reduction in sperm motility [115, 119].

In the Thomson study [97], all of the cryoprotectants, except SpermCryo and Medicult Cryosperm, included human serum albumin at an unknown concentration. Albumin has traditionally been viewed as a useful antioxidant as well as a plasma protein [120], but it is also known to be ineffective against NADPH [120], so oxidative stress by this route may still be the cause of the DNA fragmentation observed in this study.

## Recent Advances in Freeze–Thaw Protocols

### Freeze-Drying of Sperm

Long-term preservation of mouse sperm has been achieved with freeze-drying without cryoprotectants by Yanagimachi's group [121]. The sperm were plunged into liquid nitrogen for 20 s and then freeze-dried for 4 h. After storage at 4°C for periods of 1–12 months, the sperm were thawed by bringing to room temperature and hydrating with sterile water. Chromosomal stability was maintained in these sperm and embryos generated by ICSI. In another study using freeze-dried mouse sperm (new) [122], 96% of resultant zygotes had normal chromosomes and 58% developed into normal viable foetuses. Live offspring were obtained after storage of 1.5 years. Major advantages of this technique are the convenience of its short protocol and reduced need for storage space and sophisticated cryofacilities and expensive shipping procedures.

### Vitrification of Sperm

Conventional freezing techniques have been shown to cause physical–chemical damage to human sperm. Vitrification is an alternative method that can eliminate ice crystallization and, thus, decrease the cryodamage. The earliest information on vitrification comes from as far back as 1937 [123, 124]. However, vitrification lost its appeal for many years because critical speeds of cooling (~700,000°K/min) were unachievable at that time. Recently, the technique has been revisited, as rapid cooling is now possible. Two conditions must be fulfilled for vitrification to occur: an increase in the viscosity and a depression of the freezing temperature. The cryoprotectants used here have this purpose: to act like antifreeze, lowering the freezing temperature and increasing the viscosity so that instead of crystallizing, the syrupy solution turns into an amorphous ice – i.e. it vitrifies.

One of the difficult compromises faced in vitrifying cryopreservation is limiting the damage produced by the cryoprotectant. The protocol of vitrification currently used for the sperm cryopreservation involves the use of very high concentrations

(3.5–8 M) of permeating cryoprotectants and relatively high cooling rates (up to $10^{4\circ}$K/min) [81]. It is known that high concentrations of cryoprotectants have a marked toxic effect [89, 102, 103]. It is possible to decrease cryoprotectant toxicity by reducing the amount of cryoprotectant and increasing freezing and thawing rates [125]. Cryoprotectant-free vitrification has been reported [81] with promising results in that no DNA damage was observed with either vitrification or conventional slow cooling. However, this study was performed on healthy volunteers. If it were used with infertile men with more vulnerable sperm, the damage might be greater (see previous section).

## Conclusions and Future Recommendations

There is still much progress to be made in the field of semen cryopreservation. The most promising areas for research appear to be addition of antioxidants to cryomedia and sperm vitrification.

## References

1. Mortimer D. Sperm recovery techniques to maximize fertilizing capacity. Reprod Fertil Dev. 1994;6:25–31.
2. Donnelly ET, Lewis SE, McNally JA, et al. In vitro fertilization and pregnancy rates: the influence of sperm motility and morphology on IVF outcome. Fertil Steril. 1998;70:305–14.
3. Donnelly ET, McClure N, Lewis SE. Glutathione and hypotaurine in vitro: effects on human sperm motility, DNA integrity and production of reactive oxygen species. Mutagenesis. 2000;15:61–8.
4. Sakkas D, Manicardi GC, Tomlinson M, et al. The use of two density gradient centrifugation technique and the swim up method to separate spermatozoa with chromatin and nuclear DNA anomalies. Hum Reprod. 2000;15(5):1112–6.
5. Kanwar KC, Yanagimachi R, Lopata A. Effects of human seminal plasma on fertilizing capacity of human spermatozoa. Fertil Steril. 1979;31:321–7.
6. Rogers BJ, Perreault SD, Bentwood BJ, et al. Variability in the human–hamster in vitro assay for fertility evaluation. Fertil Steril. 1983;39:204–11.
7. van Loon AA, Den Boer PJ, van der Schans GP, et al. Immunochemical detection of DNA damage induction and repair at different cellular stages of spermatogenesis of the hamster after in vitro or in vivo exposure to ionizing radiation. Exp Cell Res. 1991;193:303–9.
8. van Loon AA, Sonneveld E, Hoogerbrugge J, et al. Induction and repair of DNA single-strand breaks and DNA base damage at different cellular stages of spermatogenesis of the hamster upon in vitro exposure to ionizing radiation. Mutat Res. 1993;294:139–48.
9. Drost JB, Lee WR. Biological basis of germline mutation: comparisons of spontaneous germline mutation rates among drosophila, mouse, and human. Environ Mol Mutagen. 1995;25:48–64.
10. Shekarriz M, DeWire DM, Thomas AJ, et al. A method of human semen centrifugation to minimize the iatrogenic sperm injuries caused by reactive oxygen species. Eur Urol. 1995;28:31–5.
11. Shekarriz M, Thomas AJ, Agarwal A. Incidence and level of seminal reactive oxygen species in normal men. Urology. 1995;45:103–7.

12. Griveau JF, Le Lannou D. Influence of oxygen tension on reactive oxygen species production and human sperm function. Int J Androl. 1997;20:195–200.
13. Whittington K, Ford WC. The effect of incubation periods under 95% oxygen on the stimulated acrosome reaction and motility of human spermatozoa. Mol Hum Reprod. 1998;4:1053–7.
14. Aitken RJ, Buckingham DW, West KM. Reactive oxygen species and human spermatozoa: analysis of the cellular mechanisms involved in luminol- and lucigenin dependent chemiluminescence. J Cell Physiol. 1992;151:466–77.
15. Aitken RJ, Clarkson JS. Significance of reactive oxygen species and antioxidants in defining the efficiency of sperm preparation techniques. J Androl. 1998;9(6):367–76.
16. Sharma RK, Agarwal A. Role of reactive oxygen species in male infertility. Urology. 1996;48:835–50.
17. Agarwal A, Makker K, Sharma R. Clinical relevance of oxidative stress in male factor infertility: an update. Am J Reprod Immunol. 2008;59:2–11.
18. Mahfouz R, Sharma R, Thiyagarajan A, et al. Semen characteristics and sperm DNA fragmentation in infertile men with low and high levels of seminal reactive oxygen species. Fertil Steril. 2010;94:2141–6.
19. Abd-Elmoaty MA, Saleh R, Sharma R, et al. Increased levels of oxidants and reduced antioxidants in semen of infertile men with varicocele. Fertil Steril. 2009;94:1531–4.
20. Hughes CM, Lewis SE, McKelvey-Martin VJ, et al. The effects of antioxidant supplementation during Percoll preparation on human sperm DNA integrity. Hum Reprod. 1998;13:1240–7.
21. Twigg JP, Irvine DS, Aitken RJ. Oxidative damage to DNA in human spermatozoa does not preclude pronucleus formation at intracytoplasmic sperm injection. Hum Reprod. 1998;13:1864–71.
22. Tremellen K. Oxidative stress and male infertility–a clinical perspective. Hum Reprod Update. 2008;14:243–58.
23. Halliwell B, Gutteridge JMC. Free radicals in biology and medicine. 2nd ed. Oxford: Clarendon; 1989.
24. Agarwal A, Said TM. Oxidative stress, DNA damage and apoptosis in male infertility: a clinical approach. BJU Int. 2004;95:503–7.
25. Donnelly ET, McClure N, Lewis SE. Antioxidant supplementation in vitro does not improve human sperm motility. Fertil Steril. 1999;72:484–95.
26. Menezo YJR, Hazout A, Panteix G, et al. Antioxidants to reduce sperm DNA fragmentation: an unexpected adverse effect. Reprod Biomed Online. 2007;14(4):418–21.
27. Rolf C, Cooper TG, Yeung CH, et al. Antioxidant treatment of patients with asthenozoospermia or moderate oligoasthenozoospermia with high-dose vitamin C and vitamin E: a randomized, placebo-controlled, double-blind study. Hum Reprod. 1999;14:1028–33.
28. Li ZL, Lin QL, Liu RJ, et al. Reducing oxidative DNA damage by adding antioxidants in human semen samples undergoing cryopreservation procedure. Zhonghua Yi Xue Za Zhi. 2007;87:3174–7.
29. Lewis SE, Boyle PM, McKinney KA, et al. Total antioxidant capacity of seminal plasma is different in fertile and infertile men. Fertil Steril. 1995;64:868–70.
30. Kessopoulou E, Powers HJ, Sharma KK, et al. A double-blind randomized placebo cross-over controlled trial using the antioxidant vitamin E to treat reactive oxygen species associated male infertility. Fertil Steril. 1995;64:825–31.
31. Baker HW, Brindle J, Irvine DS, et al. Protective effect of antioxidants on the impairment of sperm motility by activated polymorphonuclear leukocytes. Fertil Steril. 1996;65:411–9.
32. Battista N, Rapino C, Di Tommaso M, et al. Regulation of male fertility by the endocannabinoid system. Mol Cell Endocrinol. 2008;286:S17–23.
33. Sanger WG, Olson JH, Sherman JK. Semen cryobanking for men with cancer – criteria change. Fertil Steril. 1992;58:1024–7.
34. Sherman JK. Current status of clinical cryobanking of human semen. In: Paulson JD, Negro-Vlar A, Lucena E, Martini L, editors. Andrology: male fertility and sterility. Orlando: Academic; 1986. p. 517–47.

35. Anger JT, Gilbert BR, Goldstein M. Cryopreservation of sperm: indications, methods and results. J Urol. 2003;170:1079–84.
36. Borges E, Rossi LM, de Freitas CVL, et al. Fertilization and pregnancy outcome after intracytoplasmic injection with fresh or cryopreserved ejaculated spermatozoa. Fertil Steril. 2007;87:316–20.
37. Centola GM, Raubertas RF, Mattox JH. Cryopreservation of human semen. Comparison of cryopreservatives, sources of variability, and prediction of post-thaw survival. J Androl. 1992;13:283–8.
38. Nijs M, Ombelet W. Cryopreservation of human sperm. Hum Fertil. 2001;4(3):158–63.
39. Donnelly ET, McClure N, Lewis SE. Cryopreservation of human semen and prepared sperm: effects on motility parameters and DNA integrity. Fertil Steril. 2001;76:892–900.
40. Esteves SC, Sharma RK, Thomas AJ, et al. Suitability of the hypo-osmotic swelling test for assessing the viability of cryopreserved sperm. Fertil Steril. 1996;66:798–804.
41. Cross NL, Hanks SE. Effects of cryopreservation on human sperm acrosomes. Hum Reprod. 1991;6:1279–83.
42. Mazur P, Rall WF, Leibo SP. Kinetics of water loss and the likelihood of intracellular freezing in mouse ova. Influence of the method of calculating the temperature dependence of water permeability. Cell Biophys. 1984;6:197–213.
43. Lewis SEM, McKinney KA, Thompson W. Influence of pentoxifylline on human sperm motility in asthenozoospermic individuals using computer-assisted analysis. Arch Androl. 1994;32(3):175–83.
44. Glenn DRJ, McVicar CM, McClure N, et al. Sidenafil citrate improves sperm motility but causes a premature acrosome reaction in vitro. Fertil Steril. 2007;87:1064–70.
45. Sharma RK, Wang JH, Wu Z. Mechanisms of inhibition of calmodulin-stimulated cyclic nucleotide phosphodiesterase by dihydropyridine calcium antagonists. J Neurochem. 1997;69(2):845–50.
46. Tournaye H, van der Linden M, van den Abbeel E, et al. Mouse in vitro fertilization using sperm treated with pentoxifylline and 2-deoxyadenosine. Fertil Steril. 1994;62:644–7.
47. Glenn DR, McClure N, Cosby SL, et al. Sildenafil citrate (Viagra) impairs fertilization and early embryo development in mice. Fertil Steril. 2009;91(3):893–9.
48. Fjällbrant B, Ackerman DR. Cervical mucus penetration in vitro by fresh and frozen-preserved human semen specimens. J Reprod Fertil. 1969;20:515–7.
49. O'Connell M, McClure N, Lewis SEM. The effects of cryopreservation on sperm morphology, motility and mitochondrial function. Hum Reprod. 2002;17:704–9.
50. Rossato M, La Sala GB, Balasini M, et al. Sperm treatment with extracellular ATP increases fertilization rates in in-vitro fertilization for male factor infertility. Hum Reprod. 1999;14:694–7.
51. Verheyen G, Nagy Z, Joris H, et al. Quality of frozen thawed testicular sperm and its preclinical use for intracytoplasmic sperm injection into in vitro-matured germinal-vesicle stage oocytes. Fertil Steril. 1997;67:74–80.
52. Sabanegh ES, Ragheb AM. Male fertility after cancer. Urology. 2009;73(2):225–31.
53. Watson PF. Recent developments and concepts in the cryopreservation of spermatozoa and the assessment of their post thawing function. Reprod Fertil Dev. 1995;7:871–91.
54. Duru NK, Morshedi MS, Schuffner A, et al. Cryopreservation-thawing of fractionated human spermatozoa is associated with membrane phosphatidylserine externalization and not DNA fragmentation. J Androl. 2001;22(4):646–51.
55. Virro MR, Larson-Cook KL, Evenson DP. Sperm chromatin structure assay (SCSA) parameters are related to fertilization, blastocyst development, and ongoing pregnancy in in vitro fertilization and intracytoplasmic sperm injection cycles. Fertil Steril. 2004;81:1289–95.
56. Smit M, Dohle GR, Hop WC, et al. Clinical correlates of the biological variation of sperm DNA fragmentation in infertile men attending an andrology outpatient clinic. Int J Androl. 2007;30(1):48–55.
57. Lin MH, Lee KKR, Li SH, et al. Sperm chromatin structure assay parameters are not related to fertilization rates, embryo quality, and pregnancy rates in in vitro fertilization and intracyto-

plasmic sperm injection, but might be related to spontaneous abortion rates. Fertil Steril. 2008;90:352–9.

58. Gandini L, Lombardo F, Lenzi A, et al. Cryopreservation and sperm DNA integrity. Cell Tissue Bank. 2006;7:91–8.

59. de Paula TS, Bertolla RP, Spaine DM, et al. Effect of cryopreservation on sperm apoptotic deoxyribonucleic acid fragmentation in patients with oligozoospermia. Fertil Steril. 2006;86:597–600.

60. Calamera JC, Buffone MG, Doncel GF, et al. Effect of thawing temperature on the motility recovery of cryopreserved human spermatozoa. Fertil Steril. 2010;93:789–94.

61. Kalthur G, Adiga SK, Upadhya D, et al. Effect of cryopreservation on sperm DNA integrity in patients with teratospermia. Fertil Steril. 2008;89:1723–7.

62. Zribi N, Chakroun FN, Euch EH, et al. Effects of cryopreservation on human sperm deoxyribonucleic acid integrity. Fertil Steril. 2010;93:159–66.

63. Thomson LK, Fleming SD, Schulke L, et al. The DNA integrity of cryopreserved spermatozoa separated for use in assisted reproductive technology is unaffected by the type of cryoprotectant used but is related to the DNA integrity of the fresh separated preparation. Fertil Steril. 2009;92:991–1001.

64. Dalzell LH, Thompson-Cree MEM, McClure N, et al. Effects of 24-hour incubation after freeze-thawing on DNA fragmentation of testicular sperm from infertile and fertile men. Fertil Steril. 2003;79(3):1670–2.

65. Pasqualotto FF, Sharma RK, Kobayashi H, et al. Oxidative stress in normospermic men undergoing infertility evaluation. J Androl. 2001;22:316–22.

66. Stanic P, Tandara M, Sonicki Z, et al. Comparison of protective media and freezing techniques for cryopreservation of human semen. Eur J Obstet Gynecol Reprod Biol. 2000;91:65–70.

67. Esteves SC, Sharma RK, Thomas AJ, et al. Evaluation of acrosomal status and sperm viability in fresh and cryopreserved specimens by the use of fluorescent peanut agglutinin lectin in conjunction with hypo-osmotic swelling test. Int Braz J Urol. 2007;33:364–74.

68. Nallella KP, Sharma RK, Allamaneni SS, et al. Cryopreservation of human spermatozoa: comparison of two cryopreservation methods and three cryoprotectants. Fertil Steril. 2004;82:913–8.

69. Sherman JK. Synopsis of the use of frozen human semen since 1964: state of the art of human semen banking. Fertil Steril. 1973;24:397–412.

70. Verheyen G, Pletincx I, van Steirteghem A. Effect of freezing method, thawing temperature and post-thaw dilution/washing on motility (CASA) and morphology characteristics of high-quality human sperm. Hum Reprod. 1993;8:1678–84.

71. Morris GJ. Rapidly cooled human sperm: no evidence of intracellular ice formation. Hum Reprod. 2006;21:2075–83.

72. Morris GJ, Goodrich M, Acton E, et al. The high viscosity encountered during freezing in glycerol solutions: effects on cryopreservation. Cryobiology. 2006;52:323–34.

73. Ablett S, Izzard MJ, Lillford PJ. Differential scanning calorimetric study of frozen sucrose and glycerol solutions. J Chem Soc Faraday Trans. 1992;88:789–94.

74. Denda M, Hosoi J, Asida Y. Visual imaging of ion distribution in human epidermis. Biochem Biophys Res Commun. 2000;272:134–7.

75. Hernandez JA, Cristina E. Modeling cell volume regulation in nonexcitable cells: the roles of the Na+ pump and of cotransport systems. Am J Physiol. 1998;275:1067–80.

76. Li LY, Tighe BJ, Ruberti JW. Mathematical modeling of corneal swelling. Biomech Model Mechanobiol. 2004;3:114–23.

77. Chen HH, Purtteman JJ, Heimfeld S, et al. Development of a microfluidic device for determination of cell osmotic behavior and membrane transport properties. Cryobiology. 2007;55:200–9.

78. Mazur P. Principles of cryobiology. In: Fuller BJ, Lane N, Benson EE, editors. Life in the frozen state. Boca Raton: CRC Press; 2004. p. 3–65.

79. Gao DY, Liu C, McGann LE, et al. Prevention of osmotic injury to human spermatozoa during addition and removal of glycerol. Hum Reprod. 1995;10:1109–22.

244 D. Yu et al.

80. Gao D, Mazur P, Critser J. Fundamental cryobiology of mammalian spermatozoa. In: Karow AM, Critser JK, editors. Reproductive tissue banking. London: Academic; 1997. p. 263–328.
81. Isachenko E, Isachenko V, Katkov II, et al. DNA integrity and motility of human spermatozoa after standard slow freezing versus cryoprotectant-free vitrification. Hum Reprod. 2004;19:932–9.
82. Baumber J, Ball BA, Linfor JJ, et al. Reactive oxygen species and cryopreservation promote DNA fragmentation in equine spermatozoa. J Androl. 2003;24:621–8.
83. Print CG, Loveland KL. Germ cell suicide: new insights into apoptosis during spermatogenesis. Bioessays. 2000;22(5):423–30.
84. Kierszenbaum AL. Transition nuclear proteins during spermiogenesis: unrepaired DNA breaks not allowed. Mol Reprod Dev. 2001;58:357–8.
85. Sakkas D, Mariethoz E, John JC. Abnormal sperm parameters in humans are indicative of an abortive apoptotic mechanism linked to the Fas-mediated pathway. Exp Cell Res. 1999;251:350–5.
86. Sakkas D, Mariethoz E, Manicardi G, et al. Origin of DNA damage in ejaculated human spermatozoa. Rev Reprod. 1999;4:431–7.
87. Huszar G, Sbracia M, Vigue L, et al. Sperm plasma membrane remodeling during spermiogenic maturation in men: relationship among plasma membrane beat 1,4 galactosyltransferase, cytoplasmic creatine phosphokinase and creatine phosphokinase isoform ratios. Biol Reprod. 1997;56:1020–4.
88. Paasch U, Sharma RK, Gupta AK, et al. Cryopreservation and thawing is associated with varying extent of activation of apoptotic machinery in subsets of ejaculated human spermatozoa. Biol Reprod. 2004;71:1828–37.
89. Wundrich K, Paasch U, Leicht M, et al. Activation of caspases in human spermatozoa during cryopreservation–an immunoblot study. Cell Tissue Bank. 2006;7:81–90.
90. Martin G, Sabido O, Durand P, et al. Cryopreservation induces an apoptosis-like mechanism in bull sperm. Biol Reprod. 2004;71:28–37.
91. Thornberry NA, Lazebnik Y. Caspases: enemies within. Science. 1998;281:1312–6.
92. Weng SL, Taylor SL, Morshedi M, et al. Caspase activity and apoptotic markers in ejaculated human sperm. Mol Hum Reprod. 2002;8:984–91.
93. Marchetti C, Gallego MA, Defossez A, et al. Staining of human sperm with fluorochrome-labeled inhibitor of caspases to detect activated caspases: correlation with apoptosis and sperm parameters. Hum Reprod. 2004;19:1127–34.
94. Agarwal A, Ranganathan P, Kattal N, et al. Fertility after cancer: a prospective review of assisted reproductive outcome with banked semen specimens. Fertil Steril. 2004;81:342–8.
95. Sharma RK, Said T, Agarwal A. Sperm DNA damage and its clinical relevance in assessing reproductive outcome. Asian J Androl. 2004;6:139–48.
96. Paasch U, Grunewald S, Agarwal A, et al. Activation pattern of caspases in human spermatozoa. Fertil Steril. 2004;81:802–9.
97. Thomson LK, Fleming SD, Aitken RJ, et al. Cryopreservation-induced human sperm DNA damage is predominantly mediated by oxidative stress rather than apoptosis. Hum Reprod. 2009;24:2061–70.
98. Perez-Sanchez F, Cooper TG, Yeung CH, et al. Improvement in quality of cryopreserved spermatozoa by swim-up before freezing. Int J Androl. 1994;17:115–20.
99. Yogev L, Gamzu R, Paz G, Kleiman S, Botchan A, Hauser R, et al. Pre-freezing sperm preparation does not impair thawed spermatozoa binding to the zona pellucida. Hum Reprod. 1999;14:114–7.
100. Royere D, Barthelemy C, Hamamah S, et al. Cryopreservation of spermatozoa: a 1996 review. Hum Reprod Update. 1996;2:553–9.
101. Hallak J, Sharma RK, Wellstead C, et al. Cryopreservation of human spermatozoa: comparison of TEST-yolk buffer and glycerol. Int J Fertil Womens Med. 2000;45:38–42.

102. Gilmore JA, Liu J, Gao DY, et al. Determination of optimal cryoprotectants and procedures for their addition and removal from human spermatozoa. Hum Reprod. 1997;12:112–8.
103. Critser JK, Huse-Benda AR, Aaker DV, et al. Cryopreservation of human spermatozoa. III. The effect of cryopreservation on motility. Fertil Steril. 1988;50:314–20.
104. Gao DY, Ashworth E, Watson PF, et al. Hyperosmotic tolerance of human spermatozoa: separate effects of glycerol, sodium chloride, and sucrose on spermolysis. Biol Reprod. 1993;49:112–23.
105. Hammerstedt RH, Graham JK, Nolan JP. Cryopreservation of mammalian sperm: what we ask them to survive. J Androl. 1990;11:73–88.
106. Padron OF, Brackett NL, Sharma RK, et al. Seminal reactive oxygen species, sperm motility and morphology in men with spinal cord injury. Fertil Steril. 1997;67:115–1120.
107. Lass A, Akagbosu F, Abusheikha N, et al. A programme of semen cryopreservation for patients with malignant disease in a tertiary infertility centre: lessons from 8 years' experience. Hum Reprod. 1998;13(11):3256–61.
108. O'Flaherty C, Hales BF, Chan P, et al. Impact of chemotherapeutics and advanced testicular cancer or Hodgkin lymphoma on sperm deoxyribonucleic acid integrity. Fertil Steril. 2010;94:1374–9.
109. Polcz TE, Stronk J, Xiong C, et al. Optimal utilization of cryopreserved human semen for assisted reproduction: recovery and maintenance of sperm motility and viability. J Assist Reprod Genet. 1998;15:504–12.
110. Rofeim O, Brown TA, Gilbert BR. Effects of serial thaw-refreeze cycles on human sperm motility and viability. Fertil Steril. 2001;75:1242–3.
111. Bandularatne E, Bongso A. Evaluation of human sperm function after repeated freezing and thawing. J Androl. 2002;23:242–9.
112. Zini A, Libman J. Sperm DNA damage: clinical significance in the era of assisted reproduction. CMAJ. 2006;175:495–500.
113. Wang X, Sharma RK, Sikka SC, et al. Oxidative stress is associated with increased apoptosis leading to spermatozoa DNA damage in patients with male factor infertility. Fertil Steril. 2003;80:531–5.
114. Gadea J, Gumbao D, Canovas S, et al. Supplementation of the dilution medium after thawing with reduced glutathione improves function and the in vitro fertilizing ability of frozen-thawed bull spermatozoa. Int J Androl. 2008;31:40–9.
115. Bilodeau JF, Chatterjee S, Sirard MA, et al. Levels of antioxidant defenses are decreased in bovine spermatozoa after a cycle of freezing and thawing. Mol Reprod Dev. 2000;55:282–8.
116. Peris SI, Bilodeau JF, Dufour M, et al. Impact of cryopreservation and reactive oxygen species on DNA integrity, lipid peroxidation, and functional parameters in ram sperm. Mol Reprod Dev. 2007;74:878–92.
117. Roca J, Rodriguez MJ, Gil MA, et al. Survival and in vitro fertility of boar spermatozoa frozen in the presence of superoxide dismutase and/or catalase. J Androl. 2005;26:15–24.
118. Beconi MT, Francia CR, Mora NG, et al. Effect of natural antioxidants on frozen bovine semen preservation. Theriogenology. 1993;40:841–51.
119. Chatterjee S, de Lamirande E, Gagnon C. Cryopreservation alters membrane sulfhydryl status of bull spermatozoa: protection by oxidized glutathione. Mol Reprod Dev. 2001;60(4):498–506.
120. Twigg J, Fulton N, Gomez E, et al. Analysis of the impact of intracellular reactive oxygen species generation on the structural and functional integrity of human spermatozoa: lipid peroxidation, DNA fragmentation and effectiveness of antioxidants. Hum Reprod. 1998;13(6):1429–36.
121. Kusakabe H, Szczygiel MA, Whittingham DG, et al. Maintenance of genetic integrity in frozen and freeze-dried mouse spermatozoa. Proc Natl Acad Sci USA. 2001;98:13501–6.
122. Ward MA, Kaneko T, Kusakabe H, et al. Long-term preservation of mouse spermatozoa after freeze-drying and freezing without cryoprotection. Biol Reprod. 2003;69(6):2100–8.

123. Luyet BJ, Hodapp R. Revival of frog spermatozoa vitrified in liquid air. Proc Meet Soc Exp Biol. 1938;39:433–4.
124. Luyet BJ. Differential staining for living and dead cells. Science. 1937;85:106.
125. Liebermann J, Tucker M, Graham J, et al. Blastocyst development after vitrification of multipronucleate zygotes using the flexipet denuding pipette (FDP). Reprod Biomed Online. 2002;4:148–52.

# Chapter 13
# Sperm Chromatin and ART
# (IUI, IVF and ICSI) Pregnancy

Mona Bungum

In Western countries, 17–25% of couples in reproductive age are seeking medical care for problems of conception [1, 2]. Thanks to the introduction of assisted reproductive technologies (ART), now, almost every involuntarily childless couple has a realistic hope of parenting. In particular, the introduction of intracytoplasmic sperm injection (ICSI) has revolutionized the area of fertility [3]. The number of ART treatments, in particular ICSI cycles, is steadily increasing [4]. While in the beginning of the era of ICSI the indication for this type of treatment was severe male infertility, now also couples whose male partners are without sperm defects request and are treated with ICSI. However, by ICSI all natural biological barriers that prevent fertilization with defective sperm are bypassed, and its increasing use has led to a growing concern of transmission of genetic and epigenetic diseases.

Although the development of ART has brought us further and led to a vast increase in our understanding of early reproductive function, ART performances have been stable and we have witnessed no net improvement in healthy term pregnancy rate during the last two decades [5]. One reason for this can be a lack of adequate methods to evaluate the fertility potential of a couple and also a lack of methods to identify the most effective type of ART treatment for a given couple.

So far, the traditional semen analysis has been a cornerstone in the diagnosis of male fertility and also used as a tool to decide which ART method to use. The sperm parameters, namely, concentration, motility and morphology, are, however, claimed to be poorly standardized, subjective [6] and not powerful predictors of fertility [7, 8]. A search for better predictors of fertility has contributed to a growing focus on the genomic integrity of the male gametes used for ART [9, 10]. During the last few decades, several methods to assess sperm DNA damage have been developed. Although still many questions remain to be answered, it is evident that sperm DNA integrity is a valuable marker of male fertility, alone or in combination with the

M. Bungum, MSc, Med Dr, PhD
Reproductive Medicine Centre, Skåne University Hospital Malmö, Lund University,
Sodra Forstadsgatan, Malmö 20502, Sweden
e-mail: mona.bungum@med.lu.se

A. Zini, A. Agarwal (eds.), *Sperm Chromatin for the Clinician*,
© Springer Science+Business Media New York 2013

conventional semen parameters, in natural conception as well as in ART. This chapter reviews the role of sperm chromatin integrity in ART.

## Assisted Reproductive Technologies

The term ART covers all reproductive technologies that involve the handling of gametes outside the body, either sperm alone as in intrauterine insemination (IUI), or oocytes, sperm and embryos as in in vitro fertilization (IVF) and ICSI [11]. ART is primarily used as a treatment of infertility/subfertility and also, to some extent, in establishing pregnancy in couples carrying inherited genetic diseases. The very first documented successful use of ART in humans was in 1978 when the world first IVF-baby was born [12]. Now, about 30 years later, ART is applied worldwide, and it is estimated that more than three million babies have been born as a result of ART since then [13]. The number of ART treatments is rising every year [14].

The first choice of treatment used in ovulatory dysfunction, minimal endometriosis, unexplained subfertility and milder forms of male subfertility is the relatively simple IUI. Following a mild controlled ovarian stimulation, prepared semen is inseminated into the woman's uterus. In tubal factors, IVF is used [11]. In IVF, oocytes are fertilized by sperm in vitro. Two to five days later the pre-embryo is replaced into the woman's uterus. In ICSI, nearly the same principles are followed, but one single spermatozoon is selected and injected directly into the cytoplasm of the oocyte.

## Traditional Markers of ART Fertility Potential

Prediction of the fertility potential of a couple has never been more crucial than now. We are facing delayed childbearing and falling sperm counts as possible threats to fertility. Various predictors of fertility have been suggested; however, none is shown to be ideal. While in the female age is the only parameter that has been shown to have the potential to predict ART outcome [15], for long it was thought that the traditional sperm parameters could predict male fertilization capability. In ART, sperm samples are prepared by methods such as swim-up or density gradient centrifugation to sort out populations of sperm believed to have the highest fertilization potential. Traditionally, concentration and motility after sperm preparation have been one of the fundaments driving clinicians decisions about the choice of the specific ART method recommended for a given couple. It has, however, not shown to be sufficient for assessing of the fertilizing capacity of a sperm.

Several other laboratory tests of sperm function have been suggested, such as antisperm antibody test, vital staining, biochemical analysis of semen, hypoosmotic swelling test, sperm penetration assay, hemizona assay, creatine kinase, reactive oxygen species (ROS) tests and computer-assisted sperm analysis (CASA) [16];

however, the clinical value of these tests has been questioned [17], and only a few of them have been implemented in routine clinical use.

Owing to the lack of tools to predict sperm fertilizing capacity, the criteria for choosing ICSI and, as a consequence, the ratio between IVF and ICSI vary from clinic to clinic. Despite the fact that, in unexplained infertility, fertilization rates are as good in IVF as in ICSI [18], many clinics now perform ICSI as their primary, if not the only, ART technique [4, 19].

## Sperm Chromatin Integrity Testing

The evidence that infertile men in general possess substantially more sperm DNA damage than fertile men [20–28] has led to a growing focus on sperm chromatin integrity testing as an adjunct tool to the traditional sperm parameters in prediction of fertility. During the past three decades, a variety of techniques to assess sperm chromatin integrity have been developed. Principles, procedures and other aspects of the different tests are reviewed in detail in other chapters of this book. Briefly, mainly four tests assessing sperm DNA damage are used in ART, namely, the comet assay (single cell gel electrophoresis) [29], the TUNEL (terminal deoxy-nucleotidyl transferase-mediated dUDP nick-end labelling) assay [30], the Sperm Chromatin Structure assay (SCSA) [31, 32] and the Sperm Chromatin Dispersion (SCD) test [33].

Comet assay is a fluorescence-microscopy-based test. In this assay, spermatozoa are mixed with melted agarose and then placed on a glass slide. Thereafter, the cells are lysed and subjected to horizontal electrophoresis. DNA is visualized with the help of DNA-specific fluorescent dyes, and DNA damage is quantified by measuring the displacement between the nuclear genetic material of the comet head and the broken DNA migrated in the tail.

TUNEL assay can be run using both bright-field/fluorescence microscopy and flow cytometry. In the TUNEL assay, terminal deoxynucleotidyl transferase (TdT) incorporates labelled nucleotides to 3'-OH at single- and double-strand DNA breaks to create a signal, which increases with the number of DNA breaks. On a microscope slide, sperm are scored and classified as positive or negative depending whether they are labelled or not. In flow cytometry, the fraction of positive sperm is represented by the cells above a threshold channel value on a relative fluorescence intensity scale.

SCSA is a flow-cytometric test that measures the susceptibility of sperm DNA to acid-induced DNA denaturation in situ, followed by staining with acridine orange [31, 32]. The level of DNA denaturation is determined by measuring the shift from green fluorescence (double-stranded, native DNA) to red fluorescence (single-stranded, denatured DNA) in a flow cytometer, followed by further analysis by a specific SCSA software. The extent of DNA denaturation is expressed as DNA fragmentation index (DFI) [32]. The fraction of high DNA stainable (HDS) cells, thought to represent immature spermatozoa, is also recorded [32].

Similar to the SCSA, the fluorescence/light microscopic SCD test determines the susceptibility of sperm DNA to acid denaturation [33, 34]. Briefly, intact spermatozoa are immersed in an agarose matrix on a slide, treated with an acid solution to denature DNA that contains breaks and then treated with lysis buffer to remove membranes and proteins. Removal of nuclear proteins results in nucleoids with a central core and a peripheric halo of dispersed DNA loops. Sperm nuclei with elevated DNA fragmentation produce very small or no halos of DNA dispersion, whereas those sperm with low levels of DNA fragmentation release their DNA loops forming large halos. The sperm nucleoids may be visualized using fluorescence microscopy, after staining with a DNA-specific fluorochrome, or bright-field microscopy.

Moderate-to-high correlations between these different tests have been reported [30, 34–36], indicating that, very likely, these tests are not addressing identical aspects of the complex processes underlying sperm nuclear packaging potentially resulting in DNA breaks [37]. The test that has been most extensively tested clinically and found to have the most stable threshold values is the SCSA [20, 24, 31, 38], and this chapter focuses mainly on the results from SCSA-based studies.

Several reports have demonstrated that the association between sperm DNA damage and the traditional semen parameters is only weak-to-moderate [39, 40]. It is also shown that infertile men may have normal standard sperm characteristics according to WHO criteria, but a high number of sperm DNA defects.

In a recent case–control study on infertile vs. fertile men, the risk of being infertile resulted increased when DFI, as measured by SCSA, was above 20% in men with normal standard semen parameters, with an odds ratio (OR) of 5.1 (CI: 1.2–23). If any one of the WHO parameters were abnormal, the OR for infertility was increased already at DFI above 10% (OR 16, CI: 4.2–60). DFI above 20% was found in 40% of men with otherwise normal standard parameters [41]. In another study of 350 Latvian men from infertile couples [42], 20% of the men with otherwise normal WHO sperm parameters had a SCSA-DFI above 20%. This is clinically relevant in counselling couples during the fertility workup, and also in couples seeking ART where the choice of treatment most often is based upon the traditional sperm parameters and where an underlying high DFI can hinder a pregnancy.

## Sperm Chromatin Integrity Testing in ART

### Intrauterine Insemination

The first study indicating an association between sperm DNA damage and reduced pregnancy chances after IUI was published by Duran et al. [43]. In a retrospective study of 154 IUI cycles, they found that pregnancy could not be achieved when DFI, as measured by the TUNEL assay, was above 12%. Similar findings have been reported by Saleh's group [28] who performed a small study where 12 of 19 couples had a DFI value as measured by SCSA above 28% and none of these

**Table 13.1**  Influence of sperm DNA damage on pregnancy rates in IUI treatment

| References | Patients (n) | Pregnancy rates impaired | Test applied | DNA fragmentation index (DFI)-threshold suggested (%) |
|---|---|---|---|---|
| Duran et al. [43] | 154 | Yes | TUNEL | 12 |
| Saleh et al. [28] | 19 | Yes | SCSA | 30 |
| Bungum et al. [48] | 131 | Yes | SCSA | 27 |
| Muriel et al. [45] | 100 | No | SCD | – |
| Bungum et al. [38] | 387 | Yes | SCSA | 30 |

*IUI* Intrauterine insemination; *SCSA* Sperm Chromatin Structure assay; *TUNEL* terminal deoxy-nucleotidyl transferase dUTP nick-end labelling; *SCD* Sperm Chromatin Dispersion test

couples achieved a pregnancy. Boe-Hansen et al. [44] used SCSA in a study on 48 IUI couples. Only two of the couples had a DFI value above 30%, and none of the couples achieved a pregnancy. Recently, in a study of 387 IUI cycles, it shown that the SCSA parameter DFI can be used as an independent predictor of fertility [38]. While the proportion of children born per cycle was 19.0% when the DFI value was below 30%, those with a DFI value above 30% only had a take-home-baby rate of 1.5%. These IUI results are in good accordance with those results obtained from natural conception. In fact, both Evenson et al. [20] and Spanò et al. [24] demonstrated that, after unprotected intercourse, time-to-pregnancy increased (fertile couples took longer to conceive) as a function of the proportion of sperm with abnormal chromatin measured by the SCSA [20, 24]. By contrast, no correlation was found between SCD results and pregnancy outcome in 100 Spanish IUI patients [45].

Normal sperm DNA integrity seems to be particularly important when the contact between the two gametes occurs in a natural way as in natural conception and IUI. It has been suggested that selective pressures operate to avoid the development of an embryo derived from sperm with a high load of genetic damage in a natural environment [29]. Additionally, spermatozoa with damaged DNA could be more prone to undergo apoptosis during the transport through the genital tract than spermatozoa with normal DNA integrity. For an overview of IUI-papers, see Table 13.1.

## In Vitro Fertilization and Intracytoplasmic Sperm Injection

Numerous of retrospective studies have examined the role of sperm chromatin damage in IVF and ICSI. In Table 13.2, an overview of studies using SCSA, TUNEL, comet or SCD assays is presented.

## Sperm DNA Damage in Relation to Pregnancy Outcome

Some of the first studies relating outcome of ART to sperm DNA damage suggested that a DFI above 27% as measured by SCSA could be used as a cut-off value for infertility. The authors reported that in couples with a DFI above 27%, no pregnancy

**Table 13.2** Influence of sperm DNA damage on fertilization, embryo development and pregnancy rates in IVF and ICSI

| References | IVF (n) | ICSI (n) | Fertilization rates impaired | Embryo development impaired | Pregnancy rates impaired | Test applied |
|---|---|---|---|---|---|---|
| Tomsu et al. [62] | 40 | 0 | No | Yes | Yes | Comet |
| Morris et al. [29] | 20 | 40 | No | Yes | NA | Comet |
| Caglar et al. [116] | 0 | 56 | No | No | No | Comet |
| Lewis et al. [64] | 0 | 77 | No | NA | Yes | Comet |
| Nasr-Esfahani et al. [66] | 0 | 28 | No | No | NA | Comet |
| Larson-Cook et al. [47] | 55 | 34 | No | No | Yes | SCSA |
| Larson et al. [46] | 24 IVF/ICSI | NA | No | No | Yes | SCSA |
| Saleh et al. [28] | 10 | 4 | Yes | Yes | Yes | SCSA |
| Bungum et al. [48] | 109 | 66 | No | No | Yes | SCSA |
| Gandini et al. [49] | 12 | 24 | No | Yes (blasto-cysts) | Yes | SCSA |
| Virro et al. [50] | 249 IVF/ICSI | NA | No | No | Yes | SCSA |
| Check et al. [117] | 0 | 106 | No | No | Yes | SCSA |
| Payne et al. [52] | 46 | 54 | No | No | No | SCSA |
| Boe-Hansen et al. [44] | 139 | 47 | No | No | Yes | SCSA |
| Bungum et al. [38] | 388 | 223 | No | No | Yes | SCSA |
| Sun et al. [67] | 143 | 0 | Yes | Yes | NA | TUNEL |
| Lopes et al. [68] | 0 | 150 | Yes | No | NA | TUNEL |
| Host et al. [22] | 50 | 61 | Yes | NA | NA | TUNEL |
| Tomlinson et al. [61] | 140 | 0 | No | No | Yes | TUNEL |
| Benchaib et al. [85] | 50 | 54 | Yes | No | Yes | TUNEL |
| Henkel et al. [63] | 208 | 54 | No | No | No | TUNEL |
| Huang et al. [65] | 217 | 86 | Yes | No | No | TUNEL |
| Seli et al. [75] | 49 | NA | NA | Yes | No | TUNEL |
| Henkel et al. [118] | 208 | 54 | No | No | No | TUNEL |
| Hammadeh et al. [87] | 26 | 22 | NA | NA | No | TUNEL |
| Borini et al. [88] | 82 | 50 | NA | NA | Only for ICSI | TUNEL |
| Benchaib et al. [86] | 88 | 234 | Only for ICSI | Only for ICSI | No | TUNEL |
| Bakos et al. [119] | 45 | 68 | Only for IVF | No | Only for ICSI | TUNEL |
| Frydman et al. [120] | 117 | 0 | NA | NA | Yes | TUNEL |
| Tarozzi et al. [121] | 82 | 50 | NA | NA | Only for ICSI | TUNEL |
| Muriel et al. [45] | 85 IVF/ICSI | NA | NA | NA | No | SCD |
| Velez de la Calle et al. [122] | 622 IVF/ICSI | NA | No | Yes | No | SCD |
| Tavalaee et al. [123] | 92 IVF/ICSI | NA | Only for ICSI | NA | No | SCD |

*IVF* In vitro fertilization; *ICSI* intracytoplasmic sperm injection; *SCSA* Sperm Chromatin Structure assay; *TUNEL* terminal deoxynucleotidyl transferase dUTP nick-end labelling; *SCD* Sperm Chromatin Dispersion test; *NA* not applicable could be obtained, regardless of the type of ART applied [46, 47]. However, in 2004 when three independent SCSA reports demonstrated that a DFI level above 27% was indeed compatible with pregnancy and delivery after both IVF and ICSI [48–50], it became evident that ART can compensate poor sperm chromatin quality.

Gandini et al. [49], in a study involving 34 couples (12 IVF and 22 ICSI), did not note any difference between patients initiating pregnancies or not. They reported healthy full-term pregnancies with levels of DFI up to 66.3%. Bungum et al. [48] investigated 109 consecutive couples undergoing IVF and 66 couples undergoing ICSI. No statistically significant difference in the pregnancy outcome was noted by dividing patients according to the DFI level of 27%. However, in the group with a DFI above 27%, the results of ICSI were significantly better than those of IVF, clinical pregnancy (52.9 vs. 22.2%), implantation (37.5 vs. 19.4%) and delivery (47.1 vs. 22.2%). Virro et al. [50] studied 249 couples undergoing IVF/ICSI and noted that men with DFI below 33% had a significantly greater chance of initiating a pregnancy, lower rate of spontaneous abortions and an increased rate of ongoing pregnancies at 12 weeks (47 vs. 28%) than those with a DFI above 33%.

These data were in agreement with other previous smaller reports using TUNEL or comet assays, showing that sperm DNA damage is more predictive in IVF and, less in ICSI [22, 51]. This was later confirmed in a larger data set including nearly 1,000 men in IUI, IVF or ICSI treatment using DFI 30% as threshold level. No statistically significant difference between the outcomes of ICSI vs. IVF in the group with DFI ≤30% was seen. In the DFI >30% group, however, the results of ICSI were significantly better than those of IVF. The odds ratios (ORs) for biochemical pregnancy (BP), clinical pregnancy (CP) and delivery (D) were 3.0 (95% CI: 1.4–6.2), 2.3 (5% CI: 1.1–4.6) and 2.2 (95% CI: 1.0–4.5), respectively. For ICSI, there was even a tendency towards higher rates of BP, CP and D with a DFI >30% vs. a DFI ≤30%, however, not reaching a statistically significant difference. Moreover, the implantation rate in the ICSI group with DFI >30% seemed to be higher than in any other subgroup. The other SCSA parameter, HDS did, however, not predict the outcome of IVF or ICSI, neither alone nor in combination with DFI [38]. By contrast, one single study had, however, reported that DFI and HDS threshold values were not valid [52]. The authors found that the poorer the integrity of sperm nuclear DNA, the better is the pregnancy outcome and suggested to "redefine the relationship between SCSA data and ART outcomes". The study was, however, based on only 100 IVF/ICSI treatments where female factor infertility not was taken into consideration.

Despite convincing data from several authors, some reports have challenged the predictive value of the SCSA test [53]. One example is a position paper from the Practice Committee of the American Society for Reproductive Medicine [54]. Although ASRM, after a meta-analysis on 14 published studies, stated that fragmented sperm DNA is more frequent in infertile than in fertile and may contribute to poor reproductive performance, but concluded that, so far, there was no proven role for routine DNA integrity testing in the evaluation of infertility. Other examples are two meta-analyses including studies using either TUNEL and SCSA assays. Both Collins et al. [55], who considered 13 IVF/ICSI studies (9 carried by SCSA and 4 by the TUNEL assay), and Zini et al. [56], who considered 9 IVF (6 carried out by TUNEL assay and 3 by SCSA) and 11 ICSI studies (6 carried by SCSA and 5 by the TUNEL assay) found only small associations between sperm DNA integrity test results and pregnancy in IVF and ICSI. Two other meta-analysis including only SCSA-studies have been performed. Based on 14 papers, Evenson and Wixon [57] reported that in IVF and ICSI, CP was closely related to DFI as measured by SCSA. By contrast, based on three papers, Li et al. [58] found that neither DFI nor HDS had an effect on the chance of CP after IVF or ICSI treatment.

## Sperm DNA Damage in Relation to Fertilization

There is conflicting evidence about the relationship between sperm DNA fragmentation and fertilization rates after IVF and ICSI. Ahmadi and Ng [59] in a mouse model demonstrated that, despite a high DNA damage load, sperm were able to fertilize an oocyte. Also, several studies in the human have shown that men with high number of sperm with damaged DNA can have the same ability to fertilize in vitro as men with a lower fraction of sperm with DNA damage as measured by SCSA [38, 46–50, 58] or by other sperm DNA integrity assays [29, 60–66].

On the contrary, the presence of damaged sperm DNA was shown to have a significant inverse relationship with fertilization in other studies [22, 67] and to contribute to a failure of fertilization even in ICSI [68]. Host et al. [22] found a negative correlation between the proportion of spermatozoa with DNA strand breaks and the fertilization rates in all groups except for those undergoing ICSI.

Also, the SCSA parameter HDS, thought to represent immature spermatozoa with incomplete protamination, was found to be related to IVF fertilization rates, but not in ICSI [50]. Consequently, the authors suggested that men with HDS >15% should be treated with ICSI. This finding has, however, not been confirmed by others, and thus, HDS does not seem to have any clinical impact.

## Sperm DNA Damage in Relation to Pre-Embryo Development

Although fertilization may be independent of sperm DNA integrity, the postfertilization development of the pre-embryo can be impaired by sperm DNA damage.

It has been speculated in if and how sperm DNA damage has impact on human embryo and foetal development as well as on offspring health [69]. Incomplete or aberrant sperm DNA repair by the oocyte is hypothesized to create mutations in the genome of the zygote, which potentially could lead to implantation failure, early miscarriages or, in worst cases, diseases in the offspring [9, 70, 71]. While the mature spermatozoon itself does not have the capability to repair DNA damage, oocytes and early embryos may have this capacity [72] to a certain degree [73].

Among the first reports to indicate that sperm DNA damage is related to poor embryo development was studies in mice by Ahmadi and Ng [73]. The human data regarding pre-embryo development in relation to sperm DNA damage is somewhat conflicting. While some authors have reported similar cleavage stage embryo developmental rates between high and low DFI groups as measured by SCSA [44, 46, 47, 52, 74], others have shown that sperm DNA damage is negatively correlated with embryo quality after IVF and ICSI [28, 29, 67]. Two studies have also reported that men with high levels of DNA fragmentation are at increased risk of low blastocyst formation compared to men with a low DFI [50, 75], and consequently, it has been suggested to practice blastocyst culture as a routine in ART.

## Raw versus Prepared Semen

In a vast majority of cases, spermatozoa used for ART are prepared by density-gradient centrifugation or swim-up methods. Both approaches aim at separating normal sperm from lymphocytes, epithelial cells, abnormal or immature sperm, cell debris, bacteria and seminal fluid. Several previous reports have shown an improvement in the sperm chromatin parameters comparing neat semen samples and samples prepared for ART [39, 49, 61, 76–82]. On the contrary, other reports showed unchanged or worse results [29, 45, 62, 65, 75, 83–87].

One study has analyzed the same semen samples before and after density gradient centrifuged considering 510 ART cycles. In contrast to what has been seen for raw semen, no predictive value of the SCSA parameters DFI and HDS, evaluated on the prepared semen, emerged in relation to pregnancy outcome [82]. These data supported the two first SCSA-ART studies where the SCSA parameters were assessed also on prepared semen, even if on a more limited number of patients, 24 and 34, respectively [46, 49]. Using the TUNEL assay, Borini et al. [88] in ICSI patients found DFI >10% in density-gradient-centrifuged semen to be discriminative for pregnancy. Also, Duran et al. [43], in a study on IUI couples, used washed semen samples and found no pregnancy if DFI, as measured by the TUNEL assay, exceeded the level of 12%. Larson et al. [46] suggested that elevated DFI in neat semen may reflect chromatin or other abnormalities within the entire sperm population interfering with the ability of the sperm to fertilize, but not completely eliminated by the sperm preparation procedure.

## Incubation of Sperm

Temperature and pH are known to influence on stability and developmental potential of gametes [89, 90], but as yet there is no developed sufficient good laboratory standards for incubation of sperm during the period between sperm preparation and fertilization. The duration and environment for sperm incubation vary from clinic to clinic. Peer et al. [91] found that a 2-h incubation of density-gradient-prepared ejaculates at 37°C led to increased nuclear degradation in terms of vacuolated nuclei in comparison to that at 21°C. Testicular sperm appear to be more susceptible to damage than ejaculated sperm, yet they are subjected to conditions under the assumption that they have similar resistance to injury. For example, incubation under aerobic conditions for 4 or 24 h at 37°C leads to marked sperm DNA damage [92, 93].

## Testicular versus Ejaculated Sperm in ART

Previous reports have shown that sperm DNA damage is significantly lower in the seminiferous tubules compared with the epididymis [94] or in ejaculated sperm [95]. Use of testicular sperm in couples with repeated pregnancy failure in ART and high sperm DNA fragmentation resulted in significant better pregnancy rates [94, 95]. Although use of testicular sperm may only have a potential of solving ROS-induced sperm DNA damage, these findings should be followed up by larger prospective, randomized studies. In the majority of cases, sperm DNA damage is believed to be ROS-induced [96].

## The Use of Cryopreserved Sperm in ART

Some studies of cryopreservation of sperm have demonstrated that freezing–thawing has a negative effect on sperm DNA integrity [74], especially in infertile men [93, 97]. Cryopreservation can induce an increased rate of lipid peroxidation in the sperm plasma membrane, causing an overall increase in the concentration of oxygen radicals in the sample. Exposure to high ROS concentrations can result in the disruption of mitochondrial and plasma membranes, causing DNA fragmentation and a reduction in sperm motility [98]. Adding antioxidants to the cryoprotection media [99] have shown to be a promising ameliorating procedure. Another strategy shown to cause less chromatin damage to sperm is freezing of density-gradient-prepared semen instead of raw semen [97]. However, larger studies are needed to clarify whether these are more effective and gentle methods compared to those in use.

## Intraindividual Variation of DFI in Relation to ART

One of the drawbacks by the conventional sperm analysis is the huge intraindividual variation reported for concentration, motility and morphology [100]. By contrast, the first SCSA reports found a lower intraindividual variation for DFI [101]. A more recent study of infertile men in ART treatment has, however, demonstrated a significant day-to-day variation of DFI with a mean coefficient of variation (CV) of 29% [102]. Data from a so far unpublished study has shown that among 616 men who had their semen analyzed by SCSA both in infertility workup and in the actual ART cycle, 85% of the men remained in the same DFI category; ≤30% or >30%

from measurement 1 to 2. This implies that only 15% had a clinical effect of repeating the SCSA measurement (Oleszczuk et al., unpublished). Also, data from Giwercman et al. [41] demonstrated that a single SCSA analysis is a strong predictor of infertility.

## Future Perspectives

Despite the growing knowledge in the field of sperm chromatin integrity testing in fertility, fundamental questions remain to be answered as part of a more detailed understanding of sperm chromatin and its packaging during spermatogenesis, sperm maturation, ejaculation and unpackaging in the oocyte. For further clinical relevance, we need to know more about the following: (1) the type of DNA damage, (2) the percentage of sperm with DNA damage, (3) the extent of DNA damage per spermatozoon, (4) whether there is combined nucleotide damage and DNA fragmentation, (5) whether DNA damage affects introns or exons and (6) the ability of the oocyte to repair sperm DNA damage in the fertilizing sperm [103]. Developing standardized sperm DNA integrity assays providing such information is of highest value.

We also know too little about the origins of the damage and what can be done to prevent or cure sperm DNA damage. Cause-related therapy in the form of antioxidants has been attempted to reduce DNA damage caused by oxidative stress [95, 104–110]. However, such studies have been rather limited in size and the data are conflicting. Further large-scale studies are needed to investigate the type, role and mode of antioxidant therapy, as well as other types of causal treatment.

Another important issue for the future should be the development of new sperm separation or sorting techniques where individual or populations of sperm with intact DNA are isolated. Currently, a number of new techniques to favour sperm with normal sperm DNA integrity have been suggested and used; however, none of them are implemented into clinical practice. These include the so-called high-magnification ICSI, a method where spermatozoa with surface vacuoles are discarded [111] and the recently introduced confocal light absorption scattering spectroscopy (CLASS) technology, which allows for the non-invasive visualization of subcellular structures [112]. Also, the use of Annexin-V columns has shown to reduce the number of sperm with DNA fragmentation [113].

Another strategy suggested to follow the role of sperm DNA damage on pre-implantation development is to assess whether a quantity of known DNA damage has been repaired by the oocyte or the embryo by analyzing DNA damage in the trophoblast cells obtained by blastocyst biopsy [103].

Data from mice show links between DNA damage in spermatozoa and defects in embryonic development as well as the long-term health of the offspring [114]. However, knowledge on if and how sperm DNA defects may influence the human offspring is lacking, and it is urgent to initiate such studies.

Lastly, the question whether sperm DNA integrity tests can be used as a tool in ART to find the most effective treatment type in a given couple is only partly solved.

Although it is clearly shown that men with a SCSA-DFI above 30% should benefit from being referred directly to IVF/ICSI, it is still questionable whether there is, in these men, a clear difference in efficacy between IVF and ICSI [38]. As all available IVF/ICSI data come from retrospective studies, prospective randomized controlled trials should be conducted.

## Conclusions and Clinical Recommendations

ART fertility is a multifactorial issue and involves factors from both partners. Sperm DNA integrity status is only one piece in this puzzle. However, it covers an important aspect of sperm quality and function and should be routinely implemented as an adjunct to the conventional sperm parameters in fertility workup and ART, especially in unexplained subfertility. Among the sperm DNA integrity tests currently available, SCSA has provided the most stabile clinical threshold values in relation to infertility.

Based on existing data, it is evident that the relevance of sperm DNA integrity testing concerns, first of all, in vivo fertilization. In addition to its role as a predictor of natural conception, the SCSA parameter DFI, as measured in raw semen, can be used as an independent predictor of success in couples undergoing IUI. The predictive role of SCSA in IVF and ICSI are, however, more doubtful and needs to be further investigated by prospective randomized studies. In IVF and ICSI, it seems clear that no association between sperm DNA damage and fertilization rates exist. The same seems to be the case for embryo development until day 3. This has, however, indicated that blastocyst development is impaired in patients with high numbers of sperm with DNA damage.

In men having standard sperm parameters that indicate ICSI, there are no therapeutic consequences of performing SCSA [38, 48–50]. Men with high numbers of DNA-fragmented sperm have similar chances of obtaining pregnancy by IVF and ICSI as men with low sperm DNA fragmentation. However, the group of men who, first of all, will benefit from SCSA assessment would be unexplained subfertile men. Roughly, 20–25% of subfertile men, one out of four, with normal WHO sperm parameters have a SCSA-DFI above 20–30%, which is the DFI level where the chance of giving rise to a spontaneous or IUI-induced pregnancy reduces significantly. In order to find men with sperm DNA damage as a hidden cause to their childlessness, where the traditional semen analysis shows one or no abnormality, a SCSA analysis should be offered [41]. In men where all standard parameters are normal, chances of in vivo pregnancy starts to reduce for DFI above 20%. In the presence of one abnormal semen quality parameter, the chance of spontaneous pregnancy is significantly reduced already at DFI above 10%. Thus, in such couples DFI should be taken into consideration and the couples should be referred directly to IVF/ICSI [38].

The SCSA parameter DFI is more stable than the conventional WHO parameters. [115] In most men, a single analysis is enough to be of clinical value for the choice of ART treatment. However, when DFI is above 20% it is recommended to repeat the test prior to the actual ART treatment. Unfortunately, couples seeking ART are only to a limited degree counselled in regard to the impact of lifestyle factors on fertility. Existing knowledge on factors contributing to sperm DNA damage as for instance smoking and obesity should to a higher degree be communicated to the couples.

Laboratory procedures can harm sperm DNA integrity. In order to prevent further sperm DNA damage and to sort out sperm with fragmented DNA, density-gradient preparation is a good choice for sperm preparation. However, one should be aware that repeated centrifugations as well as the speed of centrifugation could have negative effects on sperm chromatin. Also, to prevent further DNA damage, semen samples should be processed as close to the fertilization procedure as possible. Cryopreserved and thawed semen should be tested in regard to sperm DNA damage prior to use in ART, and the fertilization method chosen according to the DFI should be assessed post thawing.

In conclusion, more research is needed to improve our current knowledge on DNA anomalies in spermatozoa. It is necessary to standardize better the methods of DNA damage evaluation and the time to apply them as pregnancy predictors in assisted reproduction. Moreover, a greater insight into the causes of sperm DNA damage is needed to develop appropriate treatment strategies and to enhance the genomic integrity of spermatozoa, thus contributing to optimize assisted reproduction outcome. So far, available data has shown that DFI as measured by SCSA can be used as a valuable tool in ART treatment and adds to the clinical management of subfertile/infertile couples. DFI has also shown to be an independent predictor of fertility in IUI and can be used to decide which type of ART treatment is needed for a couple.

# References

1. De Kretser DM. Male infertility. Lancet. 1997;349:787–90.
2. Dunson DB, Baird DD, Colombo B. Increased infertility with age in men and women. Obstet Gynecol. 2004;103:51–6.
3. Palermo G, Joris H, Devroey P, Van Steirteghem AC. Pregnancies after intracytoplasmic injection of single spermatozoon into an oocyte. Lancet. 1992;340:17–8.
4. Andersen AN, Goossens V, Ferraretti AP, Bhattacharya S, Felberbaum R, de Mouzon J, et al. Assisted reproductive technology in Europe, 2004: results generated from European registers by ESHRE. Hum Reprod. 2008;23:756–71.
5. Andersen AN, Gianaroli L, Felberbaum R, de Mouzon J, Nygren KG. Assisted reproductive technology in Europe, 2001. Results generated from European registers by ESHRE. Hum Reprod. 2005;20:1158–76.
6 Auger J, Eustache F, Andersen AG, Irvine DS, Jorgensen N, Skakkebaek NE, et al. Sperm morphological defects related to environment, lifestyle and medical history of 1001 male partners of pregnant women from four European cities. Hum Reprod. 2001;16:2710–7.
7. Bonde JPE, Ernst E, Jensen TK, Hjollund NHI, Kolstad H, Henriksen TB, et al. Relation between semen quality and fertility: a population-based study of 430 first-pregnancy planners. Lancet. 1998;352:1172–7.
8. Guzick DS, Overstreet JW, Factor-Litvak P, Brazil CK, Nakajima ST, Coutifaris C, et al. Sperm morphology, motility, and concentration in fertile and infertile men. N Engl J Med. 2001;345:1388–93.

9. Agarwal A, Said TM. Role of sperm chromatin abnormalities and DNA damage in male infertility. Hum Reprod Update. 2003;9:331–45.

10. Erenpreiss J, Spanó M, Erenpreisa J, Bungum M, Giwercman A. Sperm chromatin structure and male fertility: biological and clinical aspects. Asian J Androl. 2006;8:11–29.

11. Edwards RG, Brody SA. Principles and practice of assisted human reproduction. Philadelphia: W.B Saunders; 1995.

12. Steptoe PC, Edwards RG. Birth after the reimplantation of a human embryo. Lancet. 1978;2:366.

13. Zegers-Hochschild F, Nygren KG, Adamson GD, de Mouzon J, Lancaster P, Mansour R, et al. The International Committee Monitoring Assisted Reproductive Technologies (ICMART) glossary on ART terminology. Fertil Steril. 2006;86:16–9.

14. Dobson R. Number of babies born by assisted reproduction rises by 12%. BMJ. 2009;338:2208.

15. Hull MG, Fleming CF, Hughes AO, McDermott A. The age-related decline in female fecundity: a quantitative controlled study of implanting capacity and survival of individual embryos after in vitro fertilization. Fertil Steril. 1996;65:783–90.

16. Aitken RJ. Sperm function tests and fertility. Int J Androl. 2006;29:69–75; discussion 105–8.

17. Muller CH. Rationale, interpretation, validation, and uses of sperm function tests. J Androl. 2000;21:10–30.

18. Bhattacharya S, Hamilton MP, Shaaban M, Khalaf Y, Seddler M, Ghobara T, et al. Conventional in-vitro fertilisation versus intracytoplasmic sperm injection for the treatment of non-male-factor infertility: a randomised controlled trial. Lancet. 2001;357:2075–9.

19. Jain T, Gupta RS. Trends in the use of intracytoplasmic sperm injection in the United States. N Engl J Med. 2007;357:251–7.

20. Evenson DP, Jost LK, Marshall D, Zinaman MJ, Clegg E, Purvis K, et al. Utility of the sperm chromatin structure assay as a diagnostic and prognostic tool in the human fertility clinic. Hum Reprod. 1999;14:1039–49.

21. Gandini L, Lombardo F, Paoli D, Caponecchia L, Familiari G, Verlengia C, et al. Study of apoptotic DNA fragmentation in human spermatozoa. Hum Reprod. 2000;15:830–9.

22. Host E, Lindenberg S, Smidt-Jensen S. The role of DNA strand breaks in human spermatozoa used for IVF and ICSI. Acta Obstet Gynecol Scand. 2000;79:559–63.

23. Irvine DS, Twigg JP, Gordon EL, Fulton N, Milne PA, Aitken RJ. DNA integrity in human spermatozoa: relationships with semen quality. J Androl. 2000;21:33–44.

24. Spanò M, Bonde JP, Hjøllund HI, Kolstad HA, Cordelli E, Leter G. Sperm chromatin damage impairs human fertility. The Danish First Pregnancy Planner Study Team. Fertil Steril. 2000;73:43–50.

25. Carrell DT, Liu L. Altered protamine 2 expression is uncommon in donors of known fertility, but common among men with poor fertilizing capacity, and may reflect other abnormalities of spermiogenesis. J Androl. 2001;22:604–10.

26. Zini A, Bielecki R, Phang D, Zenzes MT. Correlations between two markers of sperm DNA integrity, DNA denaturation and DNA fragmentation, in fertile and infertile men. Fertil Steril. 2001;75:674–7.

27. Zini A, Fischer MA, Sharir S, Shayegan B, Phang D, Jarvi K. Prevalence of abnormal sperm DNA denaturation in fertile and infertile men. Urology. 2002;60:1069–72.

28. Saleh RA, Agarwal A, Nada EA, El-Tonsy MH, Sharma RK, Meyer A, et al. Negative effects of increased sperm DNA damage in relation to seminal oxidative stress in men with idiopathic and male factor infertility. Fertil Steril. 2003;79 Suppl 3:1597–605.

29. Morris ID, Ilott S, Dixon L, Brison DR. The spectrum of DNA damage in human sperm assessed by single cell gel electrophoresis (Comet assay) and its relationship to fertilization and embryo development. Hum Reprod. 2002;17:990–8.

30. Gorczyca W, Gong J, Darzynkiewicz Z. Detection of DNA strand breaks in individual apoptotic cells by the in situ terminal deoxynucleotidyl transferase and nick translation assays. Cancer Res. 1993;53:1945–51.

31. Evenson DP, Darzynkiewicz Z, Melamed MR. Relation of mammalian sperm chromatin heterogeneity to fertility. Science. 1980;210:1131–3.

32. Evenson DP, Larson KL, Jost LK. Sperm chromatin structure assay: its clinical use for detecting sperm DNA fragmentation in male infertility and comparisons with other techniques. J Androl. 2002;23:25–43.
33. Fernandez JL, Muriel L, Rivero MT, Goyanes V, Vazquez R, Alvarez JG. The sperm chromatin dispersion test: a simple method for the determination of sperm DNA fragmentation. J Androl. 2003;24:59–66.
34. Fernández JL, Muriel L, Goyanes V, Segrelles E, Gosálvez J, Enciso M, et al. Simple determination of human sperm DNA fragmentation with an improved sperm chromatin dispersion test. Fertil Steril. 2005;84:833–42.
35. Aravindan GR, Bjordahl J, Jost LK, Evenson DP. Susceptibility of human sperm to in situ DNA denaturation is strongly correlated with DNA strand breaks identified by single-cell electrophoresis. Exp Cell Res. 1997;236:231–7.
36. Erenpreiss J, Jepson K, Giwercman A, Tsarev I, Erenpreisa J, Spanó M. Toluidine blue cytometry test for sperm DNA conformation: comparison with the flow cytometric sperm chromatin structure and TUNEL assays. Hum Reprod. 2004;19:2277–82.
37. Makhlouf AA, Niederberger C. DNA integrity tests in clinical practice: it is not a simple matter of black and white (or red and green). J Androl. 2006;27:316–23.
38. Bungum M, Humaidan P, Axmon A, Spanó M, Bungum L, Erenpreiss J, et al. Sperm DNA integrity assessment in prediction of assisted reproduction technology outcome. Hum Reprod. 2007;22:174–9.
39. Spanò M, Kolstad AH, Larsen SB, Cordelli E, Leter G, Giwercman A, et al. The applicability of the flow cytometric sperm chromatin structure assay in epidemiological studies. Asclepios. Hum Reprod. 1998;13:2495–505.
40. Giwercman A, Richthoff J, Hjollund H, Bonde JP, Jepson K, Frohm B, et al. Correlation between sperm motility and sperm chromatin structure assay parameters. Fertil Steril. 2003;80:1404–12.
41. Giwercman A, Lindstedt L, Larsson M, Bungum M, Spanó M, Levine RJ, et al. Sperm chromatin structure assay as an independent predictor of fertility in vivo: a case-control study. Int J Androl. 2010;33:221–7.
42. Erenpreiss J, Elzanaty S, Giwercman A. Sperm DNA damage in men from infertile couples. Asian J Androl. 2008;10:786–90.
43. Duran EH, Morshedi M, Taylor S, Oehninger S. Sperm DNA quality predicts intrauterine insemination outcome: a prospective cohort study. Hum Reprod. 2002;17:3122–8.
44. Boe-Hansen GB, Fedder J, Ersboll AK, Christensen P. The sperm chromatin structure assay as a diagnostic tool in the human fertility clinic. Hum Reprod. 2006;21:1576–82.
45. Muriel L, Meseguer M, Fernandez JL, Alvarez J, Remohi J, Pellicer A, et al. Value of the sperm chromatin dispersion test in predicting pregnancy outcome in intrauterine insemination: a blind prospective study. Hum Reprod. 2006;21:738–44.
46. Larson KL, DeJonge CJ, Barnes AM, Jost LK, Evenson DP. Sperm chromatin structure assay parameters as predictors of failed pregnancy following assisted reproductive techniques. Hum Reprod. 2000;15:1717–22.
47. Larson-Cook KL, Brannian JD, Hansen KA, Kasperson KM, Aamold ET, Evenson DP. Relationship between the outcomes of assisted reproductive techniques and sperm DNA fragmentation as measured by the sperm chromatin structure assay. Fertil Steril. 2003;80:895–902.
48. Bungum M, Humaidan P, Spanó M, Jepson K, Bungum L, Giwercman A. The predictive value of sperm chromatin structure assay (SCSA) parameters for the outcome of intrauterine insemination, IVF and ICSI. Hum Reprod. 2004;19:1401–8.
49. Gandini L, Lombardo F, Paoli D, Caruso F, Eleuteri P, Leter G, et al. Full-term pregnancies achieved with ICSI despite high levels of sperm chromatin damage. Hum Reprod. 2004;19:1409–17.
50. Virro MR, Larson-Cook KL, Evenson DP. Sperm chromatin structure assay (SCSA) parameters are related to fertilization, blastocyst development, and ongoing pregnancy in in vitro fertilization and intracytoplasmic sperm injection cycles. Fertil Steril. 2004;81:1289–95.

51. Hammadeh ME, Stieber M, Haidl G, Schmidt W. Association between sperm cell chromatin condensation, morphology based on strict criteria, and fertilization, cleavage and pregnancy rates in an IVF program. Andrologia. 1998;30:29–35.
52. Payne JF, Raburn DJ, Couchman GM, Price TM, Jamison MG, Walmer DK. Redefining the relationship between sperm deoxyribonucleic acid fragmentation as measured by the sperm chromatin structure assay and outcomes of assisted reproductive techniques. Fertil Steril. 2005;84:356–64.
53. Aitken RJ, DeIuliis GN. Value of DNA integrity assays for fertility evaluation. Soc Reprod Fertil Suppl. 2007;65:81–92.
54. The Practice Committee of the American Society of Reproductive Medicine. The clinical utility of sperm DNA integrity testing. Fertil Steril. 2006;86 Suppl 4:35–7.
55. Collins JA, Barnhart KT, Schlegel PN. Do sperm DNA integrity tests predict pregnancy with in vitro fertilization? Fertil Steril. 2008;89:823–31.
56. Zini A, Boman JM, Belzile E, Ciampi A. Sperm DNA damage is associated with an increased risk of pregnancy loss after IVF and ICSI: systematic review and meta-analysis. Hum Reprod. 2008;23:2663–8.
57. Evenson DP, Wixon R. Meta-analysis of sperm DNA fragmentation using the sperm chromatin structure assay. Reprod Biomed Online. 2006;12:466–72.
58. Li Z, Wang L, Cai J, Huang H. Correlation of sperm DNA damage with IVF and ICSI outcomes: a systematic review and meta-analysis. J Assist Reprod Genet. 2006;23:367–76.
59. Ahmadi A, Ng SC. Fertilizing ability of DNA-damaged spermatozoa. J Exp Zool. 1999;284:696–704.
60. Sakkas D, Urner F, Bianchi PG, Bizzaro D, Wagner I, Jaquenoud N, et al. Sperm chromatin anomalies can influence decondensation after intracytoplasmic sperm injection. Hum Reprod. 1996;11:837–43.
61. Tomlinson MJ, Moffatt O, Manicardi GC, Bizzaro D, Afnan M, Sakkas D. Interrelationships between seminal parameters and sperm nuclear DNA damage before and after density gradient centrifugation: implications for assisted conception. Hum Reprod. 2001;16:2160–5.
62. Tomsu M, Sharma V, Miller D. Embryo quality and IVF treatment outcomes may correlate with different sperm comet assay parameters. Hum Reprod. 2002;17:1856–62.
63. Henkel R, Kierspel E, Hajimohammad M, Stalf T, Hoogendijk C, Mehnert C, et al. DNA fragmentation of spermatozoa and assisted reproduction technology. Reprod Biomed Online. 2003;7:477–84.
64. Lewis SE, O'Connell M, Stevenson M, Thompson-Cree L, McClure N. An algorithm to predict pregnancy in assisted reproduction. Hum Reprod. 2004;19:1385–94.
65. Huang CC, Lin DP, Tsao HM, Cheng TC, Liu CH, Lee MS. Sperm DNA fragmentation negatively correlates with velocity and fertilization rates but might not affect pregnancy rates. Fertil Steril. 2005;84:130–40.
66. Nasr-Esfahani MH, Salehi M, Razavi S, Anjomshoa M, Rozbahani S, Moulavi F, et al. Effect of sperm DNA damage and sperm protamine deficiency on fertilization and embryo development post-ICSI. Reprod Biomed Online. 2005;11:198–205.
67. Sun JG, Jurisicova A, Casper RF. Detection of deoxyribonucleic acid fragmentation in human sperm: correlation with fertilization in vitro. Biol Reprod. 1997;56:602–7.
68. Lopes CH, Mazzini MN, Tortorella H, Konrath RA, Brandelli A. Isolation, partial characterization and biological activity of mannosyl glycopeptides from seminal plasma. Glycoconj J. 1998;15:477–81.
69. Lewis SE, Aitken RJ. DNA damage to spermatozoa has impacts on fertilization and pregnancy. Cell Tissue Res. 2005;322:33–41.
70. Aitken RJ, Baker MA. Oxidative stress and male reproductive biology. Reprod Fertil Dev. 2004;16:581–8.
71. Liu CH, Tsao HM, Cheng TC, Wu HM, Huang CC, Chen CI, et al. DNA fragmentation, mitochondrial dysfunction and chromosomal aneuploidy in the spermatozoa of oligoasthenoteratozoospermic males. J Assist Reprod Genet. 2004;21:119–26.

72. Matsuda Y, Tobari I. Chromosomal analysis in mouse eggs fertilized in vitro with sperm exposed to ultraviolet light (UV) and methyl and ethyl methanesulfonate (MMS and EMS). Mutat Res. 1988;198:131–44.
73. Ahmadi A, Ng SC. Developmental capacity of damaged spermatozoa. Hum Reprod. 1999;14:2279–85.
74. Gandini L, Lombardo F, Lenzi A, Spano M, Dondero F. Cryopreservation and sperm DNA integrity. Cell Tissue Bank. 2006;7:91–8.
75. Seli E, Gardner DK, Schoolcraft WB, Moffatt O, Sakkas D. Extent of nuclear DNA damage in ejaculated spermatozoa impacts on blastocyst development after in vitro fertilization. Fertil Steril. 2004;82:378–83.
76. Golan R, Cooper TG, Oschry Y, Oberpenning F, Schulze H, Shocha L, et al. Changes in chromatin condensation of human spermatozoa during epididymal transit as determined by flow cytometry. Hum Reprod. 1996;11:1457–62.
77. Larson KL, Brannian JD, Timm BK, Jost LK, Evenson DP. Density gradient centrifugation and glass wool filtration of semen remove spermatozoa with damaged chromatin structure. Hum Reprod. 1999;14:2015–9.
78. Donnelly ET, O'Connell M, McClure N, Lewis SE. Differences in nuclear DNA fragmentation and mitochondrial integrity of semen and prepared human spermatozoa. Hum Reprod. 2000;15:1552–61.
79. Younglai EV, Holt D, Brown P, Jurisicova A, Casper RF. Sperm swim-up techniques and DNA fragmentation. Hum Reprod. 2001;16:1950–3.
80. McVicar CM, McClure N, Williamson K, Dalzell LH, Lewis SE. Incidence of Fas positivity and deoxyribonucleic acid double-stranded breaks in human ejaculated sperm. Fertil Steril. 2004;81 Suppl 1:767–74.
81. Morrell JM, Moffatt O, Sakkas D, Manicardi GC, Bizzaro D, Tomlinson M, et al. Reduced senescence and retained nuclear DNA integrity in human spermatozoa prepared by density gradient centrifugation. J Assist Reprod Genet. 2004;21:217–22.
82. Bungum M, Spanó M, Humaidan P, Eleuteri P, Rescia M, Giwercman A. Sperm Chromatin Structure Assay (SCSA) parameters measured after density gradient centrifugation are not predictive for the outcome of ART. Hum Reprod. 2008;23:4–10.
83. Zini A, Mak V, Phang D, Jarvi K. Potential adverse effect of semen processing on human sperm deoxyribonucleic acid integrity. Fertil Steril. 1999;72:496–9.
84. Zini A, Finelli A, Phang D, Jarvi K. Influence of semen processing technique on human sperm DNA integrity. Urology. 2000;56:1081–4.
85. Benchaib M, Braun V, Lornage J, Hadj S, Salle B, Lejeune H, et al. Sperm DNA fragmentation decreases the pregnancy rate in an assisted reproductive technique. Hum Reprod. 2003;18:1023–8.
86. Benchaib M, Lornage J, Mazoyer C, Lejeune H, Salle B, Francois Guerin J. Sperm deoxyribonucleic acid fragmentation as a prognostic indicator of assisted reproductive technology outcome. Fertil Steril. 2007;87:93–100.
87. Hammadeh ME, Radwan M, Al-Hasani S, Micu R, Rosenbaum P, Lorenz M, et al. Comparison of reactive oxygen species concentration in seminal plasma and semen parameters in partners of pregnant and non-pregnant patients after IVF/ICSI. Reprod Biomed Online. 2006;13:696–706.
88. Borini A, Tarozzi N, Bizzaro D, Bonu MA, Fava L, Flamigni C, et al. Sperm DNA fragmentation: paternal effect on early post-implantation embryo development in ART. Hum Reprod. 2006;21:2876–81.
89. Hamamah S, Magnoux E, Royere D, Barthelemy C, Dacheux JL, Gatti JL. Internal pH of human spermatozoa: effects of ions, follicular fluid and progesterone. Mol Hum Reprod. 1996;2:219–24.
90. Hamamah S, Gatti JL. Role of the ionic environment and internal pH on sperm activity. Hum Reprod. 1998;13 Suppl 4:20–30.
91. Peer S, Eltes F, Berkovitz A, Yehuda R, Itsykson P, Bartoov B. Is fine morphology of the human sperm nuclei affected by in vitro incubation at 37 degrees C? Fertil Steril. 2007;88:1589–94.

92. Dalzell LH, Thompson-Cree ME, McClure N, Traub AI, Lewis SE. Effects of 24-hour incubation after freeze-thawing on DNA fragmentation of testicular sperm from infertile and fertile men. Fertil Steril. 2003;79 Suppl 3:1670–2.
93. Dalzell JA, McVicar CM, McClure N, Lutton D, Lewis S. Effects of short and long incubations on DNA fragmentation of testicular sperm. Fertil Steril. 2004;82:1443–5.
94. Steele EK, McClure N, Maxwell RJ, Lewis SE. A comparison of DNA damage in testicular and proximal epididymal spermatozoa in obstructive azoospermia. Mol Hum Reprod. 1999;5:831–5.
95. Greco E, Scarselli F, Iacobelli M, Rienzi L, Ubaldi F, Ferrero S, et al. Efficient treatment of infertility due to sperm DNA damage by ICSI with testicular spermatozoa. Hum Reprod. 2005;20:226–30.
96. Aitken RJ, De Iuliis GN, McLachlan RI. Biological and clinical significance of DNA damage in the male germ line. Int J Androl. 2009;32:46–56.
97. Ahmad L, Jalali S, Shami SA, Akram Z, Batool S, Kalsoom O. Effects of cryopreservation on sperm DNA integrity in normospermic and four categories of infertile males. Syst Biol Reprod Med. 2010;56:74–83.
98. Baumber J, Ball BA, Linfor JJ, Meyers SA. Reactive oxygen species and cryopreservation promote DNA fragmentation in equine spermatozoa. J Androl. 2003;24:621–8.
99. Taylor K, Roberts P, Sanders K, Burton P. Effect of antioxidant supplementation of cryopreservation medium on post-thaw integrity of human spermatozoa. Reprod Biomed Online. 2009;18:184–9.
100. Jorgensen N, Auger J, Giwercman A, Irvine DS, Jensen TK, Keiding N, et al. Semen analysis performed by different laboratory teams: an intervariation study. Int J Androl. 1997;20:201–8.
101. Evenson DP, Jost LK, Baer RK, Turner TW, Schrader SM. Individuality of DNA denaturation patterns in human sperm as measured by the sperm chromatin structure assay. Reprod Toxicol. 1991;5:115–25.
102. Erenpreiss J, Bungum M, Spanó M, Elzanaty S, Orbidans J, Giwercman A. Intra-individual variation in Sperm Chromatin Structure Assay parameters in men from infertile couples: clinical implications. Hum Reprod. 2006;21:2061–4.
103. Sakkas D, Alvarez JG. Sperm DNA fragmentation: mechanisms of origin, impact on reproductive outcome and analysis. Fertil Steril. 2010;93:1027–36.
104. Lewis SE, Agbaje IM. Using the alkaline comet assay in prognostic tests for male infertility and assisted reproductive technology outcomes. Mutagenesis. 2008;23:163–70.
105. Kefer JC, Agarwal A, Sabanegh E. Role of antioxidants in the treatment of male infertility. Int J Urol. 2009;16:449–57.
106. Silver EW, Eskenazi B, Evenson DP, Block G, Young S, Wyrobek AJ. Effect of antioxidant intake on sperm chromatin stability in healthy nonsmoking men. J Androl. 2005;26:550–6.
107. Song GJ, Norkus EP, Lewis V. Relationship between seminal ascorbic acid and sperm DNA integrity in infertile men. Int J Androl. 2006;29:569–75.
108. Ménézo YJ, Hazout A, Panteix G, Robert F, Rollet J, Cohen-Bacrie P, et al. Antioxidants to reduce sperm DNA fragmentation: an unexpected adverse effect. Reprod Biomed Online. 2007;14:418–21.
109. Moskovtsev SI, Lecker I, Mullen JB, Jarvi K, Willis J, White J, et al. Cause-specific treatment in patients with high sperm DNA damage resulted in significant DNA improvement. Syst Biol Reprod Med. 2009;55:109–15.
110. Greco E, Iacobelli M, Rienzi L, Ubaldi F, Ferrero S, Tesarik J. Reduction of the incidence of sperm DNA fragmentation by oral antioxidant treatment. J Androl. 2005;26:349–53.
111. Bartoov B, Berkovitz A, Eltes F. Selection of spermatozoa with normal nuclei to improve the pregnancy rate with intracytoplasmic sperm injection. N Engl J Med. 2001;345:1067–8.
112. Itzkan I, Qiu L, Fang H, Zaman MM, Vitkin E, Ghiran IC, et al. Confocal light absorption and scattering spectroscopic microscopy monitors organelles in live cells with no exogenous labels. Proc Natl Acad Sci USA. 2007;104:17255–60.
113. Said TM, Grunewald S, Paasch U, Glander HJ, Baumann T, Kriegel C, et al. Advantage of combining magnetic cell separation with sperm preparation techniques. Reprod Biomed Online. 2005;10:740–6.

114. Fernández-Gonzalez R, Moreira PN, Pérez-Crespo M, Sánchez-Martín M, Ramirez MA, Pericuesta E, et al. Long-term effects of mouse intracytoplasmic sperm injection with DNA-fragmented sperm on health and behavior of adult offspring. Biol Reprod. 2008;78:761–72.

115. World Health Organization. WHO laboratory manual for the examination of human semen and sperm-cervical mucus interaction. Cambridge: Cambridge University Press; 1999.

116. Caglar GS, Köster F, Schöpper B, Asimakopoulos B, Nehls B, Nikolettos N, et al. Semen DNA fragmentation index, evaluated with both TUNEL and Comet assay, and the ICSI outcome. In Vivo. 2007;21:1075–80.

117. Check JH, Graziano V, Cohen R, Krotec J, Check ML. Effect of an abnormal sperm chromatin structural assay (SCSA) on pregnancy outcome following (IVF) with ICSI in previous IVF failures. Arch Androl. 2005;51:121–4.

118. Henkel R, Hajimohammad M, Stalf T, Hoogendijk C, Mehnert C, Menkveld R, et al. Influence of deoxyribonucleic acid damage on fertilization and pregnancy. Fertil Steril. 2004;81:965–72.

119. Bakos HW, Thompson JG, Feil D, Lane M. Sperm DNA damage is associated with assisted reproductive technology pregnancy. Int J Androl. 2008;31:518–26.

120. Frydman N, Prisant N, Hesters L, Frydman R, Tachdjian G, Cohen-Bacrie P, et al. Adequate ovarian follicular status does not prevent the decrease in pregnancy rates associated with high sperm DNA fragmentation. Fertil Steril. 2008;89:92–7.

121. Tarozzi N, Nadalini M, Stronati A, Bizzaro D, Dal Prato L, Coticchio G, et al. Anomalies in sperm chromatin packaging: implications for assisted reproduction techniques. Reprod Biomed Online. 2009;18:486–95.

122. Velez de la Calle JF, Muller A, Walschaerts M, Clavere JL, Jimenez C, Wittemer C, et al. Sperm deoxyribonucleic acid fragmentation as assessed by the sperm chromatin dispersion test in assisted reproductive technology programs: results of a large prospective multicenter study. Fertil Steril. 2008;90:1792–9.

123. Tavalaee M, Razavi S, Nasr-Esfahani MH. Influence of sperm chromatin anomalies on assisted reproductive technology outcome. Fertil Steril. 2009;91:1119–26.

# Chapter 14
# Sperm DNA Damage and Pregnancy Loss After IVF/ICSI

**Armand Zini and Jason Matthew Boman**

Standard semen parameters that exhibit a high degree of biological variability are only fair measures of fertility potential and are poor predictors of reproductive outcomes [1]. As such, there is a need for better markers that might help distinguish fertile from infertile men and help predict pregnancy outcome and adverse reproductive events. Animal studies have shown that embryo development and implantation depend, at least in part, on the integrity of the sperm DNA and that there may be a threshold of sperm DNA damage beyond which these processes are impaired [2]. While the clinical utility sperm DNA integrity testing has yet to be firmly established, there is now clear evidence that infertile men possess substantially more sperm DNA damage than do fertile men [3–7]. In addition, sperm DNA damage is associated with lower natural, IUI, and IVF pregnancy rates [8–14].

Interestingly, sperm DNA and chromatin defects are not associated with lower ICSI pregnancy rates [15–19]. This is clinically relevant because men with severe male-factor infertility are the most likely patients to possess sperm DNA defects and are the most likely to require IVF with ICSI as a means of reproducing. While sperm DNA damage does not seem to impact pregnancy rates with IVF/ICSI, a higher level of DNA defects may infer a greater risk of losing the pregnancy once established.

The risk of pregnancy loss after IVF/ICSI has been reported in a number of studies, and these results have now been reviewed in a systematic fashion. This chapter reviews the etiology of sperm DNA damage, the tests used to measure DNA damage, and relationship between DNA damage and reproductive outcomes. In particular, the impact that sperm DNA has on pregnancy loss after using IVF/ICSI to achieve pregnancy is discussed.

A. Zini, MD (✉)
Department of Surgery, Division of Urology,
McGill University, St. Mary's Hospital Center, Montreal, QC, Canada
e-mail: ziniarmand@yahoo.com

J.M. Boman, MD, FRCS(C)
Division of Urology, Department of Surgery, Centre Hospitalier Régional du Suroît,
Montreal, QC, Canada

A. Zini, A. Agarwal (eds.), *Sperm Chromatin for the Clinician*,
© Springer Science+Business Media New York 2013

# Pregnancy Loss

## *Definitions*

Confirmation of pregnancy can be achieved either by biochemical means (serum hCG elevation) or clinically (presence of a heartbeat, confirmed by ultrasound). Pregnancy loss (spontaneous abortion or miscarriage) refers to a pregnancy that ends spontaneously before the fetus has reached a viable gestational age. The World Health Organization defines it, more specifically, as expulsion or extraction of an embryo or fetus weighing 500 g or less from its mother. This typically corresponds to a gestational age of 20–22 weeks or less.

## *Etiologies*

Female *chromosomal abnormalities* account for approximately 50% of all miscarriages. The most frequently encountered chromosomal abnormalities in decreasing order of frequency are as follows: autosomal trisomies (52%), monosomy X (19%), polyploidies (22%), and others (7%). Trisomy 16 is the most common autosomal trisomy and is always lethal [20].

*Congenital anomalies* that can result from either genetic abnormalities, extrinsic factors such as amniotic bands, or exposure to teratogens can also lead to pregnancy loss. *Trauma* resulting from invasive diagnostic procedures (e.g., amniocentesis or chorionic villus sampling) or from blunt injuries to the maternal abdomen is yet another potential cause of early loss pregnancy. A myriad of *maternal host factors* that might include anatomic uterine anomalies, acute maternal infections or endocrinopathies, hypercoagulable states, and finally immunologic rejection are all potential causes of pregnancy loss.

While the majority of pregnancy losses result from female factors, increasing evidence suggests that male factors can also play a role in miscarriage. Although, it is not known exactly how sperm defects contribute to pregnancy loss, some studies suggest that abnormal sperm DNA integrity may affect embryo development and increase miscarriage risk [2, 8, 11, 12, 14, 16–18, 21].

# Sperm DNA Damage

## *Human Sperm DNA and Chromatin Structure*

Sperm chromatin is very tightly compacted by virtue of the unique associations between the DNA and sperm nuclear proteins (histones and protamines) [22]. During the later stages of spermatogenesis, the haploid spermatid nucleus is remodeled and condensed further as a result of the sequential displacement of histones by transition proteins and then by protamines [22, 23]. The DNA strands are tightly wrapped around the protamine molecules forming tight and highly organized loops [24], and it is thought that this nuclear compaction is important to protect the sperm genome from external stresses such as oxidation or temperature elevation [25]. In humans, up to 15% of the DNA remains packaged by histones at specific DNA sequences (i.e., there is a nonrandom association between histones and DNA sequences) [26]. The histone-bound DNA sequences are less tightly compacted and more available for expression than non-histone-bound DNsA sequences. It is thought that these DNA sequences and/or genes may be involved in fertilization and early embryo development [27].

Infertile men have an increased sperm histone to protamine ratio when compared to fertile controls [28]. The spermatozoa of infertile men can also exhibit incomplete nuclear sulfhydryl group oxidation – the reaction leading to the formation of stabilizing disulfide cross-links [29, 30]. These sperm abnormalities (histone to protamine ratio and sulfhydryl group status) can potentially result in defective chromatin compaction [31] and in an increased susceptibility to DNA damage [7]. Sperm nuclear compaction or condensation may be an important determinant of sperm head morphology. Both animal and human studies have demonstrated a correlation between sperm DNA stainability and head morphology, which may, in part, be due to reduced nuclear compaction [32, 33].

## Etiology of Sperm DNA Damage

The etiology of sperm DNA damage is multifactorial. Clinically, several conditions have been associated with sperm DNA and chromatin damage (e.g., chemotherapy, smoking, genital tract infection, varicocele, etc.) [8, 34–41]. Broadly, these conditions can be categorized as primary or intrinsic defects in spermatogenesis (e.g., genetic or developmental abnormalities) and secondary or extrinsic noxious factors (e.g., gonadotoxins, hyperthermia, oxidants, endocrine disruption, etc.).

At the cellular level, a number of theories have been proposed to explain the DNA damage in human spermatozoa. Studies have suggested that protamine deficiency (with aberrant chromatin remodeling), reactive oxygen species (ROS) and abortive apoptosis may be responsible for sperm DNA damage [42–47]. Recently, De Iuliis et al. have proposed a two-step hypothesis to explain the generation of sperm DNA damage. Based on the model, oxidative stress acts on poorly protaminated cells (i.e., cells with incomplete replacement of histones by protamines) generated as a result of defective spermiogenesis [48].

## Tests of Sperm DNA Damage

Several tests of sperm DNA and chromatin damage have been described [41, 49, 50]. These tests have been developed in the hope that they may (1) help in the diagnosis of male infertility, (2) predict reproductive outcomes in the context of assisted reproductive technologies (ARTs), and (3) provide some assurance regarding the integrity of the male gamete genome. Several factors must be considered when evaluating studies of sperm DNA and chromatin integrity. First, the different assays measure different aspects of sperm DNA and chromatin. Second, the assay conditions can greatly influence the accessibility of the dye or enzyme to the sites of damaged DNA and, therefore, impact on the final results. Third, current assays are limited because they do not selectively differentiate clinically important DNA fragmentation (e.g., degree or gene specificity) from clinically insignificant damage. Finally, sample preparation and handling prior to sperm DNA and chromatin integrity testing can impact on the final test results.

The Comet (single cell gel electrophoresis) and TUNEL (terminal deoxynucleotidyl transferase-mediated dUTP nick end-labeling) assays are commonly utilized assays that detect DNA strand breaks directly. Some assays measure the susceptibility of DNA to denaturation – that is the formation of single-stranded DNA from native double-stranded DNA (e.g., SCSA-sperm chromatin structure assay) – and depend on the premise that nicked DNA will denature more readily than intact DNA. Other assays rely on the differential binding of dyes or agents to single-stranded and [50] double-stranded DNA (e.g., acridine orange) or to protamine-deficient sites (e.g., aniline blue or CMA3 test). Remarkably, the results of most sperm DNA or chromatin integrity assays correlate highly with each other – with the exception of the manual acridine orange test [50]. In order to provide clinically relevant information, an upper normal level (cutoff) of the percentage of cells with DNA fragmentation or chromatin defect has been defined for most of these assays. Samples with test results above the threshold or cutoff value are considered to have high levels of DNA damage [41].

## Relationship Between Sperm DNA Damage and Pregnancy Loss After IVF and ICSI

Several studies have reported on the risk of pregnancy loss after standard IVF and after ICSI, and we have recently carried out a systematic review of the literature and performed a meta-analysis of these studies to further evaluate the impact of sperm DNA damage on pregnancy loss after IVF without and with ICSI [51].

In our review of the literature, we found seven eligible reports (with 11 studies) that involved 1,549 cycles of treatment (808 IVF and 741 IVF/ICSI cycles), 640 pregnancies (345 with IVF and 295 with IVF/ICSI), and 122 pregnancy losses in total. The characteristics of the studies were highly variable in terms of data collection (i.e., prospective vs. retrospective), definition of pregnancy loss (biochemical vs. clinical), population characteristics (unselected vs. repeated IVF failures), female inclusion/exclusion criteria, sperm DNA damage test, and sperm DNA test cutoff. The characteristics of the studies are summarized in Tables 14.1 and 14.2. In all but one study, sperm DNA damage was evaluated on whole (unprocessed)

**Table 14.1** Selected diagnostic properties of studies on sperm DNA damage and pregnancy loss (PL) after IVF and IVF/ICSI

| Study | n | ART | Assay | PL | Ab Test* | Sens (%) | Spec (%) | PPV | NPV | OR (95% CI) |
|---|---|---|---|---|---|---|---|---|---|---|
| Check et al. [17] | 104 | ICSI | SCSA | 47 | 24 | 0.31 | 0.83 | 0.63 | 0.58 | 2.27 (0.45, 11.59) |
| Zini et al. [18] | 60 | ICSI | SCSA | 16 | 19 | 0.40 | 0.85 | 0.33 | 0.88 | 3.67 (0.46, 29.42) |
| Borini et al. [11] | 82 | IVF | TUNEL | 6 | 11 | 0.91 | 0.94 | 0.50 | 0.99 | 160 (0.18, 1,44,708) |
| Borini et al. [11] | 50 | ICSI | TUNEL | 25 | 25 | 0.97 | 0.99 | 0.97 | 0.99 | 2,700 (0.38, $2 \times 10^7$) |
| Benchaib et al. [12] | 84 | IVF | TUNEL | 15 | 15 | 0.50 | 0.91 | 0.50 | 0.91 | 10.0 (0.87, 114.8) |
| Benchaib et al. [12] | 218 | ICSI | TUNEL | 12 | 15 | 0.38 | 0.88 | 0.30 | 0.91 | 4.54 (0.89, 23.28) |
| Bungum et al. [8] | 388 | IVF | SCSA | 24 | 14 | 0.11 | 0.85 | 0.19 | 0.76 | 0.73 (0.23, 2.33) |
| Bungum et al. [8] | 223 | ICSI | SCSA | 19 | 40 | 0.50 | 0.63 | 0.24 | 0.84 | 1.69 (0.63, 4.49) |
| Frydman et al. [14] | 117 | IVF | TUNEL | 19 | 32 | 0.64 | 0.75 | 0.37 | 0.90 | 5.25 (1.31, 21.11) |
| Lin et al. [19] | 137 | IVF | SCSA | 10 | 17 | 0.29 | 0.84 | 0.17 | 0.92 | 2.16 (0.37, 12.72) |
| Lin et al. [19] | 86 | ICSI | SCSA | 18 | 23 | 0.50 | 0.83 | 0.40 | 0.88 | 5.00 (0.97, 25.77) |

*ART* assisted reproductive technology; *Abn Test* proportion of abnormal sperm DNA test among documented pregnancies; *PL* pregnancy loss; *Sens* sensitivity; *Spec* specificity; *PPV* positive predictive value; *NPV* negative predictive value; *OR* odds ratio

semen. In the Borini et al. [11] study, sperm samples were washed prior to assessing DNA damage. This needs mentioning because there may a difference in sperm DNA damage between whole and prepared semen, and the sperm DNA damage cutoffs may not be reliable when evaluating washed semen in predicting outcome of ART [52].

Our meta-analysis of the evaluable studies demonstrated a combined OR of 2.48 (95% CI; 1.52, 4.04, $p < 0.0001$), indicating an important association between sperm DNA damage and the rate of pregnancy loss after IVF and ICSI [51]. Repeating the meta-analysis with the Borini et al. [11] study excluded also demonstrated a significant OR estimate (OR = 2.37), which was not significantly different from the overall meta-analysis.

We found no significant difference in the OR according to the type of ART (IVF or ICSI) However, there was a significant difference in the OR estimates between

**Table 14.2** Characteristics of studies on sperm DNA damage and pregnancy loss (PL) after IVF and IVF/ICSI

| Study | $n$ | ART | Assay | Population | Study design | PL-Def | Female Dx |
|---|---|---|---|---|---|---|---|
| Check et al. [17] | 104 | ICSI | SCSA | Failed IVFx2 | Unspecified | Per CP | Unspecified |
| Zini et al. [18] | 60 | ICSI | SCSA | Unspecified | Prospective | Per CP | <40 |
| Borini et al. [11] | 82 | IVF | TUNEL | Unspecified | Unspecified | Per CP | Unspecified |
| Borini et al. [11] | 50 | ICSI | TUNEL | Unspecified | Unspecified | Per CP | Unspecified |
| Benchaib et al. [12] | 84 | IVF | TUNEL | Unspecified | Prospective | Per CP | Unspecified |
| Benchaib et al. [12] | 218 | ICSI | TUNEL | Unspecified | Prospective | Per CP | Unspecified |
| Lin et al. [21] | 137 | IVF | SCSA | Unspecified | Prospective | Per CP | <40, FSH <15 |
| Lin et al. [21] | 86 | ICSI | SCSA | Male factor | Prospective | Per CP | <40, FSH <15 |
| Bungum et al. [18] | 388 | IVF | SCSA | Female factor | Prospective | Per BP | <40, FSH <12 |
| Bungum et al. [8] | 223 | ICSI | SCSA | Male factor | Prospective | Per BP | <40, FSH <12 |
| Frydman et al. [14] | 117 | IVF | TUNEL | Unspecified | Prospective | Per CP | <38, FSH <10 |

$n$ number of IVF or ICSI cycles; *ART* assisted reproductive technology; *PL-Def* pregnancy loss definition; *CP* clinical pregnancy; *BP* biochemical pregnancy; *Female Dx* female diagnosis; <40 or <38 = <40 or <38 year-old; FSH <15 (<12, <10) = day 3 serum FSH < 15 (<12, <10) IU/L

the TUNEL and the SCSA studies (the combined OR of the studies using TUNEL assay (OR = 7.04) was significantly higher than that of the studies using SCSA (OR = 1.77)).

The finding of an association between sperm DNA damage and pregnancy loss provides a mechanism by which sperm defects may impact pregnancy loss, particularly after IVF and IVF/ICSI, where the barriers to natural selection are bypassed.

Although it is uncertain whether knowledge of one's level of sperm DNA damage will influence a couple's decision to proceed with ARTs, assessing sperm DNA damage may still provide clinically valuable information. In our analysis of the 11 studies discussed previously, there was a positive predictive value (PPV) of 37% and a median negative predictive value (NPV) of 90% (with a median pregnancy loss rate of 18%). In other words, in populations with an overall pregnancy loss rate of 18%, the risk of pregnancy loss is estimated at 37% with an abnormal test result and 10% with a normal one. In this scenario, the clinician might want to discuss the effect of DNA damage with the patients, since testing could discriminate between pregnancy loss rates of 10 and 38%.


## Conclusion

Sperm DNA damage has been associated with reproductive difficulties in the male. While not yet routine, sperm DNA damage testing appears to be securing a place in the evaluation of the infertile male and infertile couple. The demonstration of a relationship between sperm DNA damage and pregnancy loss after IVF and ICSI provides yet another potential clinical application of this type of testing. At the very least, this relationship highlights the need to find ways to reduce sperm DNA damage in men and provides further rationale for ongoing research in this field. We believe that sperm DNA integrity testing may now be justified in the context of IVF and ICSI to help understand the possible cause of pregnancy loss and to provide prognostic information regarding a couple's potential risk of pregnancy loss following these ARTs.


## References

1. Guzick DS, Overstreet JW, Factor-Litvak P, National Cooperative Reproductive Medicine Network, et al. Sperm morphology, motility, and concentration in fertile and infertile men. N Engl J Med. 2001;345(19):1388–93.
2. Ahmadi A, Ng SC. Fertilizing ability of DNA-damaged spermatozoa. J Exp Zool. 1999;284(6):696–704.
3. Evenson DP, Darzynkiewicz Z, Melamed MR. Relation of mammalian sperm chromatin heterogeneity to fertility. Science. 1980;210(4474):1131–3.
4. Irvine DS, Twigg JP, Gordon EL, Fulton N, Milne PA, Aitken RJ. DNA integrity in human spermatozoa: relationships with semen quality. J Androl. 2000;21(1):33–44.
5. Shen H, Ong C. Detection of oxidative DNA damage in human sperm and its association with sperm function and male infertility. Free Radic Biol Med. 2000;28(4):529–36.
6. Spanò M, Bonde JP, Hjøllund HI, Kolstad HA, Cordelli E, Leter G. Sperm chromatin damage impairs human fertility. The Danish First Pregnancy Planner Study Team. Fertil Steril. 2000;73(1):43–50.
7. Zini A, Kamal KM, Phang D. Free thiols in human spermatozoa: correlation with sperm DNA integrity. Urology. 2001;58:80–4.
8. Bungum M, Humaidan P, Axmon A, Spano M, Bungum L, Erenpreiss J, et al. Sperm DNA integrity assessment in prediction of assisted reproduction technology outcome. Hum Reprod. 2007;22:174–9.
9. Larson-Cook KL, Brannian JD, Hansen KA, Kasperson KM, Aamold ET, Evenson DP. Relationship between the outcomes of assisted reproductive techniques and sperm DNA fragmentation as measured by the sperm chromatin structure assay. Fertil Steril. 2003;80(4):895–902.
10. Henkel R, Kierspel E, Hajimohammad M, Stalf T, Hoogendijk C, Mehnert C, et al. DNA fragmentation of spermatozoa and assisted reproduction technology. Reprod Biomed Online. 2003;7(4):477–84.

11. Borini A, Tarozzi N, Bizzaro D, Bonu MA, Fava L, Flamigni C, et al. Sperm DNA fragmentation: paternal effect on early post-implantation embryo development in ART. Hum Reprod. 2006;21:2876–81.
12. Benchaib M, Lornage J, Mazoyer C, Lejeune H, Salle B, Francois Guerin J. Sperm deoxyribonucleic acid fragmentation as a prognostic indicator of assisted reproductive technology outcome. Fertil Steril. 2007;87:93–100.
13. Collins JA, Barnhart KT, Schlegel PN. Do sperm DNA integrity tests predict pregnancy with in vitro fertilization? Fertil Steril. 2008;89(4):823–31.
14. Frydman N, Prisant N, Hesters L, Frydman R, Tachdjian G, Cohen-Bacrie P, et al. Adequate ovarian follicular status does not prevent the decrease in pregnancy rates associated with high sperm DNA fragmentation. Fertil Steril. 2008;89:92–7.
15. Lombardo F, Gandini L, Lenzi A, Dondero F. Antisperm immunity in assisted reproduction. J Reprod Immunol. 2004;62(1–2):101–9.
16. Virro MR, Larson-Cook KL, Evenson DP. Sperm chromatin structure assay (SCSA) parameters are related to fertilization, blastocyst development, and ongoing pregnancy in in vitro fertilization and intracytoplasmic sperm injection cycles. Fertil Steril. 2004;81:1289–95.
17. Check JH, Graziano V, Cohen R, Krotec J, Check ML. Effect of an abnormal sperm chromatin structural assay (SCSA) on pregnancy outcome following (IVF) with ICSI in previous IVF failures. Arch Androl. 2005;51:121–4.
18. Zini A, Meriano J, Kader K, Jarvi K, Laskin CA, Cadesky K. Potential adverse effect of sperm DNA damage on embryo quality after ICSI. Hum Reprod. 2005;20:3476–80.
19. Lin KQ, Fan HG, Xu H, Zhang XM. Diagnosis and treatment of complicated interstitial pregnancy. Zhejiang Da Xue Xue Bao Yi Xue Ban. 2008;37(6):638–41.
20. Sierra S, Stephenson M. Genetics of recurrent pregnancy loss. Semin Reprod Med. 2006;24:17.
21. Lin MH, Kuo-Kuang Lee R, Li SH, Lu CH, Sun FJ, Hwu YM. Sperm chromatin structure assay parameters are not related to fertilization rates, embryo quality, and pregnancy rates in in vitro fertilization and intracytoplasmic sperm injection, but might be related to spontaneous abortion rates. Fertil Steril. 2008;90:352–9.
22. Ward WS, Coffey DS. DNA packaging and organization in mammalian spermatozoa: comparison with somatic cells. Biol Reprod. 1991;44:569–74.
23. Steger K, Pauls K, Klonisch T, Franke FE, Bergmann M. Expression of protamine-1 and -2 mRNA during human spermiogenesis. Mol Hum Reprod. 2000;6:219–25.
24. Brewer LR, Corzett M, Balhorn R. Protamine induced condensation and decondensation of the same DNA molecule. Science. 1999;286:120–3.
25. Kosower NS, Katayose H, Yanagimachi R. Thiol-disulfide status and acridine orange fluorescence of mammalian sperm nuclei. J Androl. 1992;13:342–8.
26. Gatewood JM, Cook GR, Balhorn R, Bradbury EM, Schmid CW. Sequence-specific packaging of DNA in human sperm chromatin. Science. 1987;236:962–4.
27. Gineitis AA, Zalenskaya IA, Yau PM, Bradbury EM, Zalensky AO. Human sperm telomere-binding complex involves histone H2B and secures telomere membrane attachment. J Cell Biol. 2000;151:1591–8.
28. Zhang X, San Gabriel M, Zini A. Sperm nuclear histone to protamine ratio in fertile and infertile men: evidence of heterogeneous subpopulations of spermatozoa in the ejaculate. J Androl. 2006;27(3):414–20.
29. Barrera C, Mazzolli AB, Pelling C, Stockert JC. Metachromatic staining of human sperm nuclei after reduction of disulphide bonds. Acta Histochem. 1993;94:141–9.
30. Katayose H, Yanagida K, Hashimoto S, Yamada H, Sato A. Use of diamide–acridine orange fluorescence staining to detect aberrant protamination of human-ejaculated sperm nuclei. Fertil Steril. 2003;79 Suppl 1:670–6.
31. Aravindan GR, Krishnamurthy H, Mougdal NR. Enhanced susceptibility of follicle-stimulating-hormone-deprived infertile bonnet monkey (Macaca radiata) spermatozoa to dithiothreitol-induced DNA decondensation in situ. J Androl. 1997;18:688–97.
32. Beletti ME, Mello ML. Comparison between the toluidine blue stain and the Feulgen reaction for evaluation of rabbit sperm chromatin condensation and their relationship with sperm morphology. Theriogenology. 2004;62:398–402.

33. Zini A, Phillips S, Courchesne A, Boman JM, Baazeem A, Bissonnette F, et al. Sperm head morphology is related to high deoxyribonucleic acid stainability assessed by sperm chromatin structure assay. Fertil Steril. 2009;91(6):2495–500.
34. Fosså SD, De Angelis P, Kraggerud SM, Evenson D, Theodorsen L, Clausen OP. Prediction of posttreatment spermatogenesis in patients with testicular cancer by flow cytometric sperm chromatin structure assay. Cytometry. 1997;30(4):192–6.
35. Sailer BL, Sarkar LJ, Bjordahl JA, Jost LK, Evenson DP. Effects of heat stress on mouse testicular cells and sperm chromatin structure. J Androl. 1997;18(3):294–301.
36. Potts RJ, Newbury CJ, Smith G, Notarianni LJ, Jefferies TM. Sperm chromatin damage associated with male smoking. Mutat Res. 1999;423(1–2):103–11.
37. Erenpreiss J, Hlevicka S, Zalkalns J, Erenpreisa J. Effect of leukocytospermia on sperm DNA integrity: a negative effect in abnormal semen samples. J Androl. 2002;23(5):717–23.
38. Saleh RA, Agarwal A, Sharma RK, Said TM, Sikka SC, Thomas Jr AJ. Evaluation of nuclear DNA damage in spermatozoa from infertile men with varicocele. Fertil Steril. 2003;80(6): 1431–6.
39. Banks S, King SA, Irvine DS, Saunders PT. Impact of a mild scrotal heat stress on DNA integrity in murine spermatozoa. Reproduction. 2005;129(4):505–14.
40. O'Flaherty C, Vaisheva F, Hales BF, Chan P, Robaire B. Characterization of sperm chromatin quality in testicular cancer and Hodgkin's lymphoma patients prior to chemotherapy. Hum Reprod. 2008;23(5):1044–52.
41. Zini A, Sigman M. Are tests of sperm DNA damage clinically useful? Pros and cons. J Androl. 2009;30(3):219–29.
42. Cho C, Willis WD, Goulding EH, Jung-Ha H, Choi YC, Hecht NB, et al. Haploinsufficiency of protamine-1 or -2 causes infertility in mice. Nat Genet. 2001;28(1):82–6.
43. Sakkas D, Seli E, Bizzaro D, Tarozzi N, Manicardi GC. Abnormal spermatozoa in the ejaculate: abortive apoptosis and faulty nuclear remodelling during spermatogenesis. Reprod Biomed Online. 2003;7(4):428–32.
44. Aoki VW, Moskovtsev SI, Willis J, Liu L, Mullen JB, Carrell DT. DNA integrity is compromised in protamine-deficient human sperm. J Androl. 2005;26(6):741–8.
45. Aoki VW, Emery BR, Liu L, Carrell DT. Protamine levels vary between individual sperm cells of infertile human males and correlate with viability and DNA integrity. J Androl. 2006;27(6):890–8.
46. Aitken RJ, De Iuliis GN. Origins and consequences of DNA damage in male germ cells. Reprod Biomed Online. 2007;14(6):727–33.
47. Leduc F, Maquennehan V, Nkoma GB, Boissonneault G. DNA damage response during chromatin remodeling in elongating spermatids of mice. Biol Reprod. 2008;78(2):324–32.
48. De Iuliis GN, Thomson LK, Mitchell LA, et al. DNA damage in human spermatozoa is highly correlated with the efficiency of chromatin remodeling and the formation of 8-hydroxy-2'-deoxyguanosine, a marker of oxidative stress. Biol Reprod. 2009;81(3):517–24.
49. Evenson DP, Jost LK, Marshall D, et al. Utility of the sperm chromatin structure assay as a diagnostic and prognostic tool in the human fertility clinic. Hum Reprod. 1999;14(4): 1039–49.
50. Chohan KR, Griffin JT, Lafromboise M, De Jonge CJ, Carrell DT. Comparison of chromatin assays for DNA fragmentation evaluation in human sperm. J Androl. 2006;27(1):53–9.
51. Zini A, Boman JM, Belzile E, Ciampi A. Sperm DNA damage is associated with an increased risk of pregnancy loss after IVF and ICSI: systematic review and meta-analysis. Hum Reprod. 2008;23(12):2663–8.
52. Bungum M, Spanò M, Humaidan P, et al. Sperm chromatin structure assay parameters measured after density gradient centrifugation are not predictive for the outcome of ART. Hum Reprod. 2008;23(1):4–10.

# Chapter 15
# Postnatal Effects of Sperm Chromatin Damage

**Miriam Pérez-Crespo, Raúl Fernández-González, Miguel Ángel Ramírez, Eva Pericuesta, Alexandra Calle, and Alfonso Gutiérrez-Adán**

Over the past 20 years, numerous studies have identified several reproductive consequences of using sperm with damaged DNA both in animals and humans. The integrity of sperm DNA is crucial for the correct transmission of genetic information to future generations. There is evidence that sperm DNA fragmentation (SDF) may lead to conception failure, abortion, malformation, and genetic diseases [1, 2]. A significant proportion of infertile men has elevated levels of damaged DNA in their ejaculated sperm [3], and it is still unclear whether assisted reproductive technology (ART) techniques can compensate for poor chromatin packaging and/or DNA damage. Several authors have reported negative effects on pregnancy rates of increased proportions of spermatozoa with damaged DNA in sperm samples used for ART techniques [4, 5]. Developmental abnormalities arising from such chromatin damage may not be observed until postimplantation stages [6–8]. The biological impact of an abnormal sperm chromatin structure depends on the combined effects of the extent of sperm DNA or chromatin damage and the capacity of the oocyte to repair that damage [9]. In a mouse model system, spermatozoa with defective DNA have been observed to fertilize an oocyte and produce high-quality early-stage embryos, but as the extent of the DNA damage increases, the likelihood of a successful pregnancy to term decreases [10]. The authors of this report suggest that the oocyte has the capacity to repair damaged sperm DNA when less than 8% of the DNA is affected [10]. However, many situations have been described in which oocytes show a reduced capacity for repair (e.g., aged oocytes) [11]. Under these circumstances, the consequences of using sperm with fragmented DNA could be critical. Depending on the level of SDF, we would expect three possible scenarios. Thus, in some cases, the oocyte repair machinery will not be capable of repairing

M. Pérez-Crespo, PhD • R. Fernández-González, BS • M.Á. Ramírez, PhD • E. Pericuesta, PhD
A. Calle, BS • A. Gutiérrez-Adán, PhD (⊠)
Department of Animal Reproduction and Animal Genetic Resources Conservation, National Research Institute for Agriculture and Food Technology (INIA), Madrid, Spain
e-mail: agutierr@inia.es

A. Zini, A. Agarwal (eds.), *Sperm Chromatin for the Clinician*,
© Springer Science+Business Media New York 2013

the damaged sperm, and the embryo may fail to develop or implant in the uterus, or may be aborted naturally at a later stage (unrecoverable damage). In other cases, the oocyte will be able to repair the breaks in the DNA strand before initiation of the first cleavage division such that the sperm will generate normal offspring (recoverable damage). Finally, the worst scenario arises when the oocyte is able to partially repair the damaged sperm DNA, since deletions or sequence errors may be introduced possibly resulting in abnormal offspring (partially recoverable damage). In effect, some authors claim that the origin of 80% of de novo structural chromosome aberrations in humans is of paternal origin [12]. For instance, if DNA damage involves an oncogene, the result would be an increased risk of cancer in the offspring.

The routine performing of ART techniques such as intracytoplasmic sperm injection (ICSI) for sperm-related infertility problems determines a need to examine the postnatal consequences of SDF. Using this technique, full-term pregnancies are achieved despite high levels of sperm DNA damage [13]. ICSI is able to overcome the natural barriers that impede spermatozoa with a high load of damaged DNA to fertilize the oocyte and initiate a successful pregnancy, when this would hardly be possible through natural conception, intrauterine insemination (IUI), or even to some extent in vitro fertilization (IVF). Knowledge that SDF is common in infertile men, and preliminary reports on genetic and epigenetic abnormalities in children conceived through ICSI, prompted us to further address the issue of sperm DNA damage. Although the efficiency of ART techniques in humans is backed by a large body of data, some experiments designed to elucidate key mechanisms are not feasible in humans. In animals, however, DNA damage to the paternal germ line may be induced, and the long-term consequences of this damage in the offspring can then be assessed. In a mouse model, we identified a strong link between damage to the paternal genome and compromised embryo development, and more importantly, this had negative consequences on the newborns and subsequent generations [14]. Also, in mice, we detected selection mechanisms operating in nature that are able to discriminate the quality of spermatozoa DNA. Thus, the female reproductive tract and the zona pellucida (ZP) binding/penetration process play an important role in selecting sperm that, besides showing normal motility and morphology, feature intact chromatin. If we are able to understand the basis of these naturally imposed selection mechanisms that can distinguish the quality of spermatozoa, this could help clarify which of the many laboratory tests in current use are likely to be the most informative about fertility.

In this chapter, we review the findings of studies conducted in animal models, in which the offspring of males with sperm chromatin damage are characterized. First, we analyze the long-term effects on the offspring of the exposure of males to environmental or other toxic agents that affect the integrity of sperm DNA, and second, we report on various experiments that have explored the reproductive and long-term health consequences of the use of sperm with damaged DNA in natural matings, IVF, and ICSI.

DNA damage to the paternal germ line is experimentally induced by several methods: (a) using different sperm manipulation techniques such as preincubation under different conditions or freeze–thawing without cryoprotectants and (b) using physical agents such as scrotal heat stress or whole-body gamma radiation. These procedures serve to assess the long-term consequence of fertilizing oocytes using spermatozoa with different extents and types of DNA damage. Finally, we review recent experiments that have analyzed the transgenerational consequences of SDF and studies conducted in humans.

## Long-Term Effects on Progeny of Paternal Exposure to Harmful Environmental and Medical Agents That Affect Sperm Chromatin Structure in Animals

Male germ cells are targets for a wide variety of physical agents, such as radiation or heat, or chemicals including therapeutic drugs, such as chemotherapy agents and environmental pollutants (pesticides, metals, and tobacco smoke or air pollutants). Exposure to these factors may have adverse effects on sperm production and sperm function, with the risk that a damaged male genome may be transmitted to subsequent generations. Some of these agents directly target DNA, whereas others induce oxidative stress, in which case it is the reactive oxygen species generated that form DNA adducts and damage DNA [15].

The effects we have observed on the progeny of males exposed to these factors could be attributed to sperm chromatin damage, but it should be considered that these environmental agents or drugs can induce other alterations such as epigenetic modifications, which could be associated with the phenotypes observed in the progeny [16]. Table 15.1 shows the effects on the progeny of males exposed to environmental and pharmacological toxic agents that damage sperm chromatin structure. At present, three main (not mutually exclusive) hypotheses have been proposed to explain the manifestations of germ-cell genetic damage such as malformations or cancer susceptibility in the offspring [17]: (1) germ-cell mutations: mutagen–DNA interactions may fix a mutation in a spermatogenic cell line; (2) genomic stability: genetic damage in a germ cell may induce the appearance of mutations in subsequent cell generations, germ cell generations and/or embryonic cell generations [18]; and (3) apoptosis suppression: exposure to a toxic agent cousld prevent germ cells from entering apoptosis when signaled to do so, leading to the build-up of genetically damaged cells among the mature spermatozoa [19, 20].

### *Long-Term Effects on Progeny of Paternal Exposure to Radiation*

Radiation is a well-established DNA damaging agent that affects the male germ line [21, 22]. Exposure of mice to X-rays has shown that maximum DNA damage is produced in differentiating spermatogonia [22]. Currently, it is well accepted that

**Table 15.1** Postnatal consequences of paternal exposure to harmful environmental and medical agents known to affect sperm chromatin structure

| Harmful agent | Sperm quality | Species | Consequences in the offspring | Authors |
|---|---|---|---|---|
| Cyclophosphamide (chemotherapeutic agent) | Abnormalities in sperm chromatin and composition of sperm head basic proteins [29] | Rat | Pre- and postimplantation losses<br>External malformations<br>Altered behavior | [32–34] |
| Radiation | Abnormal sperm chromatin structure [54] | Mouse | Malformations | [24, 91–93] |
|  | DNA strand breaks [22] |  | Heritable chromosomal translocations<br>Heritable gene mutations<br>Genomic instability and cancer |  |
| Air pollution | DNA strand breaks [37]<br>Mutations [38] | Mouse | Inherited mutations | [38] |

preconception whole-body exposure to radiation poses a significant threat to the progeny of the irradiated parents by inducing DNA damage to sperm cells [23]. Sperm cell damage may affect fertilization and embryo development by causing numerous harmful phenotypic and genotypic effects in the offspring [23]. Phenotypic effects include reduced fertility and a variety of teratogenic effects. Genotypic alterations consist of increased mutation rates and elevated frequencies of chromosome aberrations, micronuclei formation, altered gene expression, and many other signs of transgeneration genome instability [24–26]. Such genotypic alterations may confer the progeny of irradiated parents an increased risk of genetic diseases, infertility, and cancer [24, 25, 27]. Most studies on germ-line and transgeneration radiation effects have analyzed the consequences of parental whole-body irradiation. However, this type of exposure is relatively rare compared to the localized body-part exposure that is frequently incurred during radiation diagnostics and therapy.

## Long-Term Effects on Progeny of Paternal Exposure to Chemical and Environmental Factors

A number of studies performed in humans and animal models have linked exposure to numerous environmental pollutants to sperm DNA damage (reviewed in [28]). Using animal models, it has been shown that in addition to causing increased aneuploidy rates, treatment with one or a cocktail of chemotherapeutic agents causes sperm chromatin damage (as detected using the sperm chromatin structure assay [SCSA]) and alters the sperm nuclear proteome [29]. Paternal cyclophosphamide exposure before conception induces aberrant epigenetic programming in early embryos sired by these males [30]. Likewise, this exposure has been shown to alter the expression of important DNA repair genes in preimplantation rat embryos [31]. The treatment of male rats with cyclophosphamide has been noted to give rise to preimplantation losses [32], postimplantation losses, malformed and growth-retarded fetuses [20, 33], and even to behavioral changes [34].

Air pollution has been correlated with sperm chromatin damage in humans [35, 36] and with an increase in sperm DNA strand breaks in mice [37]. Air pollution represents a mixture of genotoxic substances. Animal studies have recently provided evidence that air pollution, under ambient conditions, can induce germline mutations in vertebrate sperm at minisatellite loci and expanded simple tandem repeat loci [38]. Moreover, inherited mutations have been observed in the progeny of males exposed to air pollution [38].

The effects of many chemical and environmental factors on postnatal development vary according to the time elapsed between exposure and mating. For example, the effects of a well-known mutagen, cyclophosphamide, were observed to progressively diminish, from postimplantation losses to behavioral disorders, as a function of the time between exposure and mating [33, 34]. It, thus, seems that the longer the delay between cessation of cyclophosphamide treatment and mating, the less radical the detrimental effects on the progeny.

Using animal models, it has been possible to correlate sperm DNA damage with the traditional variables of progeny outcome used in developmental toxicity studies, such as litter size, pre- and postimplantation losses, and external or internal malformations [32–34]. Nevertheless, outcome measures, such as these, are insufficiently sensitive to predict the potential impact of exposure to drugs or environmental factors on postnatal and adult end points such as neurodevelopment, immunocompetence, or normal reproductive function, some of which may be the expected consequences of epigenetic modifications.

## Long-Term Consequences of Fertilizing Oocytes Using Spermatozoa with Different Extents and Types of Chromatin Damage Determined in Mouse Models

In this section, we review several experiments in which sperm chromatin damage is produced either by manipulating the sperm sample or by disrupting spermatogenesis using physical agents. The most outstanding experiments performed in mice are summarized in Table 15.2.

### Sperm Chromatin Damage Induced by Sperm Preincubation Conditions

During the preparation of sperm samples, nuclei can be damaged, and the developmental potential of these spermatozoa may be reduced compared to that of fresh spermatozoa. Several authors have demonstrated that the incubation conditions to which spermatozoa are subjected before ICSI can modify sperm DNA integrity [39–41]. We speculate that spontaneous DNA fragmentation during in vitro sperm incubation involves sperm endonuclease activity. Thus, when ICSI was conducted using spermatozoa incubated in a medium containing endonucleases that putatively cause sperm chromatin damage (data shown in Table 15.2), embryo implantation was significantly impaired [40]. Other authors have also shown in the mouse model that certain sperm incubation conditions prior to ICSI can produce structural chromosome aberrations in the resultant one-cell embryos. These authors described that chromosomal damage increased during sperm preincubation and that its incidence depended on the composition of the medium. They also observed that these chromosome aberrations were transmissible to offspring, with some fetuses displaying a structurally abnormal karyotype (containing reciprocal translocations, inversions, and deletions) [42]. Several authors have also suggested that chromosomal aberrations in zygotes are highly predictive of subsequent abnormal embryonic development [43].

## Sperm Chromatin Damage Produced by Freeze–Thawing in the Absence of Cryoprotectants

Recently, it has been hypothesized that the presence of double-strand DNA breaks in the spermatozoa used in ICSI procedures could give rise to embryos undergoing abnormal chromosome segregation (ACS) at the first mitotic division, depending on the spermatozoa manipulation protocol performed prior to ICSI [44]. The rate of ACS in ICSI embryos produced using frozen–thawed spermatozoa without cryoprotectants was significantly higher than among those derived from fresh sperm. Embryos showing ACS at first mitotic division appeared normal during preimplantation stages and could develop to the morula or blastocyst stage and become implanted in the uterus, yet died 7.5 days after fertilization. Accordingly, ACS during first mitosis appears to be a major cause of early pregnancy losses in ICSI-generated mouse embryos.

At our laboratory, several experiments have examined the consequences of injecting mouse spermatozoa with DNA damage following a freeze–thaw cycle in the absence of cryoprotectants into mouse oocytes. Effects were assessed in terms of the success of pregnancy and/or the health and well-being of the progeny [14] This extensive study sought to demonstrate the powerful adverse effects of using sperm with damaged DNA on embryo development, postnatal growth, and the behavior and longevity of the offspring, as well as their susceptibility to tumors. The mouse strains used were CD1 and B6D2 and DNA damage was induced by freeze–thawing the sperm in the absence of cryoprotectants prior to ICSI, since we observed higher rates of SDF in these sperm samples compared to fresh semen using the TUNEL and comet assays (data shown in Table 15.2).

We observed that ICSI using the spermatozoa with fragmented DNA produced no effects on the percentage of embryos returned by microinjection or that cleaved

**Table 15.2** Developmental and postnatal consequences of fertilizing oocytes using spermatozoa with different extents and types of chromatin damage

| DNA damage induced by | Method used to assess DNA damage | ART technique | Embryo development | Implantation rate | Effects on fetuses/newborns/adults | Authors |
|---|---|---|---|---|---|---|
| Sperm preincuba-tion conditions | TUNEL | ICSI | No difference in Bl yields (44 vs. 49% control) | Lower (21 vs. 54% control) | No difference in percentages of fetuses (33 vs. 40% control) | [40] |
| Subjecting males to γ-radiation | Comet | Natural conception | N.D. | No difference | Lower percentage of fetuses (30 vs. 92% control) | [63] |
| | | IVF | Lower Bl yields (63 vs. 96% control) | N.D | N.D | |
| | | ICSI | Lower Bl yields (43 vs. 67% control) | N.D | N.D | |
| Scrotal heat stress (42°C, 30 min) | TUNEL | Natural conception | N.D | Lower number of implantation sites (13.3 ± 2.2 vs. 24.7 ± 4 control) | Lower number of fetuses (11.2 ± 2.4 vs. 22.7 ± 4.3 control) Sex ratio distorted | [51] |
| Scrotal heat stress (42°C, 30 min) | Comet | IVF | No difference in Bl yields (90 vs. 96% control) | N.D | N.D | [63] |
| | | ICSI | Lower Bl yields (6 vs. 67% control) | N.D | N.D | |
| Freeze–thawing spermatozoa without cryoprotectant | TUNEL and Comet | ICSI | No difference in cleavage rates (71 vs. 86% control) | N.D | Lower % live pups (13 vs. 26% control) Premature symptoms of aging; increased incidence of tumors Behavioral alterations in females | [14] |

(continued)

**Table 15.2** (continued)

| DNA damage induced by | Method used to assess DNA damage | ART technique | Embryo development | Implantation rate | Effects on fetuses/newborns/adults | Authors |
|---|---|---|---|---|---|---|
| Freeze–thawing spermatozoa without cryoprotectant | ACS | ICSI | No significant difference in the incidence of ACS (38.1 vs. 26.3 control) | N.D | Lower percentage of fetuses (58.3 vs. 65% control) | [44] |
| Freeze-drying spermatozoa | SCSA | ICSI using sperm with a DFI of 46.72% | 47% Bl development | 85% | Live pups (19%) | [48] |
| | | ICSI using sperm with a DFI of 2.52% | 69% Bl development | 78% | Live pups (24%) | |
| Freeze-drying spermatozoa | N.D | ICSI | 57% Bl vs. 73% control | N.D | Lower percentage of live pups (14 vs. 33%) Viable, healthy, and genomically stable | [49] |

Studies conducted in mouse models

*Bl* blastocysts; *ART* assisted reproduction technology; *N.D* no data available; *N.C* natural conception; *ACS* abnormal chromosome segregation; *DFI* DNA fragmentation index to the 2–4 cell stage. However, the proportion of transferred embryos that gave rise to live offspring was twofold when fresh sperm cells were used for fertilization (26 vs. 13%). Immunofluorescence staining with an antibody against 5-methylcytosine (MeC) revealed a 2-h delay in the active demethylation of the male pronucleus in the embryos derived from sperm with fragmented DNA.

Twenty weeks after parturition, ICSI produced animals and in vivo produced controls were subjected to behavioral tests: locomotor activity (open field), exploratory/anxiety behavior (elevated plus maze, open field), and spatial memory (free-choice exploration paradigm in a Y maze). The female CD1 mice produced by ICSI using sperm with fragmented DNA showed general alterations in behavioral responses in both early and later stages of life. These animals suffered increased anxiety, lack of habituation patterns, deficient short-term spatial memory and exhibited age-dependent hypolocomotion in the open field test.

Anatomopathological analysis of the animals at 16 months of age revealed enlarged organs and an increased number of pathologies (33% of the ICSI-produced CD1 females developed solid tumors in the lungs or skin on the back or neck). Postmortem anatomical and histological findings indicated that ICSI using spermatozoa with fragmented DNA led to a significant increase in the number of tumors. Moreover, of the B6D2F1 mice derived from sperm with damaged DNA, 20% died before 5 months of age, 25% of those surviving showed symptoms of premature aging, and 70% died earlier than controls due to different tumors.

We suggest that, depending on the level of SDF, oocytes may be able to repair some of the fragmented DNA to produce blastocysts capable of implanting and producing live offspring. However, incomplete repair could lead to longer-term deficient phenotypes. Of most concern is that our data indicate that the use of spermatozoa with fragmented DNA in ICSI procedures can generate effects that only emerge later in life, including aberrant growth, premature aging, behavioral changes, and mesenchymal tumors. We believe that the increased incidence of tumors observed is related to DNA fragmentation in the sperm used since ICSI conducted with fresh sperm did not produce this effect. The ICSI procedure using DNA-damaged sperm could also be the cause of premature aging and the tumors associated with aging we detected. Aging and cancer are two sides of the same coin: in one case, cells stop dividing and in the other, they cannot stop dividing. DNA damage is thought to contribute to aging [45], and chromatin hypomethylation has also been related to premature aging in mice [46].

## Sperm Chromatin Damage Produced by Freeze-Drying

Freeze-drying is a very useful technique for the long-term storage and transport of viable genetic material. It is, thus, essential to check the level of DNA fragmentation in freeze-dried spermatozoa before use. Some authors have reported that mouse sperm can be freeze-dried without damaging their chromosomes [47]. Recently, Kawase et al. [48] have determined the level of DNA fragmentation in freeze-dried spermatozoa using the SCSA before undertaking ICSI. The extent of fragmentation was found to depend on the initial drying pressure and the storage temperature chosen to preserve the sperm samples. These authors observed good correlation between the DNA fragmentation index (DFI) determined by SCSA and the developmental rate to the blastocyst stage (data shown in Table 15.2). However, no correlation was detected between DFI and the percentage of live fetuses, indicating the negative consequences of using spermatozoa with fragmented DNA induced by freeze-drying affect the preimplantation period [48]. Other authors who evaluated the postnatal consequences of using freeze-dried spermatozoa in ICSI have concluded that viable, healthy, and genomically stable mice can be derived from ICSI using freeze-dried mouse sperm stored in the refrigerator for at least 2 months [49].

## Sperm Chromatin Damage Produced by Scrotal Heat Stress

Several reports have confirmed that heat applied to the scrotum leads to sperm chromatin damage [50–54]. In effect, paternal heat stress affects most protein patterns in preimplantation embryos [55], which could perhaps explain some of the negative consequences observed in embryo and fetal development. A link between paternal heat stress and embryo survival has been identified in a few studies [56–59]. Several effects on the offspring of heat-stressed males have been reported: a reduction in litter size [50, 51, 60, 61], a reduction in placental and fetus weight [50, 56, 62], and a distortion in the sex ratio toward females, when males are mated to females on the day of heat treatment [51]. We propose this shift in the sex ratio could be attributed to the different functionality of sperm carrying the X or Y chromosome.

All of the above-mentioned studies have assessed the reproductive consequences of naturally mating heat-stressed males to nonheat treated females. These consequences vary significantly depending on the moment after heat treatment when mating takes place. Some authors have observed that the most significant consequences arise when mating takes place 21–28 days after heat stress (Table 15.2). We have examined the reproductive consequences of performing IVF and ICSI using DNA-damaged spermatozoa from scrotal heat-stressed males. Spermatozoa were collected from the cauda epididymis and vas deferens of males 21–25 days after heat treatment to determine the outcome of using sperm that had developed from spermatocytes subjected to heat. In subsequent IVF experiments, a lower percentage of 2-cell embryos was recorded in the heat-stressed compared to the control group. This could be due to the lower motility of the sperm. However, blastocyst development failed to differ between the two groups, indicating a similar postimplantation development potential. However, when natural barriers of fertilization were overcome by ICSI, though the number of surviving oocytes was unaffected by the treatment, the cleavage rate decreased significantly. Moreover, the blastocyst development rate was significantly lower than for the control group, suggesting reduced DNA quality in these spermatozoa [63] (Table 15.2). Other authors conducting IVF using spermatozoa from heat-stressed males observed that the number of embryos moving into the blastocyst stage was greatly reduced (40% that recorded in controls) when sperm was obtained from mice 16 h after heat treatment. However, none of the embryos generated from sperm retrieved from males 23 days after treatment progressed beyond the 4-cell stage.

## Sperm Chromatin Damage Produced by Whole-Body Exposure to γ-Rays

The main characteristic of γ-radiation as a factor inducing SDF is the wide range of DNA damages it provokes [64]. The most likely lesion caused by γ-radiation is the presence in the DNA of double-strand breaks (DSBs). In our laboratory, γ-radiation has been used to induce SDF, which is subsequently detected by TUNEL and comet assay. Gamma radiation was applied to mice as described elsewhere [65] using a $^{137}$Cs irradiator to deliver a 4-Gy dose at a rate of 1.25 Gy/min. Our objective was to determine the reproductive consequence of mating males, both naturally and using ART techniques (IVF and ICSI), 21–25 days after irradiation treatment. After natural mating, γ-radiation did not affect the implantation rate, yet the number of fetuses conceived by irradiated males was lower than that in the control group. Radiation significantly increased the resorption rate, indicating that spermatozoa from irradiated mice, though capable of in vivo fertilization and producing blastocysts able to be implanted, give rise to an embryo viability that is somehow compromised as reflected by the lower proportion of fetuses obtained (Table 15.2).

When spermatozoa from irradiated males were used for IVF, cleavage and blastocyst rates were lower than those recorded in controls, indicating that some extent of DNA-damage induced by γ-rays allows fertilization, but compromises embryo development. When treated spermatozoa were used for ICSI, the reproductive consequences were similar to those described for the heat-stressed males. Thus, the number of surviving oocytes was unaffected by treatment, but cleavage rates were significantly reduced. In addition, blastocyst development was lower than in the control group, suggesting the reduced DNA quality of the spermatozoa [63] (Table 15.2).

## Transgenerational Consequences of the Use of Spermatozoa with Fragmented DNA

There is growing evidence that DNA damage in the fertilizing gamete as a mediator of postfertilization processes contributes to the genomic instability of subsequent generations. Transgenerational genomic instability most likely involves epigenetic mechanisms or error-prone DNA repair processes in the early embryo. Maternal and embryonic DNA repair processes during the early stages of mammalian embryonic development can have far-reaching consequences for the genomic integrity and health of subsequent generations. A series of recent studies have suggested that

DNA damage in germ cells can mediate postfertilization processes that lead to an increased risk of genomic instability in the progeny. Paternal exposure to chemical mutagens [66], ionizing radiation [67, 68], and particulate air pollution [37, 38], aside from increasing mutation frequencies in sperm, was more importantly found to induce persistent genomic instability in the F1 and F2 offspring of exposed mice [69–72]. In addition, the introduction of DNA damage by irradiated sperm triggers a genomic instability that can induce mutations in the unirradiated maternal genome [68]. These findings suggest that the mechanisms contributing to transgenerational genomic instability most likely involve epigenetic or error-prone DNA repair processes in the embryo.

There is still little experimental evidence of a transgenerational effect of sperm DNA damage. Adiga et al. have recently examined the transgenerational influence of varying the level of sperm DNA damage in both the somatic and germ-line compartment of F1 offspring in an irradiation model [73]. The data presented reveal increasing levels of genome instability in preimplantation embryos with increasing loads of damaged sperm DNA as evidenced by micronucleus analysis. Interestingly, the genetic instability is transmitted to both somatic and germ-line compartments of the F1 offspring derived from the DNA-damaged sperm. However, the extent of instability observed in embryos, somatic cells, and germ-line cells is dependent on the amount of DNA damage present in the paternal spermatozoa. Previously, Baulch et al. had observed that spermatogonial irradiation causes negative effects on embryonic cell proliferation rates and juvenile offspring protein levels in four generations [65, 74, 75]. In a later investigation, using the sperm comet assay to evaluate SDF, these authors confirmed their previous findings and clearly demonstrated heritable effects of paternal F0 spermatogonial irradiation history on chromatin [65]. This study also clearly demonstrates that the ATM (ataxia telangiectasia mutated) gene heterozygosity of the sire has a significant impact on these heritable effects.

In the same context, Dubrova et al. observed an increment and uniformity in the frequency of germ-line mutations in the F1 generation arising from different parental exposures to ionizing radiation. Dubrova found that this indirect effect leads to the destabilization of ESTR (expanded simple-tandem repeat) loci in the germ-line offspring. A significant level of mosaicism of these mutations is observed in the offspring due to early germ-line development. The uniformity observed in these increased ESTR mutation rates suggests that an epigenetic process is responsible for these alterations [70]. These observations indicate that mutation rates in the offspring of irradiated parents are substantially elevated. Also remarkable is the effect of the parental genotype on transgenerational instability. Thus, oocytes of female *scid* (severe combined immunodeficient) mice are unable to fully support the repair of double-strand breaks induced in paternal sperm which may, in turn, result in the elimination of cells/embryos containing high levels of DNA damage, thus partially preventing the manifestation of genomic instability. The suppression of mutation induced and radiation-induced genomic instability in homozygous *scid* cells can be explained by the DNA-PK-independent activation of p53 and p21, resulting in a high level of apoptosis and cell-cycle arrest in the irradiated DNA-PKcs-deficient cells [76]. Hatch et al. also demonstrated interstrain variation in responses to ionizing radiation, including the manifestation of radiation-induced genomic instability. This variation has been explained by differences in the intensity of apoptosis [77]. According to the results of Hatch et al., cells from radiation-resistant C57BL/6 mice undergo rapid apoptosis after irradiation, which could in turn suppress radiation-induced genomic instability in this strain.

Induced genomic instability can give rise to oncogenic mutations in somatic cells and malignant transformation [78]. Effectively, radiation-induced delayed transgenerational instability may have important health consequences that may become apparent in subsequent generations after the original exposure. It is clear that understanding the DNA repair capacity of the zygote and the mechanisms that contribute to transgenerational genomic instability are areas that will require significant attention in the future. The main studies that have assessed the transgenerational consequences of the use of spermatozoa with fragmented DNA are reviewed in Table 15.3.

## Postnatal Consequences of Sperm Chromatin Damage in Humans

Sperm DNA damage can affect the health of the embryo, fetus, and offspring [17, 79]. A possible consequence of sperm DNA damage is infertility in the offspring [80, 81]. A concern emerging from studies conducted in smokers is an increased risk of childhood cancer observed in the offspring of men with a high proportion of sperm with fragmented DNA in their semen. The study in question revealed that the children of these men, whose ejaculates are under oxidative stress [82] and characterized by a high level of chromatin fragmentation, are 4–5 times more likely to develop cancer in childhood than the children of nonsmoking fathers [83]. Another study has demonstrated that 15% of all childhood cancers are directly attributable to paternal smoking [84]. These studies suggest that there may be a link between sperm DNA damage and the subsequent development of childhood diseases. Moreover, because this particular mutation is fixed in the germ line, it has the potential to impact upon the health and well-being of all the future descendants of a given individual [80]. The link between sperm DNA damage and offspring abnormalities is not confined to smokers. For example, powerful associations exist between childhood disease and paternal occupation [85]. Aitken and Krausz [80] proposed that sperm DNA damage is promutagenic and can give rise to mutations after fertilization. As the oocyte attempts to repair DNA damage prior to the initiation of first cleavage, mutations occurring at this point will be fixed in the germ line and not only may be responsible for the induction of such pathologies as described above (infertility and childhood cancer), but may also confer a higher risk of disease imprinting [86, 87].

**Table 15.3** Transgenerational changes in subsequent generations of offspring derived from chromatin-damaged sperm

| Treatment | Sperm chromatin damage | Species | Time of mating after treatment | Generations affected | Alterations in the offspring | Authors |
|---|---|---|---|---|---|---|
| Gamma-irradiation of the testicular area | Denatured DNA; increased percentage tail DNA | Mouse | 18 h after irradiation | First generation | Increased genomic instability in fetal liver cells and sperm chromatin modifications in F1 males | [73] |
| WB irradiation | Increased comet tail length and percentage tail DNA assessed by neutral comet assay | Mouse | 45 days after irradiation | Third-generation descendants | Heritable chromatin effects in sperm | [65] |
| WB irradiation | Increased mutation frequencies in sperm | Mouse | 6 weeks after irradiation | F1 offspring | Transgenerational destabilization of the F(1) genome; endogenous DNA lesions | [24] |
| WB ionizing radiation | N.D | Mouse | N.D | F1 and F2 offspring | Elevated mutation rate in somatic and germinal cells. Increased cancer incidence | Reviewed in [25] |
| WB gamma radiation | N.D | Mouse | 6 weeks after irradiation | F1 offspring | Decreased fertilization rates of spermatozoa from the F1 offspring | [94] |
| Cranial irradiation | Elevated DNA strand breaks | Rat | 1 week after irradiation | F1 offspring | Epigenetic dysregulation | [95] |
| WB gamma radiation | N.D. | Rat | N.D | F1 and F2 generations | Impaired regeneration of liver tissue | [96] |
| Cyclophosphamide | Sperm DNA damage [31] Sperm chromatin alterations [29] | Rat | Immediately after treatment N.D | F2 progeny F1 and F2 progeny | Postimplantation loss and malformations Behavioral alterations | [97, 98] |

*N.D* no data available; *WB* whole-body

# Conclusions

The consequences of using sperm with fragmented DNA can be observed as early as at the preimplantational stages of development. Examples of these consequences may be found in epigenetic changes [88], chromosome aberrations observed in ICSI-produced one-cell embryos derived from spermatozoa that have been preincubated [42], or the increased embryo losses incurred after treatment of males with cyclophosphamide [32]. However, other alterations attributable to the consequences of DNA-damaged sperm could go unnoticed during embryo and fetal development and only emerge later in life. These alterations have been identified in the mouse model following the use of DNA-damaged sperm in ICSI and include aberrant growth, premature aging, behavioral changes, and mesenchymal tumors [14]. Another factor that can have long-term consequences is radiation. Radiation induces phenotypic and genotypic alterations in the progeny of treated males. Such genotypic alterations may predispose the progeny of irradiated parents to an increased risk of genetic diseases, infertility, or cancer [24, 25, 27]. Moreover, the consequences of sperm chromatin damage are not limited to the progeny of males exposed to the toxic agent, and several future generations can be affected. Most studies that have reported transgenerational damage have dealt with the harmful effects of radiation or chemotherapeutic agents [67–69, 72–75, 89].

Studies conducted in animal models in which spermatozoa with fragmented DNA are used for ART techniques such as ICSI have confirmed the negative effects on pregnancy rates already reported in humans [4, 40, 87]. However, the consequences observed in the mouse model are not restricted to reproductive failure, since several health and behavioral abnormalities are observed [14]. To avoid such undesirable consequences in the offspring when ICSI is performed, some precautions should be taken. It is advisable to check the preincubation conditions of the sperm prior to ICSI to avoid inducing sperm chromatin damage and, therefore, subsequent negative consequences on embryo development [40, 42, 90]. Further studies are needed in humans to validate the data obtained in animal models on postnatal alterations and the transgenerational genetic risks associated with DNA-damaged sperm. The long-term follow-up of children born through ICSI is also recommended. These studies will have significant implications for the growing use of ART to resolve male infertility problems.

# References

1. Sakkas D, Mariethoz E, Manicardi G, Bizzaro D, Bianchi PG, Bianchi U. Origin of DNA damage in ejaculated human spermatozoa. Rev Reprod. 1999;4(1):31–7.
2. Evenson DP. Loss of livestock breeding efficiency due to uncompensable sperm nuclear defects. Reprod Fertil Dev. 1999;11(1):1–15.
3. Irvine DS, Twigg JP, Gordon EL, Fulton N, Milne PA, Aitken RJ. DNA integrity in human spermatozoa: relationships with semen quality. J Androl. 2000;21(1):33–44.

4. Benchaib M, Braun V, Lornage J, et al. Sperm DNA fragmentation decreases the pregnancy rate in an assisted reproductive technique. Hum Reprod. 2003;18(5):1023–8.

5. Morris ID, Ilott S, Dixon L, Brison DR. The spectrum of DNA damage in human sperm assessed by single cell gel electrophoresis (Comet assay) and its relationship to fertilization and embryo development. Hum Reprod. 2002;17(4):990–8.

6. Hamamah S, Fignon A, Lansac J. The effect of male factors in repeated spontaneous abortion: lesson from in-vitro fertilization and intracytoplasmic sperm injection. Hum Reprod Update. 1997;3(4):393–400.

7. Twigg JP, Irvine DS, Aitken RJ. Oxidative damage to DNA in human spermatozoa does not preclude pronucleus formation at intracytoplasmic sperm injection. Hum Reprod. 1998;13(7):1864–71.

8. Rienzi L, Martinez F, Ubaldi F, et al. Polscope analysis of meiotic spindle changes in living metaphase II human oocytes during the freezing and thawing procedures. Hum Reprod. 2004;19(3):655–9.

9. Genesca A, Caballin MR, Miro R, Benet J, Germa JR, Egozcue J. Repair of human sperm chromosome aberrations in the hamster egg. Hum Genet. 1992;89(2):181–6.

10. Ahmadi A, Ng SC. Fertilizing ability of DNA-damaged spermatozoa. J Exp Zool. 1999;284(6):696–704.

11. Menezo Y. Oocyte capacity to repair DNA damage induced in sperm. J Gynecol Obstet Biol Reprod (Paris). 2006;35(5 Pt 2):2S19–2S23.

12. Tomar D, Magenis E, Chamberlin J, Allen L, Olson S, Donlon T, et al. Preferential paternal origin of de novo structural chromosome rearrangements. Am J Hum Genet. 1984;36(6):115s.

13. Gandini L, Lombardo F, Paoli D, et al. Full-term pregnancies achieved with ICSI despite high levels of sperm chromatin damage. Hum Reprod. 2004;19(6):1409–17.

14. Fernandez-Gonzalez R, Moreira PN, Perez-Crespo M, et al. Long-term effects of mouse intra-cytoplasmic sperm injection with DNA-fragmented sperm on health and behavior of adult offspring. Biol Reprod. 2008;78(4):761–72.

15. Aitken RJ, De Iuliis GN, McLachlan RI. Biological and clinical significance of DNA damage in the male germ line. Int J Androl. 2009;32(1):46–56.

16. Wyrobek AJ. Methods and concepts in detecting abnormal reproductive outcomes of paternal origin. Reprod Toxicol. 1993;7 Suppl 1:3–16.

17. Brinkworth MH. Paternal transmission of genetic damage: findings in animals and humans. Int J Androl. 2000;23(3):123–35.

18. Luke GA, Riches AC, Bryant PE. Genomic instability in haematopoietic cells of F1 generation mice of irradiated male parents. Mutagenesis. 1997;12(3):147–52.

19. Barnes CJ, Covington BWt, Cameron IL, Lee M. Effect of aging on spontaneous and induced mouse testicular germ cell apoptosis. Aging (Milano). 1998;10(6):497–501.

20. Brinkworth MH, Nieschlag E. Association of cyclophosphamide-induced male-mediated, foetal abnormalities with reduced paternal germ-cell apoptosis. Mutat Res. 2000;447(2):149–54.

21. Haines GA, Hendry JH, Daniel CP, Morris ID. Increased levels of comet-detected spermatozoa DNA damage following in vivo isotopic- or X-irradiation of spermatogonia. Mutat Res. 2001;495(1–2):21–32.

22. Haines GA, Hendry JH, Daniel CP, Morris ID. Germ cell and dose-dependent DNA damage measured by the comet assay in murine spermatozoaa after testicular X-irradiation. Biol Reprod. 2002;67(3):854–61.

23. Aitken RJ, De Iuliis GN. Origins and consequences of DNA damage in male germ cells. Reprod Biomed Online. 2007;14(6):727–33.

24. Barber RC, Hickenbotham P, Hatch T, et al. Radiation-induced transgenerational alterations in genome stability and DNA damage. Oncogene. 2006;25(56):7336–42.

25. Dubrova YE. Radiation-induced transgenerational instability. Oncogene. 2003;22(45):7087–93.

26. Nomura T. Transgenerational carcinogenesis: induction and transmission of genetic alterations and mechanisms of carcinogenesis. Mutat Res. 2003;544(2–3):425–32.

27. Mohr U, Dasenbrock C, Tillmann T, et al. Possible carcinogenic effects of X-rays in a trans-generational study with CBA mice. Carcinogenesis. 1999;20(2):325–32.

28. Delbes G, Hales BF, Robaire B. Toxicants and human sperm chromatin integrity. Mol Hum Reprod. 2010;16:14–22.
29. Codrington AM, Hales BF, Robaire B. Exposure of male rats to cyclophosphamide alters the chromatin structure and basic proteome in spermatozoa. Hum Reprod. 2007;22(5):1431–42.
30. Barton TS, Robaire B, Hales BF. Epigenetic programming in the preimplantation rat embryo is disrupted by chronic paternal cyclophosphamide exposure. Proc Natl Acad Sci USA. 2005;102(22):7865–70.
31. Harrouk W, Codrington A, Vinson R, Robaire B, Hales BF. Paternal exposure to cyclophosphamide induces DNA damage and alters the expression of DNA repair genes in the rat preimplantation embryo. Mutat Res. 2000;461(3):229–41.
32. Hales BF, Smith S, Robaire B. Cyclophosphamide in the seminal fluid of treated males: transmission to females by mating and effect on pregnancy outcome. Toxicol Appl Pharmacol. 1986;84(3):423–30.
33. Trasler JM, Hales BF, Robaire B. Chronic low dose cyclophosphamide treatment of adult male rats: effect on fertility, pregnancy outcome and progeny. Biol Reprod. 1986;34(2):275–83.
34. Auroux M, Dulioust E, Selva J, Rince P. Cyclophosphamide in the F0 male rat: physical and behavioral changes in three successive adult generations. Mutat Res. 1990;229(2):189–200.
35. Evenson DP, Wixon R. Environmental toxicants cause sperm DNA fragmentation as detected by the sperm chromatin structure assay (SCSA). Toxicol Appl Pharmacol. 2005;207(2 Suppl):532–7.
36. Rubes J, Selevan SG, Evenson DP, et al. Episodic air pollution is associated with increased DNA fragmentation in human sperm without other changes in semen quality. Hum Reprod. 2005;20(10):2776–83.
37. Yauk C, Polyzos A, Rowan-Carroll A, et al. Germ-line mutations, DNA damage, and global hypermethylation in mice exposed to particulate air pollution in an urban/industrial location. Proc Natl Acad Sci USA. 2008;105(2):605–10.
38. Somers CM, Yauk CL, White PA, Parfett CL, Quinn JS. Air pollution induces heritable DNA mutations. Proc Natl Acad Sci USA. 2002;99(25):15904–7.
39. Estop AM, Munne S, Jost LK, Evenson DP. Studies on sperm chromatin structure alterations and cytogenetic damage of mouse sperm following in vitro incubation. Studies on in vitro-incubated mouse sperm. J Androl. 1993;14(4):282–8.
40. Perez-Crespo M, Moreira P, Pintado B, Gutierrez-Adan A. Factors from damaged sperm affect its DNA integrity and its ability to promote embryo implantation in mice. J Androl. 2008;29(1):47–54.
41. Ward MA, Ward WS. A model for the function of sperm DNA degradation. Reprod Fertil Dev. 2004;16(5):547–54.
42. Tateno H. Chromosome aberrations in mouse embryos and fetuses produced by assisted reproductive technology. Mutat Res. 2008;657(1):26–31.
43. Marchetti F, Bishop JB, Cosentino L, Moore 2nd D, Wyrobek AJ. Paternally transmitted chromosomal aberrations in mouse zygotes determine their embryonic fate. Biol Reprod. 2004;70(3):616–24.
44. Yamagata K, Suetsugu R, Wakayama T. Assessment of chromosomal integrity using a novel live-cell imaging technique in mouse embryos produced by intracytoplasmic sperm injection. Hum Reprod. 2009;24(10):2490–9.
45. de Boer J, Andressoo JO, de Wit J, et al. Premature aging in mice deficient in DNA repair and transcription. Science. 2002;296(5571):1276–9.
46. Lopes S, Jurisicova A, Sun JG, Casper RF. Reactive oxygen species: potential cause for DNA fragmentation in human spermatozoa. Hum Reprod. 1998;13(4):896–900.
47. Kusakabe H, Yanagimachi R, Kamiguchi Y. Mouse and human spermatozoa can be freeze-dried without damaging their chromosomes. Hum Reprod. 2008;23(2):233–9.
48. Kawase Y, Wada NA, Jishage K. Evaluation of DNA fragmentation of freeze-dried mouse sperm using a modified sperm chromatin structure assay. Theriogenology. 2009;72(8):1047–53.
49. Li MW, Willis BJ, Griffey SM, Spearow JL, Lloyd KC. Assessment of three generations of mice derived by ICSI using freeze-dried sperm. Zygote. 2009;17(3):239–51.

50. Paul C, Murray AA, Spears N, Saunders PT. A single, mild, transient scrotal heat stress causes DNA damage, subfertility and impairs formation of blastocysts in mice. Reproduction. 2008;136(1):73–84.
51. Perez-Crespo M, Pintado B, Gutierrez-Adan A. Scrotal heat stress effects on sperm viability, sperm DNA integrity, and the offspring sex ratio in mice. Mol Reprod Dev. 2008;75(1):40–7.
52. Love CC, Kenney RM. Scrotal heat stress induces altered sperm chromatin structure associated with a decrease in protamine disulfide bonding in the stallion. Biol Reprod. 1999;60(3):615–20.
53. Banks S, King SA, Irvine DS, Saunders PT. Impact of a mild scrotal heat stress on DNA integrity in murine spermatozoa. Reproduction. 2005;129(4):505–14.
54. Sailer BL, Sarkar LJ, Bjordahl JA, Jost LK, Evenson DP. Effects of heat stress on mouse testicular cells and sperm chromatin structure. J Androl. 1997;18(3):294–301.
55. Zhu B, Maddocks S. The effect of paternal heat stress on protein profiles of pre-implantation embryos in the mouse. Int J Androl. 2005;28(3):128–36.
56. Jannes P, Spiessens C, Van der Auwera I, D'Hooghe T, Verhoeven G, Vanderschueren D. Male subfertility induced by acute scrotal heating affects embryo quality in normal female mice. Hum Reprod. 1998;13(2):372–5.
57. Paul C, Melton DW, Saunders PT. Do heat stress and deficits in DNA repair pathways have a negative impact on male fertility? Mol Hum Reprod. 2008;14(1):1–8.
58. Setchell BP. The Parkes Lecture. Heat and the testis. J Reprod Fertil. 1998;114(2):179–94.
59. Zhu BK, Setchell BP. Effects of paternal heat stress on the in vivo development of preimplantation embryos in the mouse. Reprod Nutr Dev. 2004;44(6):617–29.
60. Rockett JC, Mapp FL, Garges JB, Luft JC, Mori C, Dix DJ. Effects of hyperthermia on spermatogenesis, apoptosis, gene expression, and fertility in adult male mice. Biol Reprod. 2001;65(1):229–39.
61. Yaeram J, Setchell BP, Maddocks S. Effect of heat stress on the fertility of male mice in vivo and in vitro. Reprod Fertil Dev. 2006;18(6):647–53.
62. Ghasemi N, Babaei H, Azizallahi S, Kheradmand A. Effect of long-term administration of zinc after scrotal heating on mice spermatozoa and subsequent offspring quality. Andrologia. 2009;41(4):222–8.
63. Hourcade JD, Perez-Crespo M, Fernandez-Gonzalez R, Pintado B, Gutierrez-Adan A. Selection against spermatozoa with fragmented DNA after postovulatory mating depends on the type of damage. Reprod Biol Endocrinol. 2010;8(1):9.
64. Frankenberg-Schwager M, Frankenberg D, Harbich R, Adamczyk C. A comparative study of rejoining of DNA double-strand breaks in yeast irradiated with 3.5 MeV alpha-particles or with 30 MeV electrons. Int J Radiat Biol. 1990;57(6):1151–68.
65. Baulch JE, Li MW, Raabe OG. Effect of ATM heterozygosity on heritable DNA damage in mice following paternal F0 germline irradiation. Mutat Res. 2007;616(1–2):34–45.
66. Glen CD, Smith AG, Dubrova YE. Single-molecule PCR analysis of germ line mutation induction by anticancer drugs in mice. Cancer Res. 2008;68(10):3630–6.
67. Dubrova YE. Radiation-induced mutation at tandem repeat DNA Loci in the mouse germline: spectra and doubling doses. Radiat Res. 2005;163(2):200–7.
68. Niwa O, Kominami R. Untargeted mutation of the maternally derived mouse hypervariable minisatellite allele in F1 mice born to irradiated spermatozoa. Proc Natl Acad Sci USA. 2001;98(4):1705–10.
69. Barber R, Plumb MA, Boulton E, Roux I, Dubrova YE. Elevated mutation rates in the germ line of first- and second-generation offspring of irradiated male mice. Proc Natl Acad Sci USA. 2002;99(10):6877–82.
70. Dubrova YE, Plumb M, Brown J, Boulton E, Goodhead D, Jeffreys AJ. Induction of minisatellite mutations in the mouse germline by low-dose chronic exposure to gamma-radiation and fission neutrons. Mutat Res. 2000;453(1):17–24.

71. Hatch T, Derijck AA, Black PD, van der Heijden GW, de Boer P, Dubrova YE. Maternal effects of the scid mutation on radiation-induced transgenerational instability in mice. Oncogene. 2007;26(32):4720–4.
72. Dubrova YE, Hickenbotham P, Glen CD, Monger K, Wong HP, Barber RC. Paternal exposure to ethylnitrosourea results in transgenerational genomic instability in mice. Environ Mol Mutagen. 2008;49(4):308–11.
73. Adiga SK, Upadhya D, Kalthur G, Bola Sadashiva SR, Kumar P. Transgenerational changes in somatic and germ line genetic integrity of first-generation offspring derived from the DNA damaged sperm. Fertil Steril. 2010;93(8):2486–90.
74. Baulch JE, Raabe OG. Gamma irradiation of Type B spermatogonia leads to heritable genomic instability in four generations of mice. Mutagenesis. 2005;20(5):337–43.
75. Baulch JE, Raabe OG, Wiley LM. Heritable effects of paternal irradiation in mice on signaling protein kinase activities in F3 offspring. Mutagenesis. 2001;16(1):17–23.
76. Jimenez GS, Bryntesson F, Torres-Arzayus MI, et al. DNA-dependent protein kinase is not required for the p53-dependent response to DNA damage. Nature. 1999;400(6739):81–3.
77. Wallace M, Coates PJ, Wright EG, Ball KL. Differential post-translational modification of the tumour suppressor proteins Rb and p53 modulate the rates of radiation-induced apoptosis in vivo. Oncogene. 2001;20(28):3597–608.
78. Little JB. Radiation carcinogenesis. Carcinogenesis. 2000;21(3):397–404.
79. Savitz DA. Paternal exposure to known mutagens and health of the offspring: ionizing radiation and tobacco smoke. Adv Exp Med Biol. 2003;518:49–57.
80. Aitken RJ, Krausz C. Oxidative stress, DNA damage and the Y chromosome. Reproduction. 2001;122(4):497–506.
81. Silber SJ, Repping S. Transmission of male infertility to future generations: lessons from the Y chromosome. Hum Reprod Update. 2002;8(3):217–29.
82. Manicardi GC, Bianchi PG, Pantano S, et al. Presence of endogenous nicks in DNA of ejaculated human spermatozoa and its relationship to chromomycin A3 accessibility. Biol Reprod. 1995;52(4):864–7.
83. Ji BT, Shu XO, Linet MS, et al. Paternal cigarette smoking and the risk of childhood cancer among offspring of nonsmoking mothers. J Natl Cancer Inst. 1997;89(3):238–44.
84. Sorahan T, Lancashire RJ, Hulten MA, Peck I, Stewart AM. Childhood cancer and parental use of tobacco: deaths from 1953 to 1955. Br J Cancer. 1997;75(1):134–8.
85. Aitken RJ, Baker MA, Sawyer D. Oxidative stress in the male germ line and its role in the aetiology of male infertility and genetic disease. Reprod Biomed Online. 2003;7(1):65–70.
86. Cox GF, Burger J, Lip V, et al. Intracytoplasmic sperm injection may increase the risk of imprinting defects. Am J Hum Genet. 2002;71(1):162–4.
87. DeBaun MR, Niemitz EL, Feinberg AP. Association of in vitro fertilization with Beckwith-Wiedemann syndrome and epigenetic alterations of LIT1 and H19. Am J Hum Genet. 2003;72(1):156–60.
88. Barton TS, Robaire B, Hales BF. DNA damage recognition in the rat zygote following chronic paternal cyclophosphamide exposure. Toxicol Sci. 2007;100(2):495–503.
89. Dubrova YE, Plumb M, Gutierrez B, Boulton E, Jeffreys AJ. Transgenerational mutation by radiation. Nature. 2000;405(6782):37.
90. Tateno H, Kamiguchi Y. Evaluation of chromosomal risk following intracytoplasmic sperm injection in the mouse. Biol Reprod. 2007;77(2):336–42.
91. Muller WU, Streffer C, Wojcik A, Niedereichholz F. Radiation-induced malformations after exposure of murine germ cells in various stages of spermatogenesis. Mutat Res. 1999;425(1):99–106.
92. Muller WU. Radiation and malformations in a murine model. Adv Exp Med Biol. 2003;518:163–8.
93. Marchetti F, Essers J, Kanaar R, Wyrobek AJ. Disruption of maternal DNA repair increases sperm-derived chromosomal aberrations. Proc Natl Acad Sci USA. 2007;104(45):17725–9.

94. Burruel VR, Raabe OG, Wiley LM. In vitro fertilization rate of mouse oocytes with spermato-zoa from the F1 offspring of males irradiated with 1.0 Gy 137Cs gamma-rays. Mutat Res. 1997;381(1):59–66.
95. Tamminga J, Koturbash I, Baker M, et al. Paternal cranial irradiation induces distant bystander DNA damage in the germline and leads to epigenetic alterations in the offspring. Cell Cycle. 2008;7(9):1238–45.
96. Slovinska L, Elbertova A, Misurova E. Transmission of genome damage from irradiated male rats to their progeny. Mutat Res. 2004;559(1–2):29–37.
97. Hales BF, Crosman K, Robaire B. Increased postimplantation loss and malformations among the F2 progeny of male rats chronically treated with cyclophosphamide. Teratology. 1992;45(6):671–8.
98. Auroux MR, Dulioust EJ, Nawar NN, et al. Antimitotic drugs in the male rat. Behavioral abnormalities in the second generation. J Androl. 1988;9(3):153–9.

# Chapter 16
# Evaluation of Chromatin and DNA Integrity in Testicular Sperm

**Armand Zini and Naif Al-Hathal**

There is a universal agreement that the examination of conventional semen parameters alone only provides the clinician with a general sense of male reproductive health. Indeed, not infrequently, normozoospermic patients can have underlying fertilization defects [1]. Recently, sperm DNA fragmentation/damage has been studied extensively in an attempt to improve the diagnostic accuracy of the male evaluation, particularly, in couples with idiopathic infertility. However, the pathophysiology and etiology of sperm DNA damage (DD) in humans are incompletely understood, and to date, there are very few data on the treatment options for infertile men with this sperm defect.

The etiology of sperm DD is multifactorial, with the most commonly reported mechanisms being protamine deficiency, leading to defective sperm chromatin packaging, disordered apoptosis (caspase-dependent and independent pathways), and oxidative stress (secondary to the excessive elaboration of reactive oxygen species – ROS) [2, 3]. Clinically, the potential causes of sperm DNA fragmentation include varicocele, bacteriospermia, air pollution, chemotherapy, radiotherapy, drugs, cigarette smoking, cryopreservation, and advancing age [4–6].

There are several tests used to assess chromatin and/or DD in ejaculated spermatozoa. These tests include the sperm chromatin structure assay (SCSA; [7]), the acridine orange test [8], the single cell gel electrophoresis assay (COMET; [9]), the in situ nick translation assay [10, 11], and the terminal deoxynucleotidyl transferase-mediated dUDP nick-end labeling assay (TUNEL [11]) – all tailored to measure DD in ejaculated sperm. Using these assays, attempts have been made toward establishing threshold values for the percentage of sperm with DD, the values above

---

A. Zini, MD (✉)
Department of Surgery, Division of Urology,
McGill University, St. Mary's Hospital Center, Montreal, QC, Canada
e-mail: ziniarmand@yahoo.com

N. Al-Hathal, MD
Department of Surgery, Division of Urology,
Royal Victoria Hospital, McGill University, Montreal, QC, Canada

A. Zini, A. Agarwal (eds.), *Sperm Chromatin for the Clinician*,
© Springer Science+Business Media New York 2013

which fertility would be affected. Nonetheless, these assays need to be standard-ized, as there is wide variation among the various tests of sperm DD [12]. Using the SCSA, sperm DD threshold values have been established: low (≤15%), moderate (>15 and <30%), and high (≥30%) DNA fragmentation index (%DFI, proportion of cells with DD). These thresholds are associated with excellent, good, and fair to poor natural fertility potential, respectively [13–15].

There is now mounting evidence to indicate that sperm DNA integrity can influ-ence reproductive outcomes after assisted reproductive technologies – ARTs (e.g., IUI, IVF, and IVF/ICSI). Although there are few valid IUI studies, the data suggest that sperm DD is associated with lower IUI pregnancy rates [16]. A systematic review of the literature allows us to conclude that sperm DD is associated with lower IVF pregnancy rates, whereas it is not associated with ICSI pregnancy rates [17, 18]. There is also evidence to show that sperm DD is associated with an increased risk of pregnancy loss after both IVF and ICSI [19]. However, there are very few data on the influence of sperm DD on late reproductive outcomes (e.g., live birth rates, neonatal outcomes) after ARTs.

In general, cause-specific treatment of the clinical and biological factors associ-ated with sperm DD is associated with a decrease in DD. For example, repair of varicocele, treatment of genital infections, and use of oral antioxidants have gener-ally been shown to improve sperm DNA integrity [20–25]. Ultimately, these thera-pies are aimed at improving male fertility potential and reproductive outcomes after ARTs. An alternative approach to improve ART outcomes in men with high levels of sperm DD is to obtain testicular spermatozoa. This approach is based on the assumption that testicular spermatozoa generally have lower levels of DD than ejac-ulated spermatozoa because sperm DD may in part be caused by a posttesticular insult [26].

## Biological Significance of Testicular Sperm DNA Damage

Evaluation of testicular sperm DD may help us better understand the etiology (ies) of sperm DD. Experimental (animal) models with testicular DD may provide some insight into the cause(s) of the DD and its relationship with the quality of spermatogenesis. In the past two decades, several experimental studies (e.g., gene knockouts) have evaluated a number of putative genes involved in male fertility/ infertility. Some of these studies have demonstrated the relationship between male infertility and sperm DD, providing some insight into the etiology of sperm DD. For example, mice with a targeted disruption of the protamine gene produce testicular spermatozoa with poor chromatin compaction and an increased level of DD compared to wild-type animals [27]. These studies have shown that ejacu-lated (epididymal) sperm DD may in part be due to an underlying genetic defect (e.g., defective protamine expression – resulting in a relative increase in the sperm histone to protamine ratio).

Suganuma et al. conducted studies on DD in testicular and epididymal sperm to gain some insight into the influence of the posttesticular environment on DD in ejaculated spermatozoa [26]. They studied spermatozoa from wild-type mice and mice with a targeted disruption of the transition nuclear protein gene. These studies demonstrate that part of the DD observed in ejaculated spermatozoa results from an injury (e.g., oxidative stress, hyperthermia) sustained during the posttesticular transit (e.g., passage through the epididymis). These studies have shown that testicular spermatozoa with proper chromatin compaction are resistant to posttesticular stresses, whereas testicular spermatozoa with poor chromatin compaction are highly vulnerable to posttesticular insults and can sustain DNA oxidation and fragmentation.

Additional studies have evaluated fertilization rates and embryo health based on the source of surgically retrieved spermatozoa (i.e., epididymal, testicular). Suganuma et al. have observed that when sperm from the testis or caput epididymis of males were injected into enucleated mouse oocytes, the sperm chromosomes from mice with a targeted disruption of the transition nuclear protein gene showed no difference from those of wild-type mice [26]. However, the chromosomes from the sperm taken from the cauda epididymis of mutant males showed increased abnormalities. Furthermore, injection of testicular or caput epididymal sperm from males into intact mouse oocytes resulted in normal embryonic and fetal development and yields of live born equivalent to wild-type, but cauda sperm from mutant mice produced lower implantation rates and yields of live born than did those from wild-type mice [26]. Theoretically, failure to fully protect the DNA during epididymal passage may cause injury to the DNA as a result of the presence of protamine 2 precursors, slightly higher levels of residual histones, less disulfide bond formation, and decreased compaction of the sperm nuclei [28].

The results of experimental animal models allow us to conclude that testicular sperms are well protected by the microenvironment of Sertoli cells. By contrast, spermatozoa recovered from the distal epididymis may harbor DD as a result of the prolonged exposure to oxidants due to long epididymal transit and storage times [29]. Together, animal studies suggest that the primary cause of sperm DD is likely the result of a primary testicular injury (e.g., gene defect) associated with abnormal spermatogenesis and improper compaction of the chromatin. Sperm DD can then occur in the testicular and posttesticular environment as a result of the poor chromatin compaction [30].

## Clinical Significance of Testicular Sperm DNA Damage

Evaluation of testicular sperm DNA and chromatin damage may be useful in the diagnosis of male infertility. For example, establishing that a patient has high levels of testicular sperm DNA or chromatin damage would suggest an abnormal spermatogenesis, whereas the absence of such damage would be suggestive of normal spermatogenesis. Concomitant evaluation of epididymal or ejaculated sperm DNA may help identify the source of DD and more broadly the cause of the infertility. Ultimately, these types of observations may provide guidance as to the optimal treatment options.

In 2005, Greco et al. evaluated a cohort of infertile men with high levels of sperm DD in the ejaculate [31]. They performed a testicular sperm extraction in these men and observed that the percentage of testicular spermatozoa harboring DD (4.8%) was much lower than the percentage of spermatozoa with DD in the ejaculate (23.6%). They then proceeded to use the testicular sperm for ICSI (these couples had at least one previous failed ICSI cycle with ejaculated sperm). They reported an improvement in ICSI pregnancy rate with the use of testicular spermatozoa (44% ICSI pregnancy rate using testicular sperm vs. 6% pregnancy rate with ejaculated sperm). Similarly, they observed an improvement in ICSI implantation rates with the use of testicular spermatozoa, whereas fertilization rates and embryo morphology scores were similar for the treatment attempts with ejaculated and testicular spermatozoa. However, the authors do not advocate that all couples with sperm DD proceed to testicular sperm retrieval for ICSI (in view of invasiveness of testicular biopsy), but rather suggest that these cases be individualized (perhaps taking into account female age). The authors also caution that the threshold of (ejaculated) sperm DD beyond which use of testicular sperm extraction (for subsequent ICSI) should be contemplated has not been established.

Recently, Moskovtsev et al. have compared DD in ejaculated and testicular spermatozoa in patients with previously unsuccessful oral antioxidant treatment [32]. In their study, both samples (ejaculated and testicular spermatozoa) were collected on the day of ICSI (unlike the study of Greco et al., where there was a 4-month interval between the collection of the two samples). As in the Greco et al. study, ejaculated spermatozoa showed a threefold higher level of DD when compared with testicular spermatozoa (39.7% ± 14.8 vs. 13.3% ± 7.3). It is unknown whether pretreatment with antioxidant agents and vitamins had an impact on the integrity of the testicular sperm DNA.

Different established methods are available for assessment of sperm DD in the ejaculate. However, these methods have not been designed to assess testicular sperm DNA integrity or damage. Preparations of testicular tissue generally have a lower sperm concentration than semen. Moreover, unlike ejaculated sperm, testicular sperm preparations are contaminated (mixed with other cell types) and frequently testicular spermatozoa are bound to other cells (e.g., Sertoli cells). As a result of these features, testicular tissue is not suitable for sperm DNA tests that require flow-cytometry assessment (e.g., SCSA). Rather, testicular sperm DD is best assessed using slide-based techniques (e.g., terminal deoxynucleotidyl transferase-mediated deoxyuridine triphosphate nick-end labeling – TUNEL), where smears of the testicular tissue are prepared and evaluated. Another important difference between ejaculated and testicular sperm is the compactness of the DNA chromatin. When evaluating ejaculated spermatozoa, a standard nuclear decondensation step is undertaken prior to assessing DD in view of the compact nature of ejaculated sperm chromatin. By contrast, testicular sperm chromatin is less

**Table 16.1** Fertilization and embryo development after ICSI with ejaculated and testicular spermatozoa

| Sperm source | Attempts | Oocytes injected | Normal zygotes | Fertilization rate (%) | Cleaved embryos | Good-morphology embryos |
|---|---|---|---|---|---|---|
| Ejaculate | 18 | 185 | 131 | 70.8[e] | 124 (94.7%)[e] | 59 (47.6%)[e] |
| Testis | 18 | 187 | 140 | 74.9[e] | 133 (95.0%)[e] | 68 (51.1%)[e] |

e The differences in fertilization rates, cleaved embryo rates, and good-morphology embryo rates for the two sperm sources were not significant ($P > 0.05$)
Adapted from Greco et al. [31], by permission of Oxford University Press

**Table 16.2** Implantation and pregnancy after ICSI with ejaculated and testicular spermatozoa

| Sperm source | Attempts | Embryos transferred | Clinical pregnancies | Pregnancy rate (%) | Gestational sacs | Implantation rate (%) |
|---|---|---|---|---|---|---|
| Ejaculate | 18 | 56 | 1 | 5.6[e] | 1 | 1.8[f] |
| Testis | 18 | 58 | 8 | 44.4[e] | 12 | 20.7[f] |

e, f The differences in pregnancy rates and implantation rates for the two sperm sources were significant ($P < 0.05$)
Adapted from Greco et al. [31], by permission of Oxford University Press

compact, and therefore, it is unclear whether the same nuclear decondensation step is needed prior to assessing DD in these cells (testicular sperms have a lower degree of chromatin compaction and, hence, a more rapid decondensation than ejaculated sperms) [12, 33].

Assessing testicular sperm DD may be useful in the management of male infertility. Establishing that a patient has less DD in testicular compared to ejaculated sperm may provide some guidance in the choice of sperm to be used for ICSI (Tables 16.1 and 16.2). Defective sperm DNA apoptosis and alterations in the ratio of Sertoli cell to germ cells have been proposed as possible mechanisms to explain the lower levels of sperm DD in the testicular compared to ejaculated sperm. However, randomized, controlled trials are needed to define the clinical utility of testicular sperm extraction in men with high levels of sperm DD in the ejaculated sperms.

## Future Directions in the Field

Our basic understanding of the organization of the sperm chromatin and the nature of sperm DD in humans are constantly evolving (12). Nonetheless, there is an urgent need to standardize the laboratory methods for assessing DD, as there is wide variation among the various tests of sperm DD. In order to more accurately assess DD in testicular sperm, the current sperm DNA tests must be reevaluated and modified. These modified assays should also be validated by testing testicular sperm from men with different pathologies (e.g., obstructive azoospermia, nonobstructive azoospermia, oligozoospermia). Additional clinical studies are needed to better define the indications for testicular sperm retrieval in infertile men (e.g., high levels of sperm DD, unexplained ICSI failures). These studies should have parallel assessment of testicular, epididymal, and ejaculated sperm DNA integrity with subsequent assessment of ICSI outcomes in terms of fertilization rates, embryo quality, pregnancy rates, and neonatal outcomes.

# References

1. Saleh RA, Agarwal A, Nelson DR, Nada EA, El-Tonsy MH, Alvarez JG, et al. Increased sperm nuclear DNA damage in normozoospermic infertile men: a prospective study. Fertil Steril. 2002;78:313–8.
2. O'Brien J, Zini A. Sperm DNA integrity and male infertility. Urology. 2005;65:16–22.
3. Tesarik J, Ubaldi F, Rienzi L, Martinez F, Iacobelli M, Mendoza C, et al. Caspase-dependent and -independent DNA fragmentation in Sertoli and germ cells from men with primary testicular failure: relationship with histological diagnosis. Hum Reprod. 2004;19:254–61.
4. Moskovtsev SI, Mullen JB, Lecker I, Jarvi K, White J, Roberts M, et al. Frequency and severity of sperm DNA damage in patients with confirmed cases of male infertility of different aetiologies. Reprod Biomed Online. 2010;20:759–63.
5. Rubes J, Rybar R, Prinosilova P, Veznik Z, Chvatalova I, Solansky I, et al. Genetic polymorphisms influence the susceptibility of men to sperm DNA damage associated with exposure to air pollution. Mutat Res. 2010;683:9–15.
6. Sakkas D, Seli E, Bizzaro D, Tarozzi N, Manicardi GC. Abnormal spermatozoa in the ejaculate: abortive apoptosis and faulty nuclear remodelling during spermatogenesis. Reprod Biomed Online. 2003;7:428–32.
7. Evenson DP, Darzynkiewicz Z, Melamed MR. Relation of mammalian sperm chromatin heterogeneity to fertility. Science. 1980;210:1131–3.
8. Tejada RI, Mitchell JC, Norman A, Marik JJ, Friedman S. A test for the practical evaluation of male fertility by acridine orange (AO) fluorescence. Fertil Steril. 1984;42:87–91.
9. Hughes CM, Lewis SE, McKelvey-Martin VJ, Thompson W. Reproducibility of human sperm DNA measurements using the alkaline single cell gel electrophoresis assay. Mutat Res. 1997;374:261–8.
10. Gorczyca W, Traganos F, Jesionowska H, Darzynkiewicz Z. Presence of DNA strand breaks and increased sensitivity of DNA in situ to denaturation in abnormal human sperm cells: analogy to apoptosis of somatic cells. Exp Cell Res. 1993;207:202–5.
11. Sailer BL, Jost LK, Evenson DP. Mammalian sperm DNA susceptibility to in situ denaturation associated with the presence of DNA strand breaks as measured by the terminal deoxynucleotidyl transferase assay. J Androl. 1995;16:80–7.
12. Barratt CL, Aitken RJ, Bjorndahl L, Carrell DT, de Boer P, Kvist U, et al. Sperm DNA: organization, protection and vulnerability: from basic science to clinical applications – a position report. Hum Reprod. 2010;25:824–38.
13. Spano M, Bonde JP, Hjollund HI, Kolstad HA, Cordelli E, Leter G. Sperm chromatin damage impairs human fertility. The Danish First Pregnancy Planner Study Team. Fertil Steril. 2000;73:43–50.
14. Giwercman A, Lindstedt L, Larsson M, Bungum M, Spano M, Levine RJ, et al. Sperm chromatin structure assay as an independent predictor of fertility in vivo: a case-control study. Int J Androl. 2010;33(1):e221–7.
15. Evenson DP, Jost LK, Marshall D, Zinaman MJ, Clegg E, Purvis K, et al. Utility of the sperm chromatin structure assay as a diagnostic and prognostic tool in the human fertility clinic. Hum Reprod. 1999;14:1039–49.

16. Bungum M, Humaidan P, Axmon A, Spano M, Bungum L, Erenpreiss J, et al. Sperm DNA integrity assessment in prediction of assisted reproduction technology outcome. Hum Reprod. 2007;22:174–9.
17. Collins JA, Barnhart KT, Schlegel PN. Do sperm DNA integrity tests predict pregnancy with in vitro fertilization? Fertil Steril. 2008;89:823–31.
18. Zini A, Sigman M. Are tests of sperm DNA damage clinically useful? Pros and cons. J Androl. 2009;30:219–29.
19. Zini A, Boman JM, Belzile E, Ciampi A. Sperm DNA damage is associated with an increased risk of pregnancy loss after IVF and ICSI: systematic review and meta-analysis. Hum Reprod. 2008;23:2663–8.
20. Greco E, Iacobelli M, Rienzi L, Ubaldi F, Ferrero S, Tesarik J. Reduction of the incidence of sperm DNA fragmentation by oral antioxidant treatment. J Androl. 2005;26:349–53.
21. Greco E, Romano S, Iacobelli M, Ferrero S, Baroni E, Minasi MG, et al. ICSI in cases of sperm DNA damage: beneficial effect of oral antioxidant treatment. Hum Reprod. 2005;20:2590–4.
22 Moskovtsev SI. Management of patients with high sperm DNA damage. Indian J Med Res. 2008;127:101–3.
23. Moskovtsev SI, Lecker I, Mullen JB, Jarvi K, Willis J, White J, et al. Cause-specific treatment in patients with high sperm DNA damage resulted in significant DNA improvement. Syst Biol Reprod Med. 2009;55:109–15.
24. Zini A, Blumenfeld A, Libman J, Willis J. Beneficial effect of microsurgical varicocelectomy on human sperm DNA integrity. Hum Reprod. 2005;20:1018–21.
25. Zini A, Gabriel M, San Baazeem A. Antioxidants and sperm DNA damage: a clinical perspective. J Assist Reprod Genet. 2009;26:427–32.
26. Suganuma R, Yanagimachi R, Meistrich ML. Decline in fertility of mouse sperm with abnormal chromatin during epididymal passage as revealed by ICSI. Hum Reprod. 2005;20:3101–8.
27. Cho C, Willis WD, Goulding EH, Jung-Ha H, Choi YC, Hecht NB, et al. Haploinsufficiency of protamine-1 or −2 causes infertility in mice. Nat Genet. 2001;28:82–6.
28. Zhao M, Shirley CR, Hayashi S, Marcon L, Mohapatra B, Suganuma R, et al. Transition nuclear proteins are required for normal chromatin condensation and functional sperm development. Genesis. 2004;38:200–13.
29. Rajesh Kumar T, Doreswamy K, Shrilatha B, Muralidhara. Oxidative stress associated DNA damage in testis of mice: induction of abnormal sperms and effects on fertility. Mutat Res. 2002;513:103–11.
30. De Iuliis GN, Thomson LK, Mitchell LA, Finnie JM, Koppers AJ, Hedges A, et al. DNA damage in human spermatozoa is highly correlated with the efficiency of chromatin remodeling and the formation of 8-hydroxy-2'-deoxyguanosine, a marker of oxidative stress. Biol Reprod. 2009;81:517–24.
31. Greco E, Scarselli F, Iacobelli M, Rienzi L, Ubaldi F, Ferrero S, et al. Efficient treatment of infertility due to sperm DNA damage by ICSI with testicular spermatozoa. Hum Reprod. 2005;20:226–30.
32. Moskovtsev SI, Jarvi K, Mullen JB, Cadesky KI, Hannam T, Lo KC. Testicular spermatozoa have statistically significantly lower DNA damage compared with ejaculated spermatozoa in patients with unsuccessful oral antioxidant treatment. Fertil Steril. 2010;93:1142–6.
33. Kosower NS, Katayose H, Yanagimachi R. Thiol-disulfide status and acridine orange fluorescence of mammalian sperm nuclei. J Androl. 1992;13:342–8.

# Chapter 17
# Clinical Utility of Sperm DNA Integrity Tests

Armand Zini

## Clinical Utility of Sperm DNA Tests

The relationship between sperm chromatin/DNA damage and pregnancy outcomes has been examined by systematic reviews and meta-analyses [1–3]. The strength of these systematic reviews is the improved precision of the summary estimates compared with the individual study estimates of the relationship between sperm DNA defects and pregnancy outcomes. On the contrary, a weakness of meta-analyses (particularly on this topic) is the fact that it combines studies with highly variable study characteristics: data collection (prospective or retrospective), population characteristics (unselected, male factor), female inclusion/exclusion criteria, laboratory expertise in assessment of sperm DNA/chromatin damage, sperm DNA/chromatin test type, and sperm DNA test cutoff.

The recommendations for sperm DNA testing are based on (1) systematic reviews and meta-analyses of the relevant studies, (2) the characteristics of sperm DNA testing (e.g., sensitivity, positivity rate), and (3) disease prevalence (e.g., pregnancy, pregnancy loss).

## *Screening Test for First Pregnancy Planners*

The data from three studies [4–6] show that sperm DNA damage is associated with a reduced probability of natural pregnancy (combined OR 7.01, 95% CI 3.68, 13.36, $p < 0.0001$). Remarkably, the three studies [4–6] report very similar

A. Zini, MD
Department of Surgery, Division of Urology, McGill University,
St. Mary's Hospital Center, Montreal, QC, Canada
e-mail: ziniarmand@yahoo.com

A. Zini, A. Agarwal (eds.), *Sperm Chromatin for the Clinician*,
© Springer Science+Business Media New York 2013

**Table 17.1** Selected diagnostic properties of studies on sperm DNA damage and natural pregnancy

| Study | n | %hDFI | Sens | Spec | PPV | NPV | OR | (95% CI) |
|---|---|---|---|---|---|---|---|---|
| Evenson et al. [4] | 144 | 7 | 0.19 | 0.96 | 0.60 | 0.81 | 6.54 | (1.72, 24.92) |
| Spano et al. [6] | 215 | 13 | 0.23 | 0.96 | 0.86 | 0.55 | 7.59 | (2.54, 22.67) |
| Giwercman et al. [9] | 257 | 12 | 0.21 | 0.96 | 0.83 | 0.58 | 6.82 | (2.52, 18.47) |

*%hDFI* proportion of samples with high sperm DNA fragmentation index (DFI); *Sens* sensitivity; *Spec* specificity; *PPV* positive predictive value; *NPV* negative predictive value; *OR* odds ratio; *CI* confidence interval

associations between sperm DNA damage and natural pregnancy rate (with ORs of 6.54, 6.82, and 7.59, respectively, see Table 17.1). An analysis of the three studies reveals a median pregnancy rate of 53%, with a median positive predictive value (PPV) of 83% and a median negative predictive (NPV) of 58% associated with sperm DNA testing [4–6]. As such, the analysis predicts that in populations with an overall pregnancy rate of 53% (at 6–12 months of follow-up), the pregnancy rate is 17% when there is a positive test for sperm DNA damage and at 58% when the test result is normal. Therefore, testing for sperm DNA damage can discriminate between pregnancy rates of 17% and 58%. However, because the prevalence of a positive test in this context (first pregnancy planners) is low (<10%) and 17% of couples with a positive test will achieve a pregnancy, *indiscriminate sperm DNA testing in this context is not advocated. Clinicians may choose to test first pregnancy planners, but they should understand the predictive value and limitations (e.g., sensitivity, specificity) of the sperm DNA test in this context and discuss these issues with the patients.*

## Couples with Mild Male-Factor Infertility: IUI Candidates

Data from one valid IUI study show that sperm DNA damage is related to a significantly reduced IUI pregnancy rate (OR 9.9, 95% CI, 2.37, 41.51, $p < 0.0001$) [7]. In the Bungum et al. study, the overall IUI pregnancy rate is 20%, the PPV is 97%, and the NPV is 24% [7]. Therefore, in populations with an IUI pregnancy rate of 20%, a positive test for sperm DNA damage predicts the pregnancy rate to be 3% and a normal test result predicts the pregnancy rate to be 24%. Therefore, testing for sperm DNA damage prior to IUI can differentiate between pregnancy rates of 3% and 24%. *According to the Bungum* et al. *study, couples with high levels of sperm DNA damage should proceed to IVF and/or ICSI rather than IUI.* However, it is important to note that the sensitivity and prevalence of a positive test in this context (couples with mild male-factor infertility) are low (<20%) and these recommendations are derived from only one reliable study [7]. As such, *additional IUI studies are needed before routine testing is recommended prior to initiating IUI treatments.*

**Table 17.2** Selected diagnostic properties of 11 studies on sperm DNA damage and pregnancy after IVF

| Study | n | Assay | %hDD | Sens | Spec | PPV | NPV | OR | (95% CI) |
|---|---|---|---|---|---|---|---|---|---|
| Filatov et al. [11] | 176 | CC | 41 | 0.46 | 0.88 | 0.96 | 0.21 | 6.34 | (1.82, 22.08) |
| Host et al. [14] | 175 | TUNEL | 30 | 0.34 | 0.79 | 0.77 | 0.37 | 1.92 | (0.92, 4.04) |
| Henkel et al. [13] | 208 | TUNEL | 69 | 0.35 | 0.81 | 0.81 | 0.35 | 2.24 | (1.09, 4.58) |
| Huang et al. [15] | 217 | TUNEL | 19 | 0.22 | 0.83 | 0.50 | 0.57 | 1.30 | (0.66, 2.56) |
| Boe-Hansen et al. [9] | 139 | SCSA | 5 | 0.06 | 0.97 | 0.86 | 0.29 | 2.43 | (0.28, 20.83) |
| Borini et al. [10] | 82 | TUNEL | 16 | 0.17 | 0.89 | 0.85 | 0.23 | 1.66 | (0.33, 8.28) |
| Lin et al. [16] | 137 | SCSA | 16 | 0.15 | 0.83 | 0.45 | 0.51 | 0.88 | (0.35, 2.19) |
| Benchaib et al. [8] | 84 | TUNEL | 10 | 0.07 | 0.86 | 0.50 | 0.32 | 0.46 | (0.11, 2.00) |
| Bungum et al. [7] | 388 | SCSA | 16 | 0.17 | 0.86 | 0.71 | 0.34 | 1.24 | (0.69, 2.26) |
| Frydman et al. [12] | 117 | TUNEL | 44 | 0.58 | 0.68 | 0.64 | 0.35 | 2.97 | (1.39, 6.32) |
| Tarozzi et al. [17] | 82 | CMA3 | 17 | 0.22 | 0.97 | 0.97 | 0.28 | 10.86 | (0.62, 191.5) |

*%hDD* proportion of samples with high sperm DNA damage; *Sens* sensitivity; *Spec* specificity; *PPV* positive predictive value; *NPV* negative predictive value; *OR* odds ratio; *CC* chromatin compaction; *TUNEL* terminal deoxynucleotidyl transferase-mediated dUTP nick end-labeling; *SCSA* sperm chromatin structure assay; *CMA3* chromomycin A3

## Couples with Severe Male-Factor Infertility: IVF or ICSI Candidates

Data from more than 20 studies (11 evaluable – see Table 17.2) demonstrate that sperm DNA damage is associated with a modest but significant reduction in the IVF pregnancy rate (combined OR of 1.70, 95% CI 1.30, 2.23, $p < 0.05$) [7–17]. Further analysis of the 11 evaluable IVF studies (with a median pregnancy rate of 33%) reveals a median PPV of 77% and median NPV of 34%. In clinical terms, this means that in populations with an overall IVF pregnancy rate of 33%, a positive test for sperm DNA damage predicts the IVF pregnancy rate to be 23% and 34% if the test is negative. As such, couples with sperm DNA damage may choose to proceed to ICSI, where pregnancy rates are independent of test results (see below). However, *the clinical value of an 11% difference in IVF pregnancy rates (23% vs. 34%, with positive and negative test result, respectively) is modest, and it may be hard to justify routine testing in this setting.* However, clinicians may want to test select couples (e.g., with failed IVF) so as to better counsel these couples in future ART cycles.

Data from more than 20 studies (14 evaluable – see Table 17.3) have evaluated the relationship between sperm DNA integrity and pregnancy rates after IVF/ICSI. As with IVF studies, these ICSI studies are quite heterogeneous. In keeping with a

**Table 17.3** Selected diagnostic properties of 14 studies on sperm DNA damage and pregnancy after ICSI

| Study | n | Assay | %hDD | Sens | Spec | PPV | NPV | OR | 95% CI |
|---|---|---|---|---|---|---|---|---|---|
| Hammadeh et al. [20] | 60 | ABlue | 44 | 0.50 | 0.71 | 0.82 | 0.35 | 2.40 | (0.72, 7.96) |
| Host et al. [14] | 61 | TUNEL | 59 | 0.57 | 0.38 | 0.58 | 0.36 | 0.79 | (0.28, 2.25) |
| Henkel et al. [13] | 54 | TUNEL | 48 | 0.68 | 0.63 | 0.79 | 0.50 | 3.67 | (1.12, 12.0) |
| Gandini et al. [19] | 22 | SCSA | 41 | 0.31 | 0.44 | 0.44 | 0.31 | 0.36 | (0.06, 2.08) |
| Huang et al. [15] | 86 | TUNEL | 57 | 0.64 | 0.50 | 0.55 | 0.60 | 1.80 | (0.76, 4.27) |
| Zini et al. [22] | 60 | SCSA | 18 | 0.17 | 0.81 | 0.46 | 0.51 | 0.87 | (0.23, 3.22) |
| Check et al. [18] | 104 | SCSA | 28 | 0.29 | 0.76 | 0.72 | 0.34 | 1.34 | (0.52, 3.43) |
| Boe-Hansen et al. [9] | 47 | SCSA | 38 | 0.36 | 0.57 | 0.67 | 0.28 | 0.76 | (0.21, 2.72) |
| Borini et al. [10] | 50 | TUNEL | 60 | 0.71 | 0.75 | 0.90 | 0.45 | 7.36 | (1.67, 32.4) |
| Benchaib et al. [8] | 218 | TUNEL | 17 | 0.19 | 0.87 | 0.72 | 0.37 | 1.55 | (0.70, 3.41) |
| Bungum et al. [7] | 223 | SCSA | 33 | 0.29 | 0.61 | 0.52 | 0.37 | 0.65 | (0.37, 1.14) |
| Lin et al. [16] | 86 | SCSA | 24 | 0.26 | 0.77 | 0.52 | 0.52 | 1.21 | (0.45, 3.23) |
| Micinski et al. [21] | 50 | SCSA | 35 | 0.40 | 0.85 | 0.91 | 0.28 | 3.73 | (0.74, 18.77) |
| Tarozzi et al. [17] | 50 | CMA3 | 56 | 0.49 | 0.27 | 0.61 | 0.18 | 0.34 | (0.09, 1.29) |

*%hDD* proportion of samples with high sperm DNA damage; *Sens* sensitivity; *Spec* specificity; *PPV* positive predictive value; *NPV* negative predictive value; *OR* odds ratio; *ABlue* aniline blue; *TUNEL* terminal deoxynucleotidyl transferase-mediated dUTP nick end-labeling; *SCSA* sperm chromatin structure assay; *CMA3* chromomycin A3

recent analysis [1], the results of this updated meta-analysis on ICSI studies indicate that sperm DNA damage is not related to ICSI pregnancy rates (combined OR of 1.15, 95% 0.90, 1.55, $p = 0.65$) [7–10, 13–22]. *These data suggest that sperm DNA testing is not clinically valuable in predicting ICSI outcomes.* Perhaps the most concerning aspect of these findings is the unknown long-term consequence (i.e., postnatal health) of a successful pregnancy with high levels of DNA damage.

Testing couples with severe male-factor infertility enrolled in IVF or ICSI may also be valuable because sperm DNA damage is associated with a significantly higher rate of pregnancy loss after IVF or ICSI (combined OR of 2.48, 95% CI; 1.52, 4.04, $p < 0.0001$) [3]. Data derived from these studies (PPV and NPV) indicate that in populations with an overall rate of pregnancy loss of 18%, the rate of pregnancy loss is estimated at 37% when the test is positive and 10% when it is negative. The difference between a pregnancy loss rate of 37% and 10% may be valuable to patients and clinicians. Although the effect of DNA damage on pregnancy loss should be discussed with patients prior to undergoing ART, many couples will proceed with these treatments regardless of sperm DNA test results and the impact on pregnancy loss.

## Couples with Pregnancy Loss After IVF or IVF/ICSI

The prevalence of a positive test, sensitivity and specificity of sperm DNA testing in the context of pregnancy loss after IVF and ICSI are and 25, 40, and 85%, respectively [3]. This indicates that sperm DNA damage is a minor cause of pregnancy loss after IVF and ICSI (based on the low prevalence and low sensitivity). However, if the test is positive, it suggests that the sperm DNA damage (or male-factor) may be the cause of the pregnancy loss (based on the high specificity). In this setting, it may be advisable to evaluate or reevaluate the male and correct any potential male factor (e.g., varicocele) that may contribute to the DNA damage.

## Guidelines on Clinical Value of Sperm DNA Tests

The ASRM (American Society for Reproductive Medicine) has published guidelines on the clinical utility of sperm DNA integrity tests in 2006 and again in 2008 [23, 24]. Based on their evaluation of the existing literature (up to 2006 in both the 2006 and 2008 reports), they conclude the following:

1. Existing data on the relationship between abnormal DNA integrity and reproductive outcomes are limited.
2. Sperm DNA damage is more common in infertile men and may affect reproductive outcomes in selected couples, including those with recurrent spontaneous miscarriage or idiopathic infertility.
3. At present, the results of sperm DNA integrity testing alone do not predict pregnancy rates achieved with intercourse, IUI, or IVF and ICSI.
4. Currently, there is no proven role for routine DNA integrity testing in the evaluation of infertility.
5. Treatments for abnormal DNA integrity have not been shown to have clinical value.

Although these guidelines provide clinicians with a fair assessment of the value of sperm DNA tests (based on literature up to 2006), more recent studies have added to our understanding of this test and the data suggest that there may be value in testing couples prior to ARTs.

## Summary

Tests of sperm DNA and chromatin integrity are being used in the evaluation of infertile men. To date, the clinical studies on sperm DNA and chromatin defects allow us to conclude that sperm DNA damage is associated with lower natural, IUI, and IVF pregnancy rates, but not with ICSI pregnancy rates. Moreover, sperm DNA damage is associated with an increased risk of pregnancy loss in those couples undergoing IVF or ICSI. Although the clinical utility of tests of sperm DNA/chromatin damage remains to be firmly established, the data suggest that there is clinical value in testing couples with recurrent abortions or prior to initiating ART cycles.

# References

1. Collins JA, Barnhart KT, Schlegel PN. Do sperm DNA integrity tests predict pregnancy with in vitro fertilization? Fertil Steril. 2008;89:823–31.
2. Zini A, Sigman M. Are tests of sperm DNA damage clinically useful? Pros and cons. J Androl. 2009;30:219–29.
3. Zini A, Boman JM, Belzile E, Ciampi A. Sperm DNA damage is associated with an increased risk of pregnancy loss after IVF and ICSI: systematic review and meta-analysis. Hum Reprod. 2008;23:2663–8.
4. Evenson DP, Jost LK, Marshall D, Zinaman MJ, Clegg E, Purvis K, et al. Utility of the sperm chromatin structure assay as a diagnostic and prognostic tool in the human fertility clinic. Hum Reprod. 1999;14:1039–49.
5. Giwercman A, Lindstedt L, Larsson M, Bungum M, Spano M, Levine RJ, et al. Sperm chromatin structure assay as an independent predictor of fertility in vivo: a case-control study. Int J Androl. 2010;33:221–7.
6. Spano M, Bonde JP, Hjollund HI, Kolstad HA, Cordelli E, Leter G. Sperm chromatin damage impairs human fertility. The Danish First Pregnancy Planner Study Team. Fertil Steril. 2000;73:43–50.
7. Bungum M, Humaidan P, Axmon A, Spano M, Bungum L, Erenpreiss J, et al. Sperm DNA integrity assessment in prediction of assisted reproduction technology outcome. Hum Reprod. 2007;22:174–9.
8. Benchaib M, Lornage J, Mazoyer C, Lejeune H, Salle B, Francois Guerin J. Sperm deoxyribonucleic acid fragmentation as a prognostic indicator of assisted reproductive technology outcome. Fertil Steril. 2007;87:93–100.
9. Boe-Hansen GB, Fedder J, Ersboll AK, Christensen P. The sperm chromatin structure assay as a diagnostic tool in the human fertility clinic. Hum Reprod. 2006;21:1576–82.
10. Borini A, Tarozzi N, Bizzaro D, Bonu MA, Fava L, Flamigni C, et al. Sperm DNA fragmentation: paternal effect on early post-implantation embryo development in ART. Hum Reprod. 2006;21:2876–81.
11. Filatov MV, Semenova EV, Vorob'eva OA, Leont'eva OA, Drobchenko EA. Relationship between abnormal sperm chromatin packing and IVF results. Mol Hum Reprod. 1999;5:825–30.
12. Frydman N, Prisant N, Hesters L, Frydman R, Tachdjian G, Cohen-Bacrie P, et al. Adequate ovarian follicular status does not prevent the decrease in pregnancy rates associated with high sperm DNA fragmentation. Fertil Steril. 2008;89:92–7.
13. Henkel R, Kierspel E, Hajimohammad M, Stalf T, Hoogendijk C, Mehnert C, et al. DNA fragmentation of spermatozoa and assisted reproduction technology. Reprod Biomed Online. 2003;7:477–84.
14. Host E, Lindenberg S, Smidt-Jensen S. The role of DNA strand breaks in human spermatozoa used for IVF and ICSI. Acta Obstet Gynecol Scand. 2000;79:559–63.
15. Huang CC, Lin DP, Tsao HM, Cheng TC, Liu CH, Lee MS. Sperm DNA fragmentation negatively correlates with velocity and fertilization rates but might not affect pregnancy rates. Fertil Steril. 2005;84:130–40.
16. Lin MH, Kuo-Kuang Lee R, Li SH, Lu CH, Sun FJ, Hwu YM. Sperm chromatin structure assay parameters are not related to fertilization rates, embryo quality, and pregnancy rates in in vitro fertilization and intracytoplasmic sperm injection, but might be related to spontaneous abortion rates. Fertil Steril. 2008;90:352–9.
17. Tarozzi N, Nadalini M, Stronati A, Bizzaro D, Dal Prato L, Coticchio G, et al. Anomalies in sperm chromatin packaging: implications for assisted reproduction techniques. Reprod Biomed Online. 2009;18:486–95.
18. Check JH, Graziano V, Cohen R, Krotec J, Check ML. Effect of an abnormal sperm chromatin structural assay (SCSA) on pregnancy outcome following (IVF) with ICSI in previous IVF failures. Arch Androl. 2005;51:121–4.

19. Gandini L, Lombardo F, Paoli D, Caruso F, Eleuteri P, Leter G, et al. Full-term pregnancies achieved with ICSI despite high levels of sperm chromatin damage. Hum Reprod. 2004;19:1409–17.
20. Hammadeh ME, al-Hasani S, Stieber M, Rosenbaum P, Kupker D, Diedrich K, et al. The effect of chromatin condensation (aniline blue staining) and morphology (strict criteria) of human spermatozoa on fertilization, cleavage and pregnancy rates in an intracytoplasmic sperm injection programme. Hum Reprod. 1996;11:2468–71.
21. Micinski P, Pawlicki K, Wielgus E, Bochenek M, Tworkowska I. The sperm chromatin structure assay (SCSA) as prognostic factor in IVF/ICSI program. Reprod Biol. 2009;9:65–70.
22. Zini A, Meriano J, Kader K, Jarvi K, Laskin CA, Cadesky K. Potential adverse effect of sperm DNA damage on embryo quality after ICSI. Hum Reprod. 2005;20:3476–80.
23. The Practice Committee of the American Society for Reproductive Medicine. The clinical utility of sperm DNA integrity testing. Fertil Steril. 2006;86:S35–7.
24. The Practice Committee of the American Society for Reproductive Medicine. The clinical utility of sperm DNA integrity testing. Fertil Steril. 2008;90:S178–80.

# Index

A. Zini, A. Agarwal (eds.), *Sperm Chromatin for the Clinician*,
© Springer Science+Business Media New York 2013